Humanistic Wellbeing

Joar Vittersø

Humanistic Wellbeing

Toward a Value-Based Science of the Good Life

Springer

Joar Vittersø
Department of Psychology
UiT The Arctic University of Norway
Tromsø, Norway

ISBN 978-3-031-69294-9 ISBN 978-3-031-69292-5 (eBook)
https://doi.org/10.1007/978-3-031-69292-5

This work was supported by UIT The Arctic University of Norway.

This Springer imprint is published by the registered company Springer Nature Switzerland AG
The registered company address is: Gewerbestrasse 11, 6330 Cham, Switzerland

To Astrid
For everything

Competing Interests

The author declares that he has no conflict of interest. The publication charges for this article have been funded by a grant from the publication fund of UiT The Arctic University of Norway.

Preface

Walter Mischel once said that "Psychologists treat other peoples' theories like toothbrushes—no self-respecting person wants to use anyone else's" (Mischel, 2008). With the present book, introducing the humanistic theory of wellbeing (HTW), I must plead guilty as charged. Considering the overflow of existing theories and models in psychology in general, and in wellbeing studies in particular, it is fair to ask if we really need another one.

I think we do. Theories are essential to science, and it should be kept in mind that Mischel's warning was not directed against theory building as such. Rather, it was opposing what he saw as a tendency to publish premature theories created in the interest of developing careers rather than advancing knowledge. Mischel also cautioned against "turf" theories that are too narrowly directed toward "sub-fields within sub-disciplines." What we must avoid, Mischel specified, is a "Terminological Tower of Babel across the sub-fields and disciplines that cements their disconnect, carving nature at unnatural joints." Theories must be as broad as they need to be and should not be restricted by sub-field borders artificially created by organizational convenience or historical and bureaucratic traditions.

New theories must be openly and critically debated. Science makes progress by perfecting concepts, correcting flaws and weaknesses, and by gradual improvements of knowledge. In developing the HTW, therefore, I spent much time comparing and critiquing existing theories. Too much, perhaps, and I apologize if my analyses have come across as unnecessarily harsh.

But I wanted this book to follow the most promising paths toward better knowledge and I found the most inspiring recipe toward this goal in the work of Ernst Mayr. During his exceptionally long and productive career as a biologist, Mayr came to realize that "progress in the biological sciences is characterized not so much by individual discoveries, no matter how important, or by the proposal of new theories, but rather by the gradual but decisive development of new concepts and the abandonment of those that had previously been dominant. In most cases the development of major new concepts has not been due to individual discoveries but rather to novel integration of previously established facts" (Mayr, 1982, p. 856).

In writing this book I have been hard at work trying to develop new concepts. My ambition was to integrate relevant and established knowledge from a broad scientific landscape. Along the way, I have also pointed out that some of the popular concepts in the study of wellbeing should be revised or perhaps abandoned. Even core concepts in the field, such as affect, life satisfaction, hedonia, and eudaimonia, are used in vague and inconsistent ways. I have also criticized the epistemological foundation of wellbeing research and believe that the current understanding of science as objective and value-free should be replaced with a feminist epistemology that considers science to be a social activity. Feminist, or social, epistemology argues that objective observations do not exist. Hence, to deal with the subjectivity that comes with any world view, including the scientific ones, multiple perspectives must be confronted with each other. "It is through the give and take of ideas—the challenging, the questioning, the adjusting and amending—that scientists integrate their colleagues' work, offer up criticisms, and contribute to the growth of warranted knowledge" (Oreskes, 2019, p. 51).

From this vantage point, the humanistic theory of wellbeing is founded on debates of "big," existential ideas. It set sails between the biological question "What is life?" and the philosophical question "What is good?" The theory assumes that values originated with the creation of life and that all living organisms have a valuation mechanism that provides hints about what is good and bad for them. Our biology was in other words normative from the very beginning; even DNA molecules are value oriented. A science of wellbeing should therefore start by answering fundamental questions such as: How are valuations of goodness and badness possible? What are the mechanisms that make us feel good and think that our lives are good?

The HTW further suggests that the concept of wellbeing needs a normative grounding. Being well is more than a psychological description. Being well is something good in itself. As scientists we ought to be clear about that.

Researchers have the same moral responsibilities as the general population. For example, they must respect basic human rights and avoid harming others if it can be prevented. We must also assume that most scientists believe that being committed to (some) moral obligations makes the world a better place. From here, it seems like a small step to submit that a human life cannot be good unless it is committed to a set of universal moral values. The humanistic theory of wellbeing therefore suggests that it is good to like one's life, but even better to like it for the right reasons.

Tromsø, Norway
June 2024

Joar Vittersø

References

Mayr, E. (1982). *The growth of biological thought. Diversity, evolution, and inheritance*. Harvard University Press.

Mischel, W. (2008). The toothbrush problem. *APS Observer (December 1)*, *21*(11). https://www.psychologicalscience.org/observer/the-toothbrush-problem

Oreskes, N. (2019). *Why trust science? [Kindle]*. Princeton University Press.

Acknowledgments

The best story that I know of about the cooperative nature of human achievements was told by Shelly Taylor. One day, she writes in the preface of her 1989 book on *Positive Illusions*, an anthropologist from the University of Chicago was carrying his granddaughter on his shoulder when he encountered a colleague. The friend, who had not seen the little girl for a while, looked up at her and said: "My, my! How you have grown!" The child responded: "Not all of this is me."

In the years that have passed since Springer offered me a book contract in 2011, I have been carried forward on many shoulders. I am thankful to my first editor, Esther Otten, who kicked the project off, and to my current editor, Shinjini Chatterjee, who helped me pass the finishing line.

I am also grateful to students and colleagues at the UiT The Arctic University of Norway for the many hours we have spent together, discussing the good life and how it can be grasped by means of a scientific rationality. I am particularly thankful to my PhD students, Robert Biswas-Diener, Karoline Kopperud, Gunvor Marie Dyrdal, Lisa Vivoll Straume, Helga Synnevåg Løvold, Audun Hetland, Kjærsti Thorstensen, Benedicte Langseth-Eide, and Marie Seberg Primdahl.

Many people have given me their thoughts, reactions, criticism, and suggestions on various drafts of the book, and for that, I am grateful. Anders Barstad at Statistics Norway (SSB) kindly offered comments on a draft of the first chapter of the book. Thanks also to Ulrich Schimmack at the University of Toronto, Canada, for the thoughtful remarks and criticism that he gave on parts of an earlier draft. His profound knowledge about wellbeing and sharp eye for conceptual inconsistencies have been most helpful.

In Tromsø, I have had the fortune of interacting with my inspiring colleague Tove Dahl. In addition to our numerous discussions about the good life, and all sorts of gifts she offers to make the lives of those around her better, Tove has also read and commented on parts of this book. Thank you, Tove.

In Oslo, two academic environments have been excellent company. The first is PROMENTA, which is a research center working in the fields of mental health and wellbeing. One of its research groups, the "Happiness lab," has kindly invited me to present parts of this book at their meetings. I thank Thomas Nielsen, Thomas

Hansen, Lilian Mayerhofer, Maja Eilertsen, Kristian Krogshus, Heidi Marie Umbach Hansen, Maud Edvoll, Monica Beer Prydz, and Live Skow Hofgaard. Four members of the Happiness lab, Irene Teulings, Jinrui Liu, Ragnhild Bang Nes, and Espen Røysamb, have been particularly good allies of my book project. They also constitute the psychological ensemble of my second Oslo-based home, a research consortium named "Modeling Human Happiness," or ModHap for short. ModHap is an interdisciplinary research project that integrates insights from philosophy and psychology to develop scientific models of happiness to inform research, public debate, and policymaking. It is financed by the Norwegian Research Council (grant no. 325898) and has been a very stimulating source of inspiration and learning in the final period of my book writing. I would like to thank the philosophers at ModHap for their inspiring and insightful reflections and feedback on some of the topics discussed in the book: Thomas Kjeller Johansen, Franco Trivigno, Eyjólfur Kjalar Emilsson, Gry Oftedal, Paal Fredrik Skjørten Kvarberg, and Derk van Zoonen.

Ragnhild Bang Nes and Espen Røysamb have been my friends for many years, and I am grateful for their continuous encouragement and support. I am thankful for the back-up I have received from Henning Bang, who is also a psychology professor at the University of Oslo. The four of us have frequently debated the big questions in life, and I have benefited from, and much enjoyed, our conversations. Espen is a particularly dear friend who means a lot to me both privately and professionally. He has read and commented on parts of the manuscript and for this, and for his friendship, inspiration, and profound insights into wellbeing and its measurements, I am deeply indebted. Due to the countless occasions he has offered me to sit on his broad and generous shoulders, my work on wellbeing looms larger than it otherwise would have done.

Finally, and above all else, my warmest thanks go to my wife, Astrid Musland, soulmate and lifelong partner. Since we met as undergraduate students in the early 1980s, she has patiently conversed with me about so many things, including the psychology of wellbeing. She has frequently corrected my ideas when they have gone astray or been inconsistently formulated. During the years that I have been occupied with this book, she has always cheered me up and encouraged me to carry on. Thank you for believing in me when the going was rough! Astrid has thoroughly read the entire manuscript and detected many shortcomings in my reasoning. For the most part, I have gratefully taken her advice. Without Astrid and her continuous support, the book would be much poorer.

Contents

About the Author

Joar Vittersø is a professor of social psychology at the UiT The Arctic University of Norway, with a secondary appointment at the University of Oslo. He holds an MS in social anthropology, an MS and a Ph.D. in social psychology, all from the University of Oslo. Vittersø's research includes studies of conceptual developments in the science of wellbeing, and he has published extensively on topics such as life satisfaction, positive emotions, personal growth, and eudaimonic wellbeing. He is the editor of the "Handbook of Eudaimonic Well-Being."

Abbreviations

EWB	Eudaimonic wellbeing
HFM	Hedonic fluency model
HTW	Humanistic theory of wellbeing
HWB	Hedonic wellbeing
LS	Life satisfaction
NA	Negative affect
PA	Positive affect
PWB	Personal wellbeing
SDT	Self-determination theory
SGBE	Spontaneous good-bad evaluations
SWB	Subjective wellbeing

List of Figures

List of Tables

Chapter 1
A World of Values

Introduction

> Our brains are quite literally valuation machines.
> [They are] "values all the way down."
> (Montague, 2007, pp. x and 247)

Life invented values. Before life, during the first 10 billion years after the Big Bang, the Universe just existed; it followed the laws of nature without any purpose or meaning. Then, about 4 billion years ago, the chemical structure we call life appeared on the face of Earth. From the very beginning, these structures were able to not only reproduce themselves but also differentiate between good and bad. Biology began. Valuation was born. Everything changed.

The new chemical structure enabled organisms to be active, self-organizing, and purposive. Once life started to move, survival and reproduction became important, and a valuation mechanism was the unavoidable consequence. Values, roughly defined as things we care about, have therefore pervaded our existence since its very beginning, and the reason is simple: Nothing would have survived if it mixed nourishment with poison, safety with hazards, or the "good stuff" with the "bad stuff," as Haidt calls it (Haidt, 2012, p. 64). And that, I shall argue in this book, explains why we humans care so much about happiness.

To get there, however, some premises must be clarified. I am, for example, not suggesting that everything we value is automatically and solely oriented toward survival and reproduction. To say that the earliest forms of life kick-started a valuation process is not to say that primitive valuation is all we need to know about values. Humans are cultural beings with intricate value structures and sophisticated moral beliefs. Indeed, with this book, I intend to examine the complexity of values and human goodness at great length. But biological valuation is the mechanism that explains how and why we started to care about what happens to us. The phenomenon of goodness might have begun as a primitive valuation mechanism, but for humans, it certainly did not end as one. Values are about survival, Damasio tells us,

J. Vittersø, *Humanistic Wellbeing*, https://doi.org/10.1007/978-3-031-69292-5_1

but for humans, "value also relates to the quality of that survival in the form of well-being" (Damasio, 2010, loc. 812). The most essential possession of any living being, Damasio argues, "is the balanced range of body chemistries compatible with healthy life. It applies equally to an amoeba and to a human being. All else flows from it. Its significance cannot be overemphasized" (Damasio, 2010, loc. 779). This evolutionary perspective also justifies a scientific investigation of values, morality, and wellbeing. If values start with life and are a part of it, we do not need metaphysics to understand them.

The principle behind the biologically rooted valence orientation is not complicated. According to Montague (2007, p. 55), a valuation mechanism simply indicates the value of the current state of affairs. These valuation mechanisms, or value functions, "can be seen at every level in biological systems, from molecules all the way up to strategies for social exchange" (p. 2). Montague uses the warmer-colder game as an analogy. An object is hidden by one of the players, and the others are guided toward it by a message that things are becoming "warmer" if they approach the object and "colder" if they move away. Thus, the "warmer message" is a value signal that intensifies as the distance decreases and weakens as the distance increases. Biologists seem to agree that even the most primitive life-forms have this ability to identify and reach out for what appears to be the better option. All organisms are prewired to aim for things that are good for them. Plants, for example, evaluate stimuli in their environments, reacting to the presence of alien plants by increasing their own root profusion (Clore & Schiller, 2016). Even genes are value-laden in the sense of providing a kind of normative information (Damasio, 2018; Lane, 2015; Mayr, 2004).

Consider bacteria, small creatures that have inhabited our planet for almost 4 billion years. By means of an intriguing driving force called chemotaxis, this oldest and simplest form of life searches for goodness by stretching out toward benign environments and shrinking down when meeting unhealthy ones (Montague, 2007). When a bacterium is placed in an environment with a variable concentration of glucose, it "swims" toward the high concentration region (Pross, 2016). The process can even be observed in collaborative, almost moral-like, behaviors. For example, in affluent environments, bacteria live relatively independently, but when resources become scarce, they cluster together in clumps (Damasio, 2018). This is an intriguing example of how bacteria are goodness-seeking cells capable of joining others in their striving toward some sort of a common good. They even seem to "punish" noncooperating "cheaters" by isolating them (Jousset et al., 2013).

The essence of these insights was to some extent realized by Aristotle. In the *Nicomachean Ethics*, he went straight out and said: "Every art and every inquiry, and similarly every action and pursuit, is thought to aim at some good; and for this reason, the good has rightly been declared to be that at which all things aim" (Aristotle, trans. 1908, p. 7). Aristotle was wrong about nonliving things aiming for the good, however. Rocks and planets do not search for anything—and certainly not for goodness. But even if Aristotelian epistemology did not sufficiently separate biology and physics, his teleology was "remarkably modern" in regard to living organisms (Mayr, 2004, p. 44). Every organism pursues goals, De Waal (2013,

p. 164) tells us, and Erwin Schrödinger could reveal life's deepest secrets when the laureate physicist realized that a piece of matter becomes alive "when it goes on 'doing something', moving, exchanging material with its environment, and so forth" (Schrödinger, 2010/1946, p. 62).

Aristotle was uninformed about chemical details and biological valuation mechanisms. However, he had a rough idea about goals, or telos as he called them, and how they regulate behavior. Aristotle moved rather freely between speaking of the "goal of something" and "the good of something," which is how many psychologists think of goals today as well (e.g., Fishbach & Ferguson, 2007; Oatley, 1992). A goal is something we care about; it can be defined as a standard for evaluation (Baron, 2024), and as we have seen, science confirmed how such value-oriented activity is built into the very structure of biological life. But Aristotle did not stop with the description of life as being driven by goals. He went normative and wanted to understand which goals we humans ought to follow and which we should abhor. Extensive examinations led Aristotle to believe that happiness, eudaimonia in Greek, was the ultimate good, the "summum bonum." And happiness, he suggested, is "activity of the soul in accordance with virtue" (Aristotle, trans. 1908, p. 14).

An ancient thinker, Aristotle saw the world differently than us. He did not know about evolution by natural selection. He had no notion about universal human rights. He thought that the brain was a fairly useless organ. His philosophy was partly mythological, and his attitudes toward women, slavery, minority issues, and cultural diversity are no longer acceptable. Scientifically, Aristotle's idea that our ultimate telos must be happiness is also problematic. Evolutionary speaking, no animate organism has happiness as its final goal since that role is delegated to reproduction. "Happiness is not a goal left unaccomplished by some bungling designer, it is an aspect of a behavioural regulation mechanism shaped by natural selection" (Nesse, 2005, p. 10). Although the happiness that Nesse refers to is not the same happiness as Aristotle had in mind, the notion of a good life as laid out in the *Nicomachean Ethics* is not consistent with the idea that life is fundamentally oriented toward survival and reproduction (see Chap. 6).

Yet, there might be elements in Aristotelian theorizing still appealing to us moderns. As a general principle, his reasoning about goodness as fulfillment could have relevance for scientific theories of wellbeing. The idea will at least be pursued in the theory to be developed in this book, which I have named the humanistic theory of wellbeing (HTW). An Aristotelian inspiration central to the HTW can therefore be formulated as a slogan: *A life is good to the extent that it allows us to perform our humanness well.*

It is important to note that the term "our humanness" conveys a different meaning than the term "our nature." After all, human nature "has enough diversity to fit almost any ethical taste" (Kagan, 1998, p. 188), and Damasio reminds us that it is cultures, not human nature by itself, that "can decide when natural things are good—and determine the degree of goodness—and when they are not. Greed is just as natural as profit but is not culturally good, contrary to what Gordon Gekko famously affirmed" (Damasio, 2018, p. 237). A general appeal to our human nature therefore has limited utility. The concept of humanness is more constrained and, in the HTW, embedded in an explicit normative framework, referred to as "basic humanistic values."

Admittedly a vague phrase, the slogan that life is good to the extent that it allows us to perform our humanness well will be expanded throughout the book. I will start by examining the concept of good and how it can be analyzed within the framework of scientific reasoning. It should further be noted that the terms happiness, wellbeing, and a good life are used interchangeably in this chapter. Throughout the book, however, they will be supplied with more distinctive and differentiated meanings.

What Is Good?

The philosophical literature on goodness is vast. It spans millennia of critical thinking and covers approaches such as axiology, value theories, and meta-ethics. The texts are often technical, and they certainly expand far beyond the limits of this book. However, three important distinctions made in the field will be briefly mentioned. The first separates absolute goodness from relational goodness, and the second divides instrumental from noninstrumental goodness. The third dichotomy is between prudential and moral goodness.

Absolute goodness refers to the inherent or intrinsic moral value of something; it means that something is good regardless of context and consequences. Absolute goodness is in other words not good for someone, not good of a kind, but nonetheless good (Kraut, 2012). The analytical "Trinity philosopher" G. E. Moore is probably the best-known defender of this perspective. In his *Principia Ethica* (1993/1903), Moore claimed that "theree is *a sui generis* property of absolute goodness that is not reducible to any other properties. The term 'good' designates that property and that property is shared by all good things" (cited in Kazemi, 2023). That something can be good absolutely is also called good *simpliciter;* and friendship, justice, and the appreciation of beauty are often taken to be examples of such goodness. Relative goodness, by contrast, is good in relation to a context, circumstance, or the consequences of actions or decisions. Something is good relative to a standard such as a goal, skill, or function. We can, for instance, say that eating vegetables is good for health or that a knife is good because it cuts well. Grammatically oriented philosophers refer to the distinction between absolute and relative goodness as predicative versus attributive goodness (Geach, 1956; Ross & Ross, 2002; Turp, 2016). Adjectives such as "red" and "blue" are predicative because an object can be plainly red or plain blue. To say that "A is red" makes sense. This is not the case for attributive adjectives. We can, for instance, not say that "A is tall" without referring to a context. "Things can only be said to be tall for something or qua something" (Kazemi, 2023, p. 2).

Instrumental values or goods are contrasted with noninstrumental goods. Something is instrumentally good when it is good as a means to something else that is good. By contrast, a noninstrumental value is an end in itself (Huemer, 2021). Aristotle (trans. 1908) discusses the issue in his *Nicomachean Ethics,* where we can read that some goods must be good in themselves, such as happiness, whereas others are good because of these, such as money or fame (p. 11). Another illustration of the distinction between intrinsic and instrumental values comes from David Hume (2006). He tried to unpack the true sources of our values by asking—hypothetically rather than empirically—why people truly want something. Why do, for instance, people want money? The answer, he assumed rather than tested, is that we want it because it leads us to something else, something that is valuable in itself. Following this reasoning to its logical end leads us to the realization that the true and only noninstrumental value is pleasure. "And beyond this it is an absurdity to ask for a reason" (Hume, 2006, cited in Moen, 2012, p. 8).

The third distinction to be reviewed is between prudential and moral goodness (e.g., Griffin, 1986; Hirata, 2011; Zimmerman, 2015). Prudential goodness concerns individuals' lives, whereas moral goodness deals with social life. Something is prudentially good if it is valuable for the person whose life it is, whereas something is morally good if respecting others is explicitly valued. The distinction says that being well is not the same as being moral; my goodness is not necessarily your goodness or our goodness. This seems reasonable as far as it goes, but it is also plausible that the two value domains overlap and more so than commonly assumed in the literature on values and wellbeing. The notion of prudential values comes uncomfortably close to an individualistic model of humans as rational actors whose primary goal is to maximize the satisfaction of their own interests. Sayer (2011), for example, duly asks why theories of wellbeing are so strongly influenced by the idea that individuals should be free to decide on their conception of the good, and confronted with the philosophical wellbeing literature, it often strikes me that much of their thinking does not fully recognize the genuine "we-ness" embedded in our human nature. Searle (1995) made the same point and accused philosophers of overestimating individual intentionality at the expense of social and collective intentionality. That rationality, and intentionality, is located in individual minds does not mean that their respective foci are limited to the individual in whose head it exists. Many philosophers, I suspect, fall prey to such an individualistic reductionism and consider humans to primarily be self-sufficient and rational beings. Social scientists, by contrast, more often think of us as cooperative and relational beings. Insights from moral psychology and social psychology make it clear that we will not fully understand our humanness unless we see how fundamentally oriented humans are toward one another. It is not merely a matter of being "social animals" in the sense that we constantly orient ourselves toward others and integrate our own lives with the lives of those around us. Being cultural means that our humanness would not have existed if our sociability was, miraculously, stripped away—if we were to look at "pure individuality," if you like. For example, were they not cultural beings, humans would not have had language or the ability to think abstractly and logically. A "pure" individual would not understand mathematics or concepts such as subjectivity, objectivity, and justice. Neither would a noncultural, "pure" individual understands the concept of wellbeing nor be able to articulate a sophisticated idea about "my interests." It is not that these capacities would be completely absent without our "we-ness," but they would have been very rudimentary and different from what we observe in *Homo sapiens*. If we can imagine a human individual growing up in complete isolation, their mental life will likely be similar to that of a chimpanzee (Tomasello, 2019).

Although this knowledge does not speak directly to the distinction between prudential and moral goodness, it would be strange if the human we-ness that we only are beginning to understand have no bearing on the conceptualization of the two kinds of goodness. If the model of a human being as a rational, self-sufficient, independent, autonomous, and self-interested individual is wrong, it makes little sense to target a certain kind of goodness exclusively toward such a nonexistent entity. Moreover, the birth of an ethics of care has contributed to a new comprehension of how individual identities are relational in the sense of reflecting a mutual kind of autonomy. For example, Held (2006) argues that "those who conscientiously care for others are not seeking primarily to further their own individual interests; their interests are intertwined with the persons they care for" (p. 12). In these instances, the concept of prudential goodness seems misleading.

The Good, the Bad, and the Scientist

Science has a good grip on the mechanisms that make feelings and reflections about goodness possible. But scientists are often uneasy in front of normative claims and are seldom willing to award goodness an ascendant influence in their work (e.g., Kagan, 1998). The term good will typically endure an unscientific airing, and most researchers are uncomfortable talking professionally about it. Jerry Fodor's opinion is mainstream: "Science is about facts, not norms; it might tell us how we are, but it couldn't tell us what is wrong with how we are. There couldn't be a science of the human condition" (Fodor, 2007, p. 19). Scientists are thus at home when discussing factual statements and can readily make claims such as "the cat is on the mat." To state that "the cat on the mat is a good cat," by contrast, is a different matter. There are important reasons for this practice, even if, as we shall see in the "Values in Science" section, the separation of factual statements and value statements is not as clear-cut as it once seemed (e.g., Douglas, 2009; Elliott, 2017; Putnam, 1993).

It is not that scientists never use the term good, but they often do it with some care. For instance, when Seligman (1998) as the president of the American Psychological Association announced his ambition that psychologists should study the "good life," he put the phrase in brackets. Diener has also followed the same practice, as in explaining that scientists of subjective wellbeing "hope to further our understanding of the age-old questions of what composes the 'good life' and the 'good society'" (Diener, 1998, p. 312). A similar reluctance to use the term goodness in scientific prose can be observed in Sapolsky's *Behave* (Sapolsky, 2017). In this book, Sapolsky provides a comprehensive analysis of how human behavior can be improved, and to me, he appears to have clear opinions about good and bad ways of leading a life. However, he is reluctant about the word good. It is too "hot-blooded

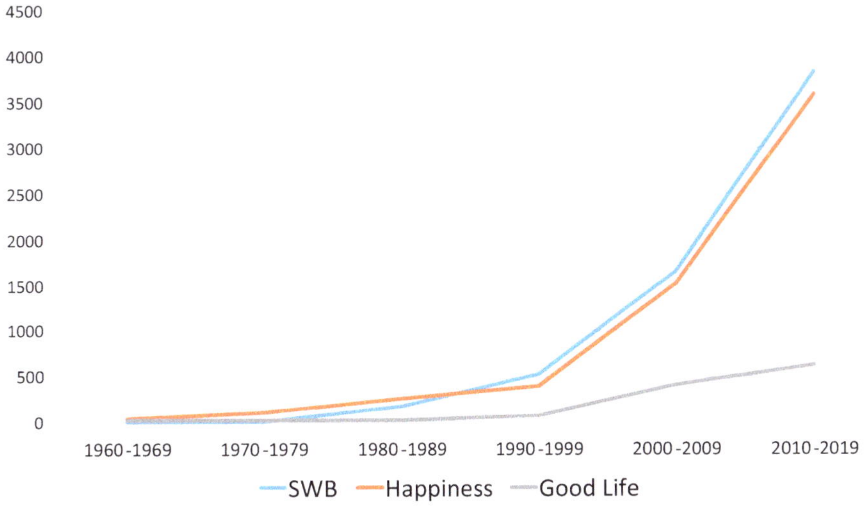

Fig. 1.1 Use of the terms subjective wellbeing (SWB), happiness, and good life between 1960 and 2019 according to PsycINFO

and frothy" he tells us (p. 25). Rather than talking about goodness, Sapolsky admits that he prefers to speak of our best behavior rather than our good behavior.

My impression is that terms such as goodness and the good life are more frequently used without brackets in recent literature. Oishi et al. (2018) claim, for instance, that "a good society is a society that makes its citizens happy" (p. 164). Oishi and Westgate have even proposed a definition of a good life, which, according to the two authors, is "a life well lived from the perspective of the person living it" (Oishi & Westgate, 2022, p. 790).

As illustrated in Fig. 1.1, however, terms such as subjective wellbeing and happiness are currently the dominant terms in the psychological literature on wellbeing. The term "a good life" is older; however, and according to the PsycINFO database, it was used twice in the period from 1860 to 1900. It then appeared 41 times between 1900 and 1960. By contrast, subjective wellbeing appeared for the first time in the 1960s, but since the 1980s, it has taken over as the preferred wellbeing nomenclature, together with happiness.

The Psychology of Good and Bad

It is now commonly agreed that evaluations of goodness and badness are among the first, quickest, and most frequent assessments humans make (Arnold, 1960; Bargh, 1994; Barrett, 2006; Gilovich et al., 2005; Kahneman, 1999; Lazarus & Folkman, 1984). It has even been proposed that the significant role that evaluations play in our lives justifies the name "homo evaluaticus" (Winkielman et al., 2003). We continuously evaluate the stream of sensations and perceptions we take in and are "chronically engaged in ascertaining the goodness or badness of stimuli in our environments" (Pratto, 1994, p. 116). The judgments of goodness and badness are probably the most fundamental building blocks of a conscious mind and a sense of self (Damasio, 1999, p. 30). Jarvis and Petty even refer to the constant evaluation of goodness and badness as a need (Jarvis & Petty, 1996). Our ubiquitous concern with spontaneous evaluations can be observed throughout human history and across cultures. All languages, for example, can express the feeling of goodness (Wierzbicka, 1999, pp. 279–282), and the words good and bad are among the first words that children learn (Baumeister, 1991, p. 38). Philosopher Ralph Perry (1926) noted a hundred years ago that living minds tend to view their surroundings with favor or disfavor. This bias toward or away from things "appears in many forms, such as liking and disliking, desire and aversion, will and refusal, or seeking and avoiding" (cited in Sumner, 1996, p. 35). In reviewing influential ideas in the history of psychology, Kagan (1998) investigates what he considers to be a universal desire to regard self as good. One consequence of this desire for goodness, he argues, is that humans generally "think and act in ways that support rather than disconfirm that evaluation." Kagan is "even tempted to suggest that the continuous seeking of evidence to prove one's virtue is, like Darwin's notion of natural selection, the most potent condition sculpturing each person's trait over the lifetime" (p. 157). Among the arguments Kagan drew on to make this proposal is a quote from the historian Hayden White, who has observed that it is next to impossible to communicate about human doings and whereabouts outside a normative framework. "Novels, critical reviews, plays, autobiographies, historical treatises, and most essays in social science journals implicitly assume that certain states of affairs are good and others are bad" (cited in Kagan, 1998, pp. 157–158).

Thorndike was an early analyst of these omnipresent good-bad evaluations. Somewhat surprisingly, he saw them as a "constant error" (Thorndike, 1920, p. 25). Thorndike got the error idea from a study of two large industrial corporations in which workers who were asked to describe their colleagues tended to generalize them "as rather good or rather inferior." Thorndike complained that this inclination made it difficult to obtain precise information about the specific qualities each employee truly possessed and considered the tendency to evaluate others as either good or bad as an "error toward suffusing ratings of special features with a halo belonging to the individual as a whole" (p. 25).

Spontaneous good-bad evaluations may not be "erroneous" in the capacity to be judgments, however. Ambady and Rosenthal (1993) reported that strangers who rated unknown teachers' nonverbal behavior, based on very brief video clips, accurately predicted the ratings of the same teachers by people who had substantial interactions with those teachers (e.g., students and supervisors). This research not only shows how quickly and spontaneously good-bad evaluations are made but also that they can be surprisingly precise. Ambady and Rosenthal's study showed that judgments based on 30-s exposures (three 10-s clips of each teacher) were not significantly more accurate than judgments based on 6-s exposures (three 2-s clips of each teacher). More recent and comprehensive studies in social cognition have corroborated the universal display of Thorndike's so-called "halo" effect, although under a different label. Fiske et al. (2007) summarized the field of social perceptions and concluded that evolutionary pressures have honed us to immediately evaluate others along two dimensions of goodness: warmth and competence. To function well socially, Fiske and colleagues argue, social animals must determine "whether the 'other' is friend or foe (i.e. intends good or ill) and then, whether the 'other' has the ability to enact those intentions" (p. 77). The authors found that the basic dimensions of warmth and competence account for 82% of the variance in perceptions of everyday social behaviors people we encounter.

Interestingly, people we perceive as warm and competent uniformly elicit positive emotions (Fiske et al., 2007, p. 77), indicating that a fundamental feeling component is involved in the perception of someone else. The feeling element in good-bad evaluations is probably something humans share with other sentient beings. But the valuation mechanism also functions in organisms that almost certainly have no feelings (Damasio, 2018) and can basically be conceptualized as a guidance signal rather than a subjective feeling (Montague, 2007, p. 123). However, the fact that valuations can be made without a feeling component does not mean that feelings are unimportant. Hogan (2003) found, for example, that stories that can be regarded as universals are appealing to emotions. Two emotions are particularly important: the love story and the story of angry conflict. Studies that explore the underlying structure of emotions further confirm that good-bad evaluations are essential for human psychology. Wilhelm Wundt, for example, memorably found that pleasantness was the most salient among his so-called mental elements. When participants in his laboratory in Leipzig were asked to describe their experiences, of colors, music, odors, and more complex objects, the feelings were typically reported to involve an element of pleasure or displeasure (Ruckmick, 1925). These evaluations came easily and naturally, even if it was difficult to specify them more concretely (Frijda, 2010). Wundt concluded that feelings not only are irreducible mental elements but are also evaluative in the sense that they imply acceptance or nonacceptance of the stimulus or the experience itself. The doctrine of "affective primacy" was formulated to account for the instant liking and disliking of subjects attached to either approach or avoid a stimulus (see Haidt, 2012).

In North America, William James also reasoned that feelings reflect a comment on the favorability or unfavorability of the environment. Without this ability, James argued, nothing in the universe would have importance. In other words, meaning and values are essentially linked to the feelings of goodness in James' thinking (Wessman & Ricks, 1966, p. 2). Similarly, Gustav Jung believed that humans continuously judge their environment along a goodness-badness dimension, and he associated these judgments with feelings. To Jung, feeling good or bad constitutes a subjective criterion of acceptance or rejection (Denton, 2005, p. 218). Work by psychologists such as Beebe-Center (1932) and Young (1961) further contributed key insights to the study of pleasure and human goodness.

Sigmund Freud was no stranger to good and bad feelings and viewed pleasure-seeking as a fundamental human drive, one that motivates the "id" to seek immediate gratification of our needs and wishes (Freud, 1930, 2012/1920). Basically, the principle is hedonic in the sense of suggesting that people seek pleasure and avoid pain, first and foremost by satisfying their biological and psychological needs. Freud assumed that the unconscious was constantly scanning the environment for potential threats or benefits. Another of the early psychologists, Charlotte Bühler (1928, 1951), developed an interesting evaluative concept called "function lust" or "function pleasure." In contrast to the homeostatic explanation Freud applied to justify his pleasure principle, Bühler's idea is that the behavior itself, the movements of a body, produces pleasure. This kind of pleasure comes from the experience of being able to do things and is not identical to the pleasure, or satisfaction, that comes with the fulfillment of biological needs. The "function pleasure" can be seen most clearly in children's play but it does operate throughout the entire life span.

As a final example of early contributions to the psychology of goodness, Thorndike's "law of effect" can be mentioned (Thorndike, 1927). The law of effect is crucial because it postulates that behavior that is followed by a pleasant feeling is more likely to be repeated. Hence, good-bad feelings are functionally important because they explain how behavior is shaped and maintained. They are at the core of reinforcement learning.

These early ideas continued to attract new generations of psychologists. Good-bad evaluations have, for instance, been referred to as a human drive (Festinger, 1954) and the dominating force in life (Allport, 1961). From the perspective of motivational psychology, Schneirla (1959) suggested that approach and avoidance are rooted in good-bad evaluations that are highly functional and evolutionarily beneficial: "The high road of evolution has been littered with the remains of species that have failed to acquire one or more mechanisms for accurately determining the beneficial or harmful potential of environmental stimuli" (cited in Elliot & Covington, 2001, p. 77). An important step toward our current understanding was taken when Zajonc (1968, 1980) introduced the concept of the mere exposure effect (for a review, see Bornstein, 1989). The idea that "preferences need no inferences" points out the automatized nature of good-bad evaluations: "When we meet a stranger, we know within the fraction of a second whether we like the person or not. The reaction is instantaneous and automatic. Perhaps the feeling is not always precise; perhaps we are not always aware of it, but the feeling is always there. If our later experience with the stranger conflicts with the first impression, we are terribly surprised. We consider it an exception" (Zajonc, 1980, p. 157).

Accumulated evidence for snap and universal good-bad judgments includes the observation that individuals who encounter a new situation need less than 250 milliseconds to obtain a rough idea about whether the new condition is good or bad (Bargh, 1997; Bargh et al., 1995). Other studies, using electrophysiological responses, revealed that good-bad evaluations occur within 300–600 ms when measuring the earliest onset (Leuthold et al., 2015) and within 1000 ms when measuring facial electromyogram responses ('t Hart et al., 2018). Even shorter response times have been found by Willis and Todorov (2006) and Van Berkum et al. (2009). Based on photographs of unfamiliar faces, these authors asked participants to judge traits such as attractiveness, likeability, and trustworthiness. They found that judgments made with a 100-ms time limit correlated strongly with judgments made in the absence of time constraints. This result suggests that exposure times as short as 100 ms could be sufficient to form an impression of another person, which aligns with literature reviews concluding that the brain is wired to distinguish good from bad stimuli, and it is able to do so very quickly (e.g., Malle, 2021). The core of these good-bad evaluations is well captured by Barrett (2006, p. 36), who considers them to be "a simple form of meaning analysis in which something is judged as good or bad, helpful or harmful." Similarly, review studies show that a single good-bad evaluation item used in large surveys reveals an impressive predictive power for a range of health and life quality outcomes, such as longevity, hospital visits, partnership dissolution, and job changes (Kaiser & Oswald, 2022).

Spontaneous Good-Bad Evaluations

I shall refer to the quick and automatized tendency to evaluate things in terms of goodness and badness as spontaneous good-bad evaluations (SGBE). They constitute a kind of information processing that can be distinguished from nonevaluative processing, such as computations, perception, and memory, and are probably very close to what Kahneman (1999) refers to as "a running affective commentary" or an evaluative good-bad dimension. An elegant illustration of the SGBE is the so-called "good guy/bad guy" study by Tranel and Damasio (1993), in which the evaluative capacities of a patient called Boswell was examined. Boswell suffered severe memory deficits and was, for instance, unable to learn new facts. Yet, he seemed to hold some preferences and avoidance for people in his surroundings. In this experiment, Boswell met regularly with three different people. One of them was instructed to meet with Boswell in an extremely pleasant and welcoming way (the "good guy"), and another person, a beautiful woman, interacted systematically in a harsh and rude way (the "bad guy"). A third person was told to appear in an emotionally neutral way. After a period of 5 days of encountering these three individuals, Boswell was repeatedly asked to look at photographs of each. Boswell could not tell anything about the three persons in the photos, but when asked who he considered to be his friend, he chose the "good guy" over 80% of the time, significantly above chance. The "bad guy" was rarely chosen and significantly below chance. In other words, Boswell revealed an unconscious preference for the "good guy," suggesting that the evaluation of goodness and badness is fundamental in the sense that it needs no "cognitive" inferences.

A related story is told by Jill Bolte Taylor, a neuroanatomist who suffered a stroke in 1996, at the age of 37. Her gem of a book, entitled *My Stroke of Insight* (Taylor, 2008), provides a detailed story of what a stroke looks like from within, "trapped inside the perception of a meditation that I could neither stop nor escape" (p. 38). During the most acute phase of her attack, Taylor was unable to execute even the most basic cognitive skills, such as interpreting the telephone number in front of her to call for help. But her feelings of goodness and badness were intact, and some of her experiences during the stroke were surprisingly positive (see also Chaps. 3 and 4). For example, as a patient at the hospital, Taylor was mostly unable to understand what happened to her. Nevertheless, she was emotionally informed about good and bad things in her surroundings, such as caregivers who treated her with warmth and respect. With these nurses and doctors around, Taylor felt taken care of and safe. She felt like a human being. In contrast, other staff members were inattentive to her needs, and these health workers gave her a bad feeling and a sense of being unsafe. Like Boswell's responses to the confederates in the "good guy/bad guy" study by Tranel and Damasio, Taylor was not capable of interpreting her surroundings with cognitive clarity, yet she did not lose her ability to sense goodness and badness.

Factor Analyses

Another approach to documenting the dominance of spontaneous good-bad evaluations in the human mind comes from studies using factor analysis of self-reported feeling states. A factor analysis is a statistical technique used to identify and analyze the underlying structure (or factors) that may be influencing a set of observed variables. When the method gained momentum in the 1950s, the attempts to find the basic dimensions of subjective experiences became remarkably similar to the descriptions offered by Wundt half a century earlier. The introspective analyses of the contents of feelings that Wundt pioneered in Leipzig typically resulted in an experiential model that comprised a three-dimensional structure. The pleasure-displeasure dimension was the most dominant and stable, but two other and separate dimensions were also identified: an excitement-inhibition/quiet dimension and a tension-relaxation/relief dimension (e.g., Reisenzein, 1992). This three-dimensional structure of human feelings was later reproduced in a series of factor analytic studies. Schlosberg (1954) is an early example, although the results from Osgood et al. (1957) are more exhaustive and well-known. The three bipolar dimensions that Osgood and his colleagues identified as constituting the "meaning space"—what Osgood later specified to be "affective meaning"—were evaluation (liking), potency (control), and activity (arousal) or EPA for short (Osgood, 1969). Among the three dimensions, evaluation was most dominant. In the hundreds of factor analyses conducted by Osgood and others, the evaluation dimension accounted for between 50% and 75% of the variance (Tesser & Martin, 1996). In a cross-cultural study in which data from bipolar adjective scales translated to 21 languages were factor analyzed, the equivalent to the evaluative "good-bad" dimension appeared in all but one analysis—the exception being Thai (Osgood et al., 1975, pp. 160–162). Among all the adjectives tested in the project, good—together with big—was the most "productive qualifier" of the entire semantic space (p. 391). Veenhoven (1984) also mentions some factor analytic studies conducted before 1970 that support the existence of a dominant evaluation factor, or a "general satisfaction factor," as Veenhoven calls it (p. 297). Similarly, many analyses of the so-called affect circumplex (Russell, 1980) also testify to the hypothesis that people are chronically engaged in ascertaining the goodness or badness of stimuli in their environments. Good-bad evaluations, often referred to as a valence dimension that runs from unpleasant to pleasant, are typically found to be more dominant than arousal, which is the other major dimension in the affect circumplex (Barrett, 1995; Lang, 1995).

In fact, it has been argued that the evaluative factor is the only truly general trait, a "mega" disposition reflecting a bias toward positive self-evaluation (Davies et al., 2015; Kim & Rosenberg, 1980). Data collected by Wessman and Ricks (1966) provide solid evidence for the dominating role of the valence dimension. In their factor analyses of 16 mood scales, distributed across measures of daily peaks, daily averages, and what they referred to as "daily trough," the authors found that a first factor accounted for most of the variance. This factor was described as "a pervasive overall level of 'good mood-bad mood' that tended to hold across subjects on most of the scales" (p. 70).

More recently, when a wellbeing module was included in the third round of the European Social Survey (ESS; Huppert et al., 2009), the factor structure of 45 items intended to measure a broad variety of wellbeing dimensions could be analyzed. As expected, the items had a very dominant first- factor, as illustrated by the scree plot in Fig. 1.2.

Similarly, a higher-order factor identified as goodness was observed in Peterson and Seligman's (2004) strength and virtue approach (see McGrath, 2015). In this study, a second factor, labeled inquisitiveness, was also found.

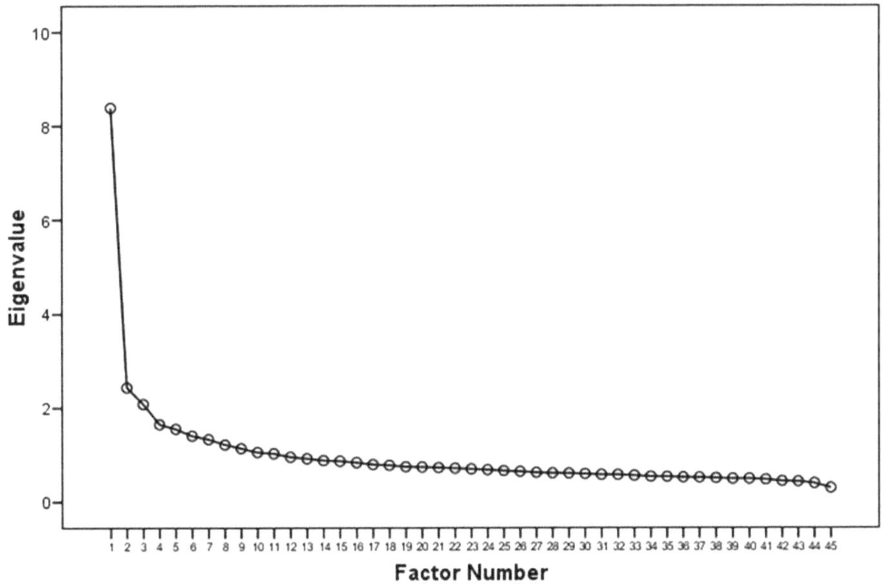

Fig. 1.2 A scree plot [A scree plot illustrates how much of the variance in the analyzed variables the factors explain, successively. The amount of explained variance is referred to as eigenvalues] from a factor analyses of the wellbeing module from the European Social Survey Round 3

The existence of a strong good-bad evaluation factor in self-reported wellbeing may help explain why so many of the instruments in the wellbeing literature correlate strongly with each other, even when they were designed to measure distinct dimensions of wellness (e.g., Disabato et al., 2016). The so-called Ryff scales, for instance, have a clear one factor structure at the second-order level (Springer & Hauser, 2006; Springer et al., 2006), and the scale also correlates highly with the traditional measures of SWB (Chen et al., 2013). Seligman's PERMA model, assumed to account for five unique wellbeing factors (i.e., positive emotions, engagement, relationships, meaning, and accomplishment), seems to be properly accounted for by a single second-order factor as well. This dimension also correlates almost perfectly with mainstream measures of happiness and life satisfaction (Goodman et al., 2018). In a recent and comprehensive analysis of self-reported wellbeing, Bjørndal et al. (2023) identified six wellbeing factors. Across three studies, these six factors all loaded on a single higher-order factor, referred to by the authors as a general "happiness factor," or h-factor, akin to the p-factor in psychopathology research. My interpretation of the h-factor is slightly different, however, since I believe that it reflects a more basic element than happiness, namely, the omnipresent good-bad evaluation I refer to as SGBE. It contributes variance to many psychological measures, both within the field of wellbeing research and beyond.

The Good in Positive Psychology

The positive psychology movement is one of several scientific communities devoted to researching wellbeing, what Seligman, as we have seen, introduced as the study of the "good life" (Seligman, 1998). The idea of categorizing things according to their positivity or negativity is not new, of course. The pre-Socratic philosopher Parmenides aimed, for instance, at creating a taxonomy of "all the elements of the world," and he organized them into two broad and overarching clusters: positive parts and negative parts (Rickless, 2012).

The term "positive" in relation to psychology can be traced back to commentators of Auguste Comte's positivism in the beginning of the twentieth century. As known from the history of science, Comte proposed that knowledge develop through three phases: the theological phase, the metaphysical phase, and the positive phase. In this scheme, scientific knowledge was positive because it was reliable, i.e., referred to indisputable facts (e.g., Suppe, 1977). Comte further assumed that psychological knowledge could never become positive because psychology is about "the soul," and our understanding of the soul will forever remain metaphysical. Consequently, Comte never used the term positive psychology. Others did, however, and the term was first launched in the USA approximately a hundred years ago by defenders of logical positivism. Positive psychology, such understood, was a psychology practiced in accordance with logical positivism. Even today, some use the term with this meaning. For example, Jensen (2008, p. x) claims that a positive analysis means "the analysis of the way the world is, how it behaves, independently of any normative value judgments about its desirability or undesirability."

However, some scholars have suggested that Comte did develop a notion of positive psychology in the sense that was later adopted by Maslow (1954) and Seligman (1998, 2002), i.e., positive psychology as the study of the good life. Comte formed a taxonomy of character traits, with vanity and pride[1] deemed as lower dispositions, and attachment, veneration, and goodness (or universal love) considered as higher propensities. Comte was criticized for making these value statements, which appeared metaphysical rather than positive (e.g., Hollander, 1901). In contrast, commentators such as Heyd (1989) have argued that Comte's positive psychology[2] applies both to his philosophical work (positivity as reliable knowledge) and to wellbeing theories (positivity as the good life). The reason is that happiness in Comte's theory was identified as a feeling that rested on truth—in other words, something that could be related to the truthfulness of a positive science. From this assumption, Comte appears to have envisioned the idea that the final stage of scientific and political development was nothing less than happiness.

Whether the two meanings of positive psychology—as reliable knowledge and as a theory of a good life—were truly united in Comte's own work will not be further examined here.[3] What follows is rather a more general investigation of the term positive in the sense of reflecting something good.

Modern Positive Psychology

As with most other concepts, positivity has been ascribed a multitude of meanings (Primdahl, 2024). Etymologically, the word "positive" is derived from the Latin verb *pono,* which had to do with setting up or building something. Although we can easily narrow the meaning of positive from its broad etymological origin, positive psychologists agree that the term still refers to a host of different concepts (Delle Fave et al., 2011; Sheldon, 2011; Wong, 2011). Symptomatically, Hart and Sasso (2011) identified 53 published definitions of positive psychology, although many were somewhat overlapping.

The most comprehensive analysis of the term positive in modern positive psychology is probably provided by Pawelski (2016a, 2016b). After reviewing documents central to the foundation of positive psychology (e.g., Seligman, 1999; Seligman & Csikszentmihalyi, 2000; Sheldon et al., 2000), Pawelski identified five

[1] The transformation of pride from a vise to a virtue is relatively recent. For example, the ancients classified pride as one of the seven "deadly sins," and the positive connotations attributed to pride in modern speech tends to overlook the negative consequences that also attests to this trait, like selfishness and lack of sympathy (Oveis et al., 2010).

[2] Comte's refusal to associate his ideas with a science termed psychology forced him to talk about positive *physiology* rather than positive *psychology*. Some of his successors, however, used the phrase positive psychology.

[3] Interested readers may consult (Plé, 2000) for further details about Comte's theory of happiness.

"common elements" of positivity, i.e., ways in which positive psychology is claimed to be positive:

1. Orientation—A call for a focus on the positive to complement the hegemonic emphasis on the negative.
2. Typography—Specific areas, such as optimism, courage, and social responsibility, should be studied.
3. Target population—The context in which positive psychology is to be applied.
4. Process—Identifying the kind of processes to be used.
5. Aim—The good life as a key object.

A sixth, referred to as simple preference, was added later in the article. Note that all but the last element was already included in the "old positive psychology," particularly the version articulated by Maslow. Pawelski concludes his analysis by arguing that it is not the endeavor to understand and cultivate positive outcomes that distinguishes modern positive psychology from other approaches, "but the particular way in which it seeks to do so."

Barbara Fredrickson is another leading authority in the positive psychology movement and is known to have mothered the influential broaden-and-build theory (e.g., Fredrickson, 2001; Fredrickson, 2013). To Fredrickson, positivity is basically about emotions, and she presents six claims about it: (1) Positivity feels good. (2) Positivity changes how your mind works. (3) Positivity transforms your future. (4) Positivity puts the brakes on negativity. (5) Positivity obeys a tipping point. (6) You can increase your positivity (Fredrickson, 2009, pp. 8–11). She also lists ten forms of positivity: joy, gratitude, serenity, interest, hope, pride, amusement, inspiration, awe, and love (p. 39). According to the broaden-and-build theory, however, all ten emotions seem to be collapsed into one general positive emotion category (Smith et al., 2014).

The broaden-and-build theory excludes sensory pleasures from the domain of positive emotions, basically because they operate on a different time frame than positive emotions. Sensory pleasures are about payoffs in the moment, which set them apart from the true positivity of emotions. It is emotions, not sensations, that broaden your mind and eventually pay off as building resources further down the road (Fredrickson, 2009). Fredrickson also excludes happiness from her model, because happiness is too vague a concept to be useful.

Positive Emotions

The science of emotions is broad and includes a rich variety of terms, concepts, and theories, such as appraisal theories (Lazarus & Folkman, 1984; Scherer et al., 2001), communicative theories of emotions (Oatley, 1992), affective neuroscience (Adolphs & Anderson, 2018; Panksepp, 1998; Rolls, 2005), emotional expression theories (Ekman, 2003), affect theories (Izard, 1977; Tomkins, 1962), core affect theories (Russell, 2003; Russell & Barrett, 1999), and others (Fox et al., 2018; Frijda, 1986). These concepts will be surveyed in Chap. 3.

Suffice it for this section to mention that some scholars believe that the notion of positivity is difficult to pin down as an emotional referent. Positivity, it is argued, is rather a term that links up with a series of very different things, both in terms of their physiologies, thoughts, phenomenology, and schemas. For example, Kagan (2002) argues that the convention of dichotomizing emotional responses as either good or bad—i.e., positive or negative—lacks a sound scientific origin. The members of such a positivity category do not share a common referent but constitute a semantic network that links together a variety of signs of something praiseworthy or normatively good. Similarly, Frijda (2007) accuses the concept of positive emotion, indeed the entire movement of positive psychology, of being confusing and untenable. Positivity is nothing more than an artifact, he argues (Frijda, 2007, p. 87). Alas, it is difficult to consistently dissociate oneself from words that are as useful as positive and negative. Just a few pages before Frijda scolded colleagues who use the term positive in emotion research, he defined pleasure as "the positive outcome of constantly monitoring one's functioning, and competences are doing what they are for" (Frijda, 2007, p. 82).

In contrast to the position taken by Kagan and Frijda, it can be argued that, ontogenetically, humans develop their emotions from a rudimentary yet bipolar emotional life. Thus, Lewis (2016, p. 282) claims that "on the one hand, there is a general distress marked by crying and irritability. On the other hand, there is pleasure marked by satiation, attention, and responsivity to the environment." This suggests that an overarching and rudimentary positivity may be defended in the early stages of emotional development.

Another argument against Kagan's perspective comes from Oatley (1992), who points out that the term positive emotions makes sense if emotions are associated with action tendencies and linked with the regulation of goals. Thus, emotions can be called positive when they are associated with behaviors that make goal achievement more likely. In this context, Oatley reminds us, goals are typically considered as a psychological term for what classical Greeks call "good" (Oatley, 1992, p. 30). Within such a framework, emotions are kinds of value judgments. Negative emotions signal that one's wellbeing is threatened, and positive emotions signal that one's wellbeing has increased or is about to be increased (see Chap. 3).

Oatley's idea of positivity comes close to a claim made by Rawls (1971), which states that human goodness can be equated with reaching major life goals. In Rawls phrasing: "a person is being happy when he is in the way of successful execution (more or less) of a rational plan of life drawn up under (more or less) favorable conditions, and he is reasonably confident that his plan can be carried through" (cited in Feldman, 2010, p. 148). Oatley's perspective is also related to an argument Lazarus (1991) forwarded to defend a distinction between positive and negative emotions. Lazarus suggested that an emotion may be categorized as positive if it (1) is produced by a situation that is appraised as goal congruent, (2) produces positive consequences, or (3) feels subjectively positive. Appraisal theorists thus define an emotion as positive when it is produced by a situation or event that is appraised as goal-congruent or consistent with one's desires (cited in Harmon-Jones & Harmon-Jones, 2021).

Yet, there might be something more to concepts such as positivity and a good life than reaching a goal of individual importance—regardless of what the goal is about. As pointed out by Nussbaum, an emotion can only be termed positive in relation to normative thinking:

> For all the ancient thinkers, a necessary and sufficient condition of an emotion's being truly positive—in the sense of making a positive contribution toward a flourishing life—is that it be based on true beliefs, both about value and about what events have occurred. (…) Pleasure is only as good as the thing one takes pleasure in: if one takes pleasure in harming others, that good-feeling emotion is very negative; even if one takes pleasure in shirking one's duty and lazing around, that is also quite negative. (Nussbaum, 2008, p. s93)

One can argue then that the notion of positivity needs a value basis to be meaningful. How such a conceptualization can be carried out scientifically is discussed next.

Values in Science

Scholars regularly claim that science is, or at least should be, value-free (e.g., Elliott, 2017; Merton, 1938; Sayer, 2011). This is neither a precise description nor a good ideal, since scientists rely more on values and background beliefs than are commonly admitted (Brown, 2020; ChoGlueck & Lloyd, 2023; Longino, 2002). Hence, in suppressing their normative grounding and insisting on their value neutrality, Oreskes (2019, p. 155) argues that "scientists have gone down a wrong road."

There are several reasons why the notion of a value-free science is misleading, one of which is simply that science cannot by itself instruct us to believe in it. To believe in science means, for instance, to accept empirical arguments, but there is nothing in the observations themselves that justify their importance. This limitation was principally formulated in Kurt Gödel's incompleteness theorems, which explain how every logical system of some complexity is incomplete by itself. All knowledge structures are thus relational in the sense that there will always be statements in the structure that cannot be proven within the system (e.g., Raatikainen, 2022). The relational nature of science is further articulated in the thesis dubbed by Willard Quine as underdetermination of scientific theory by evidence or empirical underdetermination for short (Stanford, 2021). Briefly, empirical underdetermination means that no empirical evidence is sufficient to choose a theory or determine what beliefs we should hold in response to it. According to Longino (1979), it is not the relation between a fact and a hypothesis that determines whether the hypothesis is correct. It is the background beliefs we hold about that relation that determine whether an empirical fact is taken as evidence for a hypothesis.

For example, we cannot conclude that the Earth spins around its axis at a steady rate from the observation that day and night roughly alternate at a steady rate (when perceived from the equator). This observation only becomes evidence when related to a particular cosmology such as the heliocentric theory. In light of a geocentric cosmology, by contrast, the observation would be evidence that the sun is moving around the Earth. The same principle applies for experimental results, since they also become evidence only in the context of a set of background beliefs or assumptions (Longino, 1979, p. 42).

Some of the background beliefs that help scientists to get going are called epistemic values. Epistemic values are directly related to knowledge and have to do with things such as theoretical reasoning, logical consistency, and, as already mentioned, respecting empirical data. Hence, to say that science is grounded in epistemic values is not controversial. However, scientists disagree about which values to count as epistemic. For example, some epistemic values are related to the criteria used to evaluate the adequacy of a theory, and Kuhn (2002, p. 422) suggested that accuracy, consistency, scope, simplicity, and fruitfulness serve this purpose. Others have highlighted that science must be fallible (Popper, 1963) or that explanatory power is the core feature of a theory (Borsboom et al., 2021; Thagard, 2012). Some scholars suggest that openness and novelty are important (Longino, 2008), whereas others argue that novelty contributes to the so-called replication crises and theory crises in (some) scientific disciplines (e.g., Eronen & Bringmann, 2021).

However, not all the values and assumptions that scientists hold are epistemic, and these background beliefs are often referred to as non-epistemic values (e.g., Douglas, 2009; Elliott, 2017; Kendler, 2000; Oreskes, 2019). Non-epistemic values can be further separated into ethical values and social values. Following the taxonomy proposed by Douglas (2009), ethical values include concern for human life, a reduction in suffering and political freedom, whereas social values include privacy, social stability, and even dress codes.

A too strict separation of epistemic and non-epistemic values runs the risk of overlooking the interactions between them. Rooney (1992) has, for instance, pointed out how non-epistemic values may affect epistemic values in a critical manner, thus making the demarcation between them permeable. One of her examples is the disagreement between Niels Bohr and Albert Einstein regarding the acceptability of quantum theory. Einstein was reluctant to accept the randomness underlying the theory, whereas Bohr defended it. Rooney elaborates how metaphysical beliefs influenced the arguments used by the two giants. Einstein was a religious man who trusted that "God does not play dice." Bohr, an atheist, replied "Einstein, stop telling God what to do." Analyzing the debate in detail enabled Rooney to conclude that the epistemic standards used by Einstein and Bohr were clearly influenced by the non-epistemic values held by the two scientists.

Yet, it is important to acknowledge that a theory cannot be accepted on the grounds that some scientists like them or because they support a political ideology. An example in case is Trofim Lysenko from the Stalin era, a well-known Soviet "barefoot scientist," i.e., a person without a university degree. Lysenko was a Lamarckian who believed that crops would rapidly adapt to environmental factors. Stalin fell for Lysenko's non-academic and "anti-bourgeois" style and secured him a career as a top scientist and decision-maker in the Soviet political establishment. Although it was not completely without merit, Lysenko's theory was basically wrong and contributed to a severe famine that caused the death of millions of Soviet people in the 1930s (e.g., Elliott, 2017).

No Ought from an Is

In David Hume's so-called first law, the Scottish thinker states that facts and values are distinct: To observe that a person feeds someone in hunger is different from saying that this person is kind. Reporting an act of feeding is descriptive, whereas labeling the act as kindness is normative. As noted infinitely since Hume introduced his law, there is no association between descriptive and normative statements; the fact does not explain the value. According to Hume, that is because facts are reducible either to simple impressions or to the logical relations among ideas. In contrast, values are based on passions. It is the feeling, not the fact, that makes valuations possible.

But Hume also introduced a second law, with stronger moral connotations than the first. It concerns the impossibility of analytically deriving an "ought claim" from an "is statement." The fact that something is does not imply that this something is right in the sense that it should or ought to be like it is. The fact that social and economic inequalities are currently increasing in the Western world cannot be taken, for instance, as an argument that we ought to increase inequalities. The ought part of this proposition is not only normative but also prescriptive, i.e., it contains a moral judgment (Kristjánsson, 2013). I will return to this issue in the section Values in the Science of Wellbeing below.

From a modern perspective, several aspects of Hume's fact/value dichotomy are misleading. First, Hume's understanding of perceptions and knowledge was incomplete. As demonstrated in the Psychology of Good and Bad section above, evaluations are more integrated into human cognition than Hume foresaw. Evaluations are not "an icing on the cake of hard facts" (Kristjánsson, 2013, p. 99). Second, although an ought cannot be deduced logically from an is, factual knowledge may have relevance for normative thinking. Sauer (2017) argues, for instance, that "It is rather clear that, though even if empirical research has no direct normative implications, there are ways to make empirical research normatively relevant" (p. 21). He claims that empirical observations can undermine the presuppositions of various normative ethical theories make about our human nature. Moreover, data can weaken the justifications used to support a moral argument. For example, a normative theory might assume that a moral judgment is generated by a particular cognitive process. If it turns out that the assumption is empirically wrong, the justification is undermined. Finally, empirical information can improve a moral theory by stimulating "reflexive judgment and agency." By reflexive judgment and agency Sauer seems to mean an informed examination of implicit biases that philosophers have when they work out their moral models. Factual knowledge about these biases might inform theorists about when and how the tools they wish to "deploy in moral cognition and action are unsuitable or likely to be broken" (Sauer, 2017, p. 23).

One could also add to Sauer's list that scientific reasoning is not restricted to deductive logic. Scientists use a range of techniques and argumentative reasoning in their attempts to understand the world, which gives science more methodological leeway than the restrictions implied in Hume's first law suggest. Oreskes (2019) insists that scientific reasoning is possible only as a social practice. To handle the subjectivity that unavoidably comes with any world view, multiple perspectives must be considered. "It is through the give and take of ideas—the challenging, the questioning, the adjusting and amending—that scientists integrate their colleagues' work, offer up criticisms, and contribute to the growth of warranted knowledge" (Oreskes, 2019, p. 51). Scientific fallibility—its self-correcting nature—is also more of a cultural than an individual undertaking. It is not so much that scientists correct themselves; it is more that scientists correct each other. Thus, scientific objectivity can be established through critical, discursive interaction and building consensus out of an assembly of subjective perspectives. Such reasoning is only possible within a cultural practice comprising institutions such as universities, research institutes, peer-reviewed journals, conferences, etc. The consensus developed by scientific communities not only includes agreements about empirical facts but also embraces epistemic and non-epistemic values. This is important because value neutrality is no longer the guarantor of scientific objectivity—value pluralism is. The trust we have in science, Oreskes claims, is "based on the social character of scientific inquiry and the collective critical evaluation of knowledge claims" (p. 68).

In a readable review of these issues, Anderson (2004) explains that "Even if we grant that no substantive value judgment logically follows from any conjunction of factual statements, this merely puts value judgments on a logical par with scientific hypotheses. For it is equally true that there is no deductively valid inference from statements of evidence alone to theoretical statements. Theories always logically go beyond the evidence adduced in support of them. The question of neutrality is not whether factual judgments logically entail value judgments, but whether they can stand in *evidentiary relations* (italics added) to them" (p. 5). Consequently, scientists both utilize and revise value judgments in light of empirical evidence, which is to say that the link between evidence and hypotheses is mediated by background assumptions. Anderson uses studies of divorce and its consequences to illustrate how value-laden beliefs can affect a study field. Traditionally, divorce was only seen as something negative, and studies of its consequences were one-sidedly focused on what was lost. In the 1970s, however, feminist thinkers and psychologists started to conceive of divorce not only as a loss but also as an opportunity for personal growth (Anderson, 2004, p. 14).

We might also see something slightly similar in wellbeing research, for instance, in the emerging trend that considers family wellbeing to be equally or even more important than individual wellbeing. In other words, an approach not only considers family wellbeing as a predictor of an individual's wellbeing but also suggests that the family itself should be the subject of wellbeing (e.g., Krys et al., 2021). The family wellbeing perspective might be related to an argument presented by Held (2006, p. 12), which claims that being well in a caring relationship is a matter of the cooperative wellbeing of those in the relationship. It is a wellbeing associated with the relation itself, and not with isolated individuals.

A value revision can also enter the background assumptions of a research field and change how it interprets empirical data. An example comes from a feminist approach to the psychological study of moral development. Carol Gilligan (2023) worked with Lawrence Kohlberg (e.g., Kohlberg, 1975) but offered an alternative interpretive approach to evaluating the answers children gave to moral problems. In the "Heinz dilemma," for example, Heinz's wife will die from cancer unless she gets some expensive medicine. Heinz can't afford the medicine, so should he steal it? Kohlberg says yes and expects the children to justify this answer with the argument that a life is more valuable than the drugs. However, some of the girls whom Gilligan interviewed suggested that Heinz should not steal the drugs, because he then risked ending up in jail. Being away and unable to take care of his wife, she will die anyway. Perhaps Heinz could get the money from somewhere else, some of the girls suggested, for example, by a loan? This is an example of what Gilligan refers to as a "different voice," a way of reasoning that Kohlberg would not accept as a correct answer. He only accepted responses grounded in abstract logic and universal moral principles. But regardless of the empirical data, a reasoning grounded in care ethics can provide different answers to a moral dilemma than an ethic of rule-based justice, or "a math problem with humans," as Gilligan describes Kohlberg's approach (Gilligan, 1993, p. 2).

Another fine illustration of the impact of value is the "tending instinct," which was discovered by Shelly Taylor (2002, 2006). It turns out that most of what we know about stress, including the "fight or flight" metaphor, was until recently based on male biology and perhaps even a "male ideology." Many of the accepted conclusions in the field cohere with a "kill-or-be-killed" perception of the world. Hence, when Taylor started to study stress, she was surprised to see that almost all the data were from males. It was male rats, male mice, and male humans that had provided the field with its empirical basis. When Taylor and her colleagues examined how females react to stress, they discovered that the typical response was to intensify care and form alliances with social groups. In other words, stress leads not only to combatting or running away but also, particularly among women, to tending and befriending. Hence, the most important way to cope with stress might not be through fights and flights but through interaction and social support. Caregiving, Taylor suggests, seems to be a human instinct, no less natural than selfishness and aggression.

The Naturalistic Fallacy

We will now turn to the philosophical tradition of nonnaturalism and the notion of a naturalistic fallacy. Very roughly, nonnaturalism is the idea that moral philosophy is fundamentally autonomous from the natural sciences (Ridge, 2014). George Edward Moore is the prototypical nonnaturalist, known for defending the idea that the property of goodness is simple and unanalyzable, particularly in non-moral terms (Hurka, 2015, p. 5). Ethics thus understood is an autonomous enterprise, irreducible to natural science or even to metaphysics (Baldwin, 2010, p. 9). Accordingly, it is not possible to compare things that exist in the world with things that are good. Those who try fall for the naturalistic fallacy.

The nonnaturalistic way of thinking is grounded in a distinction between synthetical and analytical propositions (e.g., Putnam, 2004). Synthetic propositions are true by how their meaning relates to the world, for example, that the cat is on the mat. Analytic propositions are true by virtue of their meaning, as in defining a bachelor as an unmarried, adult man. Moore argued that statements about good and bad belong to the realm of analytical propositions. Theories that derive goodness from synthetic propositions, such as natural facts, therefore confuse the property of goodness with the things that possess it. Such theories are in other words submitted to the "naturalistic fallacy."

Moore used a thought experiment known as the open question to illustrate his point. Hurka (2015) explains that an open question is one it makes sense to ask. For example, it makes sense to ask if the cat is on the mat. However, it does not make sense to ask if a bird is a bird or a square is a circle. Birds are birds and circles are not squares by analytical definition. Thus, if a definition identifies a moral property with a natural property, Moore's thought experiment suggests that it should be obvious that something moral cannot be identified with something we can observe. For example, if someone says that "X is good" and that "X is pleasure," then the judgement "pleasure is good" must be equivalent to "pleasure is pleaseure" (Hurka, 2015, p. 3). Yet, it still makes sense to ask if pleasure really is good. The fact that the question remains open suggests to Moore that goodness is not simply reducible to pleasure.

Hence, to determine if something is good, the identity between goodness and the thing one wants to define as good must be confirmed. Casebeer (2003) explains that to verify that X is good means that X and good must have the same meaning; they must be identical in an analytical sense. The principle is known from logical systems such as mathematics, where it can be proven that 2 + 2 is the same as 4. Moore wanted to apply this logic as a proof in his nonnaturalistic argument. For something good to be analyzed naturalistically, something (A) in the natural world must be identical to something (B) in the nonnatural world. Moore considered such a conclusion to be impossible.

However, Moore's way of reasoning is weird. Humans rarely use or analyze concepts as identities. Rather, we tend to understand the world conceptually, as mental representations of categories of things (Murphy, 2002). These representations are most likely organized as knowledge structures that gradually increase as the result of interactions between observations and interpretations of the world. As our empirically grounded comprehension of the world develops, increased precision can be added to our concepts (Mayr, 1982; Thagard, 1992). The idea of analytically derived concepts has therefore little to do with how humans understand things.

To illustrate the limitations of Moore's nonnaturalistic analysis, Churchland (2018) points out how scientific concepts typically evolve, which is in accordance with the perspectives presented by scholars such as Murphy, Mayr, and Thagard in the previous section. Churchland takes temperature as her example. Temperature is scientifically defined as molecular kinetic energy, but to claim that temperature and kinetic energy are identical makes no sense. When temperature is scientifically conceptualized as kinetic energy, it is because measures of temperature correspond with measures of kinetic energy: "the property measured one way was found to be the same as the property measured another way" (Churchland, 2018, p. 188). To see the flaw of Moore's identity argument more clearly, Churchland offers a thought experiment. Suppose you find out that your neighbor is the head of the CIA. This discovery does not imply that the terms "head of CIA" and "your neighbor" are identical.

If the synonymy of terms is a poor model for concept development in general, why should it be necessary for a proper understanding of the concepts of good and bad? Although an analytic symmetry applies to mathematical statements such as $2 + 2 = 4$, it does not prove that ethics must be analyzed according to the same logic (Thagard, 2010; Turp, 2016). Indeed, upon further—posthumously published—reflections, Moore seems to have rejected his ideas about how goodness can be understood only within the framework of a closed, analytical rationality (Casebeer, 2003). Yet, Moore's legacy has promoted an unfortunate reluctance to include scientific theories in debates about normativity and ethics. By segregating goodness from anything else we know about the world, Moore's orthodoxy has, as I see it, impeded a fruitful understanding of how facts about the world can contribute to a better understanding of human goodness.

Without the bite from Hume's first law and Moore's naturalistic fallacy, a better take on the fact-value dichotomy is gradually evolving (e.g., Brinkmann, 2011a; Brown, 2020; Hicks, 2014; Holman & Wilholt, 2022; Marchetti & Marchetti, 2016; Putnam, 2004). How some of these insights might be integrated into the science of wellbeing will be discussed next.

Values in the Science of Wellbeing

In terms of an academic division of labor, philosophers are traditionally supposed to perform normative work, and scientists are supposed to perform descriptive work. This practice is also commonly observed in studies of wellbeing (e.g., Mitchell & Alexandrova, 2021; Prinzing, 2021; Sumner, 1996; Tiberius, 2013b, p. 220). For example, when Haybron (2008, p. 32) proclaimed that Aristotle had a theory of wellbeing, but not a theory of happiness, Haybron basically referred to the moral dimension in Aristotle's theory and the lack thereof in scientific theories. However, the terminology is a bit confusing, because Haybron uses the word wellbeing when referring to normative theories and the word happiness when referring to descriptive theories. As will be discussed in Chap. 2, most scientists and some philosophers use the words happiness and wellbeing interchangeably, and then, of course, Haybron's distinction appears confusing. But conceptually, Haybron's taxonomy is widely accepted since most scholars agree that philosophers operate with value-loaden theories, while scientists operate with value-free theories.

For instance, in his seminal article from 1984, Diener maintained that the field of subjective wellbeing should be descriptive, and he advised researchers to renounce from the philosophical tradition of making normative statements about wellbeing. Regarding Aristotelian eudaimonism, Diener noted that "when Aristotle wrote that eudaemonia is gained mainly by leading a virtuous life, he did not mean that virtue leads to feelings of joy. Rather, Aristotle was prescribing virtue as the normative standard against which people's lives can be judged. Therefore, eudaemonia is not happiness in the modern senses of the word, but a desirable state judged from a particular value framework" (Diener, 1984, p. 543). Similarly, Phillips et al. (2014) declared that the scientific concept of subjective wellbeing (SWB) is purely descriptive. All a scientist needs to know about someone's SWB "is an accurate list of all the psychological states the person experiences" (p. 2). A third example can be found in Seligman (2002), who writes that "I completely agree that science must be descriptive and not prescriptive. It is not the job of Positive Psychology to tell you that you should be optimistic, or spiritual, or kind or good-humored; it is rather to describe the consequences of these traits (for example, that being optimistic brings about less depression, better physical health, and higher achievement, at a cost perhaps of less realism). What you do with that information depends on your own values and goals" (p. 175).

Diener's remark points out that philosophical theories of wellbeing are substantially different from scientific theories of wellbeing. Here, Diener expresses sympathy with the position defended by Haybron and other philosophers. The comment from Phillips and coauthors also regards the notion of a value-free science and maintains that lists of psychological states can be generated as "pure description." However, as spelled out in the Values in Science section, the idea of a pure description is hardly sustainable; descriptions are always embedded in a set of values and background assumptions. For example, how should scientists know which psychological state to include in the concept of wellbeing? Not all mental states are indicative of wellbeing; thus, some value-laden background assumptions are necessary to identify the relevant states as dimensions of SWB.

Seligman citations could be interpreted as being slightly different. He clearly defends the idea that science should be descriptive, but he does not contrast the descriptive with the normative. He contrasts it with the prescriptive; thus, we may ask whether Seligman distinguishes between the term normative and the term prescriptive. Kristjánsson (2013) explains that some makes such a distinction whereas others do not. In the former case, normativity is defined as having to do with evaluations, while prescriptions is defined as having to do with morality. There is a difference between claiming that something is good and claiming that this something is the right thing to do. The evaluative claim, Kristjánsson maintains, relates to Hume's first law, and the prescriptive claim relates to his second law (p. 110). However, most psychologists do not seem to make the distinction between normative as something good or bad and prescriptive as something we ought/ought not to do (e.g., Brinkmann, 2011b).

Dual-Character Concepts

When philosophers such as Longino (2002) argue that all concepts are value-loaded in an epistemological sense, they do not mean that all concepts have a moral or prescriptive element. However, for some concepts, such as happiness and wellbeing, a moralistic connotation may be actively involved. For example, when Phillips et al. (2014) were cited above on subjective wellbeing being a descriptive concept, they contrasted their scientific value neutrality with an ordinary, or folk theoretical, conceptualization of happiness. In most people's minds, these authors argue, happiness seems to be a so-called dual-character concept, which means that they jointly entails descriptive and normative qualities (e.g., Knobe et al., 2013). Empirical studies suggest that the core concepts of wellbeing are dual-character concepts. People associate, for example, the term happiness with concrete psychological features, such as certain feeling qualities, and at the same time with a deeper, more abstract meaning of value and morality (e.g., King & Napa, 1998; Phillips et al., 2017). Thus, happiness and other dual-character concepts are both descriptive and embedded in a deeper meaning of value. For instance, Phillips et al. (2014) found in a series of vignette studies that participants include normative judgments when asked to judge how happy a person in a short story seems to be. In one study, the fictive character Richard was introduced as a Red Cross field doctor and described with a set of mental attributes. In a different version, Richard was introduced as working in a Nazi death camp and then described with the identical set of mental attributes as in the Red Cross version of the story. When asked (on a 1 to 7 scale) if Richard was happy, participants rated Red Cross Richard as significantly happier than Nazi Richard, suggesting that people consider happiness to be more than the mere sum of a person's psychological states. Such a normative effect has been found in several studies and indicates that folk theories of happiness comprise both moral goodness and psychological indicators of wellbeing (e.g., Carlquist et al., 2017; Nafstad et al., 2009). Folk theories, or ordinary happiness as Phillips et al. (2011) call it, are in other words closer to the value-laden Aristotelian notion of wellbeing than to the value-free scientific understanding. There is also some cross-cultural evidence for a normative aspect of happiness. The social anthropologist Jean Briggs offers, for instance, an interesting analysis of the moral aspects of happiness. Her monograph, *Never in Anger* (Briggs, 1970), is grounded in 17 months of fieldwork among a small, remote Inuit tribe in the Canadian Arctic, called Utkuhikhalingmiut, or Utku for short. Briggs' work is best known for analyzing anger, and the book is sometimes interpreted as a statement about the Utku's never being angry, which is something it never claimed. But Briggs aimed wider than analyzing anger, and the monograph demonstrated her skills as a sharp observer of other emotions. Hence, in contrast to anger, which was the most disapproved emotion among the Utku, Briggs also noted that happiness (*quvia*) was a highly valued emotion in the tribe. Briggs interpreted Utku happiness as a morally laden emotion, in the sense that happy people are good people. Happy behavior is decent behavior because a happy person is safe and not frightening. This is one of Briggs' accounts of Utku happiness: "The term occurs frequently in spontaneous speech, both as an expression of a person's own feeling and as a judgment on other people's behavior. People who laugh, smile, joke, and enjoy telling stories are described as happy are judged to feel *quvia*, and they are said to rouse *quvia* feelings in others. Enjoyable experiences as diverse as listening to music, dancing, playing, fishing, chasing lemmings or stoning ptarmigans, traveling (under good conditions), visiting with pleasant company or being with a loved person, being physically warm, and eating are all described as 'making one feel happy' (quvianaqtuq)" (pp. 327–328).

Philosophers also operate with a kind of dual-character concept, referred to as a distinction between thick and thin concepts (Kirchin, 2013b; Williams, 2011/1985). Thick concepts have both descriptive and normative meanings, and Anderson (2002) calls a concept thick if (a) its application is guided by empirical facts, (b) it licenses normative inferences, and (c) interests and values guide the extension of the concept (cited in Alexandrova & Fabian, 2022, pp. 2–3). Courage is an example of a thick concept because it comprises descriptions such as being good at facing danger, but it is also normative in the sense that it is something we admire (Tiberius, 2013b, p. 220). The notion of being a caring person is similarly describing a person who looks after others and helps fulfill their needs, while these practices at the same time are traits we tend to admire in a person (Held, 2006). In contrast, thin concepts have only evaluative content or are at least "thought not to have much or any descriptive conceptual content" (Kirchin, 2013a, p. 2). Good and right are examples of thin concepts because their contents are not further specified.

The philosophical literature on thick and thin concepts is large and sometimes rather technical. However, in several papers, Tiberius has offered understandable explanations of thickness and thinness and made them relevant for wellbeing research. She argues that these concepts invite a renewed integration of scientific and philosophical perspectives of wellbeing (e.g., Tiberius, 2013b, 2017a; Tiberius, 2017b).

Division of Labor

Tiberius supports the idea that academic work should be separated according to a normative/descriptive demarcation line and that only philosophy should address normativity. Such a division of labor will stimulate cooperation among students with different perspectives on wellbeing and facilitate an alliance between philosophers and scientists.[4] Somewhat simplified, the setup suggests that philosophers start by constructing theories of wellbeing, which they then turn over to the scientists

[4] For some reason, Tiberius uses psychology as the only example of a wellbeing science, thus ignoring the contributions from economy, sociology, anthropology, geography, history, biology, neuroscience, and other disciplines. I will instead follow the practice of contrasting philosophy with science, and not only psychology. The exception would be when psychology/psychologists appear in a citation verbatim.

for empirical testing (Tiberius, 2013b, p. 220). Philosophers could, for example, "defend an informed preference theory of well-being and psychologists could tell us what things people prefer when informed" (p. 218).

In more details, the argument implies that a theory about wellbeing must answer two different questions. The first concerns the content of wellbeing and is often accounted for by lists of elements that define the field of study. For example, the mainstream theory of subjective wellbeing defends a list comprising three elements: life satisfaction, positive affect, and negative affect (Diener, 1984). Such lists aim to explain what a person needs to be well and comprise a descriptive part of wellbeing theories. The list provides answers to what philosophers call the enumerative (Crisp, 2006b) or substantive question (Crisp, 2017; Griffin, 1986; Haybron, 2008; Nussbaum, 2001; Sumner, 1996). Then a different query asks what it is about these elements that make them prudentially good. How can the list of elements be justified as a theory of wellbeing? Why are these elements good for you? This challenge is often referred to as the formal question. Tiberius (2013a) illustrates the difference between substantive and formal questions with an analogy to the recipe for a cake. The substantive theories align with the question of what goes in the batter, and the formal theories are associated with the question of why we need just these ingredients to make a good cake.

Tiberius presumes that the justification of formal questions must be undertaken by "the tools of philosophy: wide reflective equilibrium, conceptual or reconstructive analysis, thought experiments, counter-exampling and other methods are designed to defend philosophical theories of normative concepts" (Tiberius, 2013b, p. 220). Elsewhere, she has also declared that scientists have little to say about the formal question and that empirical wellbeing research should be restricted to investigating "particular aspects or components of it" (Tiberius, 2015, p. 178). The reason is that wellbeing is "too vague and broad" for scientists to study. Thus, Tiberius suggested that when philosophers have worked out a theory, on hedonism about wellbeing, for instance, scientists can pick it up and start testing it empirically. "Once we know that the target is pleasure, psychologists can investigate the causes of it without the help of philosophers" (Tiberius, 2013b, p. 224). Similarly, Feldman (2010) claims that the aim of philosophy in the study of wellbeing "would be to discover the nature of happiness" and that such conceptual analyses "are traditionally done by philosophers" (pp. 7–8). Feldmann further asserts that the philosophical projects of discovering the true nature of happiness should have priority over the scientific project, which, he believes, has the restricted aim of uncovering the causes and correlates of happiness. Unless the empirical researchers have a clear idea about what happiness is, Feldman argues, their results will not be very informative: hence, the philosophical priority. A final example is from Prinzing (2021) who charges that it is impossible for wellbeing scientists to know where to direct their empirical attention unless they have philosophers to point out a direction for them. After all, Prinzing argues, only a philosophical theory can reveal the ingredients of wellbeing and identify what is ultimately good for a person. After being told what wellbeing is, the task of science is then to "identifying the correlates, causes, and consequences of observable phenomena" (p. 152).

One critique against these recommendations is that philosophers such as Tiberius, Feldman, and Prinzing construe a rigid image of scientific practice that mischaracterizes the relation between the conceptual and the factual. These authors make the interplay between philosophers and scientists look like a "20 questions game," in which philosophical ideas are reiteratively thrown into a yes or no procedure of strict empirical experimentation and hypothesis testing conducted by scientists (see Newell, 1973, about the 20 questions analogy). For example, Tiberius writes that "if empirical evidence bears on philosophical analysis, once we've settled on the right analysis the remaining work is empirical. This would be true if our analysis makes well-being, for example, something purely empirical" (Tiberius, 2013b, p. 224). However, the business of science is not restricted to being "purely empirical." Science is seriously involved in developing concepts, and not at least in improving them. This is excellently illustrated by Ernst Mayr in his classic book *The Growth of Biological Thought* (1982). Here, Mayr writes that "it seems to me that progress in the biological sciences is characterized not so much by individual discoveries, no matter how important, or by the proposal of new theories, but rather by the gradual but decisive development of new concepts and the abandonment of those that had previously been dominant. In most cases the development of major new concepts has not been due to individual discoveries but rather to novel integration of previously established facts" (Mayr, 1982, p. 856). Similarly, Thagard (1992) provides a thorough analysis of the major conceptual developments that have ensued since the dawn of the scientific revolution, and he details the procedures of how concepts are worked out scientifically. Clearly, empirical testing is not the only device in the scientific tool kit.

These comments may appear irrelevant for the claims philosophers want to make about wellbeing, since wellbeing is a thick concept and the concepts discussed by Mayr and Thagard are not. However, it is still unclear to me how useful philosophical contribution is, even when it comes to developing and analyzing thick concepts. Take philosophical hedonism about wellbeing as an example. The doctrine claims that "all and only pleasure intrinsically makes people's lives go better *for them* and all and only pain intrinsically makes their lives go worse *for them*" (Weijers, 2021, italics in original). How helpful is it for scientists to be told that some philosophers think like this? Not very, I would say, because the core premises of hedonism are most likely wrong. As will be further detailed in Chaps. 3 and 5, practically everything we know scientifically about pleasure speaks against philosophical conceptualizations of the term and against the assumption that pleasure is "the only 'good-for-making' property there is," as Crisp (2006a, p. 623) has expressed the hedonic dictum. Humans are complex beings with complex, multiple, and intricate value structures; thus, the idea that only one of them should be "intrinsic" is not liable. Moreover, from the perspective of evolution, pleasure cannot be the ultimate goal, or value, since that role is taken by survival and reproduction. We are not born to feel pleasure, but pleasure helps us navigate our lives (Damasio, 2018; Nesse, 2005). Finally, the idea that pain is ultimately bad for us is also uncanny. Although pain can be a source of intense suffering, it is essentially a functional psychological mechanism. Without the ability to feel pain, humans would not have survived (e.g., Eregowda et al., 2016).

Hedonism is not the only philosophical wellbeing theory around; others are both more popular and more complex. For these approaches, the division of philosophical and scientific labor becomes more interesting, Tiberius argues, and points to Sumner's authentic happiness theory (Sumner, 1996) for illustrative help. The authentic happiness theory considers wellbeing—or welfare as Sumner also calls it—to have "both an affective component (experiencing the conditions of your life as fulfilling or rewarding) and a cognitive component (judging that your life is going well for you, by your standards for it)" (Sumner, 1996, p. 172). Sumner also maintains that people's wellbeing should be determined by self-reports. What the theory suggests looks pretty much like what scientific wellbeing research already have been doing for decades, except that inauthentic happiness must be excluded from the analyses. Unless self-reports are authentic, they "do not accurately reflect the subject's own point of view. Welfare therefore consists of authentic happiness, the happiness of an informed and autonomous subject" (Sumner, 1996, p. 172).

How should an authentic and accurate reflection of a subject's point of view be identified? Sumner is vague on this important part of his theory, but he seems to suggest that authenticity can be jeopardized either from manipulation and indoctrination or from identifying oneself with the wrong values. Hence, "to decide whether someone's happiness is non-autonomous, we have to decide whether the causal history of that person being made happy by that is a history that involves injustice, or whether the person's identity is represented by that happiness" (Tiberius, 2013b, p. 225). Sumner admits that the endeavor of figuring authenticity out would be "a complex, and probably endless, task" (Sumner, 1996, p. 176). To uncover a person's life story and true identity is indeed a complex task, and I don't quite see how scientists should integrate this part of Sumner's theory in empirical studies of wellbeing. Hence, I doubt that scientists will benefit much from accepting Tiberius' invitation to let philosophers such as Sumner do the conceptual work and "all the heavy lifting" and leave science as "the handmaiden to philosophy" (Tiberius, 2013b, p. 225).

To the contrary, I suggest that scientists will be better off by providing the conceptual heavy lifting themselves. According to Thagard (2010), philosophy seems no more successful at sorting out normative truths than religion has been. Compared with religion and philosophy, Thagard maintains, science offers a more promising way of reasoning about fundamental questions "concerning the nature of reality, knowledge, and morality" (p. 2). If knowledge about the world is in the minds of human beings, studying psychology is a promising path to improving our understanding of the structure and growth of knowledge (Thagard, 1992, p. 17). The same reasoning could be applied to enhance our knowledge about what it means to lead a good life as well.

Summing up, I do not believe that the science of wellbeing will benefit much from having philosophical debates on normativity "handed over" to them for empirical testing. Rather, scientific knowledge about wellbeing should basically evolve like scientific knowledge in general develops. This is achieved by gradual improvements in core concepts and the abandonment of concepts that no longer appear fruitful. This procedure, I suggest, can also be applied to normative analyses. The ambition of the present book is to take some steps toward an integration of value statements in scientific reasoning about wellbeing. The underlying normativity of the humanistic theory of wellbeing will be elaborated throughout the text, particularly in Chap. 7. But to briefly advance the game, the normative part is summarized as the last part of HTW's definition of wellbeing as *to like one's life for the right reasons*.

A Preview of the Humanistic Theory

The humanistic theory of wellbeing suggests that a life is good to the extent that it allows us to perform our humanness well. This slogan-like formulation is much too vague for scientific prose and must be further constrained to be useful. The term humanness is therefore defined as the fulfillment of three universal needs within a normative framework. The needs are for stability, change, and care, whereas the normative framework is grounded in three so-called humanistic values: respecting basic human rights, avoiding preventable harm, and accepting an ethics of care. This is not to say that our humanness can only be well performed if all our activities are aimed toward these values. The idea is rather that what we do in a life well lived cannot severely violate these values.

Universal Human Needs

Stability

Life depends critically on the preservation of a stable organic structure, a fact recognized already by the ancient Greeks. For instance, Hippocrates believed that a healthy mind and body were regulated by a harmonious balance of the "elements" (Lercher, 2018). The Greek referred to this stability as homeostasis, their word for "standing still" (Pross, 2016, p. 6). Walter Cannon reintroduced the term in his book *The Wisdom of the Body* (Cannon, 1932), a work strongly influenced by Claude Bernard, the French genius who first worked out the principle of stability maintenance in its modern form. Bernard realized that the homeostatic principle, the "milieu interieur" in his vocabulary, is one of the greatest achievements in our evolutionary past and that it can essentially be seen as the primary condition for freedom and independence of existence (see Denton, 2005). Currently, homeostasis is considered the most important biological mechanism for regulating stability, and the term typically refers to any process that living organisms use to actively maintain the fairly stable conditions necessary for survival (Rodolfo, 2000; Billman, 2020). Much of humans' physiological, psychological, and social lives are—more or less stringently—regulated according to these principles. The dynamics of homeostatic regulation often correspond to experiences of pleasure and pain (e.g., Damasio, 2021; Denton, 2005), and this concept will be further elaborated upon in Chaps. 3 and 5.

Change

At a fundamental level, life is chemical. As such, biological organisms are regulated by a balance between stability and instability, which means that everything alive must operate in a continuous interplay between their need for stability and their need for change (e.g., Pross, 2016). Some changes involved in the grander scheme of life are obvious, such as when a larva turns into an insect, an egg becomes a chicken, or a human baby grows up to become an adult. Large transformations are not the only changes necessary for the preservation of life. Numerous "small" changes in our everyday lives are also vital, which is why the developmental psychologist Augusto Blasi bluntly argued that an organism must either die or change (Blasi, 1976, p. 35). Maslow's hierarchy of needs represents another psychological change theory, and his model will be carefully reviewed in Chap. 6. For now, the following point will hopefully suffice to nail the argument I am trying to make about change and wellbeing.

If both stability and change are needed in our lives, we must expect that separate mechanisms have evolved to help us secure their respective fulfillments. Hence, it would be strange if the feelings and thinking related to stability needs were identical to the feelings and thinking related to change needs. How would we then be guided about the different kinds of actions needed to fulfill the respective needs? The two needs are regulated by different behaviors, and it is thus reasonable to suggest that they will also be accompanied by different experiences. Consequently, the humanistic theory of wellbeing suggests that both in terms of phenomenology and functioning, the feelings and judgments that assist in managing the need for stability must be somewhat different from the feelings and judgments that help regulate the need for change (Vittersø, 2016). A theory of wellbeing should therefore be able to identify and acknowledge differences associated with indicators of stability needs and indicators of change needs.

Care

The caring need has two separable but overlapping aspects. One is the need *to* care, the other the need *for* care. Both elements are grounded in the biological valuing mechanism, but they play different roles in the human life cycle.

The focal inspiration for the need *to* care is Tomasello's ontogenetic theory of human development (e.g., Tomasello, 2016, 2019 #19015). The theory emphasizes the importance of cooperation and communication in human development in general and in the development of moral behavior in particular. Environmental changes in our evolutionary past, approximately 200,000 to 400,000 years ago, forced our ancestors to become more cooperative. As a consequence, new cognitive skills evolved, first and foremost the ability to share attention, intentions, and goals with others. Tomasello refers to these skills as shared intentionality, and with shared intentionality came a genuine concern for others' health and wellbeing. This happens because advanced forms of cooperation require not only the ability to understand that my wellbeing depends on your wellbeing, but more remarkably that it also requires the realization that *our* wellbeing depends on *us* taking care of *one another* (Tomasello, 2018, p. 72). Additionally, Tomasello's theory suggests that it is our cultural nature that makes the distinction between subjectivity and objectivity possible. The concept of an objective perspective developed because of sophisticated role-taking across various collaborative projects. Some facts and values are not mine, or yours, but universal in the sense of applying to "all." Such a third-person perspective provides stability and objectivity to a cultural group and ensures that notions of right and wrong, justice, and fairness can be established as universal (within-group) truths that prompt us to take care of each other in dyads, in families and small groups, and on a more general basis. Taken together, this cultural capacity for caring is just as much an ability to care for others, as a need to be cared for by others (Tomasello, 2016). Although logically the one presupposes the other, the need to care goes beyond what is typically articulated as caring in the literature on care ethics.

All humans need to be cared *for*. Invariably, every one of us has been taken care of as a child and should thus see the value in caring relations. Yet, the grand theories of ethics have basically been silent about the role of care as an interpersonal relation. Kantian ethics, utilitarianism, and Aristotelian virtue ethics offer, according to Held (2006), no satisfactory formulation of the idea that attending to and meeting the needs of a particular other should be a moral responsibility. A consistently articulated ethics of care is therefore only a few decades old. Some attempts have been made to integrate an ethics of care with virtue ethics (e.g., Slote, 2007; Steyl, 2019) or Kantian ethics (e.g., Darwall, 2002). However, the tensions between the abstract, rational, and impartial elements of traditional ethics and the moral value of private, particular, and family- and friend-oriented relationships emphasized by care ethics make these positions difficult to integrate. Virtue ethics focuses, for instance, on individual characteristics, whereas the ethics of care concerns caring relations (Held, 2006, p. 19). Care ethics also departs from the universal and impartial principles of utilitarianism and deontology because the reason why we care for someone close to us is not that they are like everyone else but rather that they are special to us (Held, 2006, p. 93). Without care, we cannot have life, and there could be no societies. As a description of our existence, it thus seems correct to say that without care and morality, humans would not have been humans. According to the HTW, these insights are included in the background assumptions we need to develop scientific knowledge about wellbeing.

Humanistic Values

The appeal to perform our humanness well is normative. This notion is inspired by Aristotelian philosophy, which, as we have seen, defines the good life as rational activity[5] in accordance with virtue. Hence, for Aristotle, wellbeing is a moral concept. The HTW also takes a moral standpoint, as it assumes that our humanness will become more fully developed and expressed when performed in accordance with certain values. These values are not grounded in Aristotelian ethics, but in what roughly can be referred to as humanism. Note that humanism is not a precisely defined ideology, but can loosely be understood as a nondogmatic, ethical stance that emphasizes human's rights and responsibilities to shape their own lives. The organization Humanists International suggests, for instance, that humanisms "stands for the building of a more humane society through an ethic based on human and other natural values in the spirit of reason and free inquiry through human capabilities. It is not theistic, and it does not accept supernatural views of reality."[6] Some key principles associated with humanism are human rights and dignity, reason and science, education, knowledge, social justice and cultural expression (e.g., Beauregard, 2022; Butler, 2021; Fredman, 2008; Pinker, 2018; Shue, 2020).

Three values originating in humanism are of particular importance to the humanistic theory of wellbeing. The first is grounded in the idea of basic human rights as articulated in the First Article in the UN's Declaration of Human Rights: "All human beings are born free and equal in dignity and rights" (UN, 1948). A second humanistic value is the so-called principle of beneficence, which states that one should avoid harming others if it can be prevented. A third value commitment in the HTW is related to an ethics of care (e.g., Held, 2006; Noddings, 2013; Robinson, 2011; Slote, 2007). From this perspective, human life is seen as relational and organized in networks of caring relations. As such, we are morally obliged to provide care to those who need it. In addition to these three basic values, the humanistic theory of wellbeing also rejects the idea of absolute value relativism. Briefly, the theory assumes that a life embedded in mutualistic cooperation, solidarity, freedom, peace, and democracy is better than a life of ruthless competition, selfishness, serfdom, war, and tyranny.

I will loosely refer to the values just described as basic humanistic values, well aware that no consensus exists as to how such a category should be precisely defined. The HTW readily admits that a care ethics works better within groups than between groups and that one of today's most pressing challenges is to establish institutions that contribute to enlarging the "circle of care." Our lives can only be sustainably good when we realize that all humans belong to the same moral community.

---

[5] The exact wording in the Nicomachean Ethics is "activity of the soul." Many philosophers seem however to translate this phrase into "rational activity," for reasons further explored in Chap. 6.

[6] https://humanists.international/policy/iheu-minimum-statement-on-humanism/

Justifying Values

A challenge for the HTW is to integrate humanistic values in a scientific framework. Here, the theory trusts that, fundamentally speaking, science is value-laden. One of the arguments highlighted in this chapter is the thesis that scientific theories by necessity are empirically underdetermined. It is therefore impossible to logically deduce the elements in a scientific theory from empirical observations. Consequently, the relation between value judgments and scientific knowledge is in principle no different from the relation between factual judgments and scientific knowledge. You cannot deduce an ought directly from an is, but you cannot deduce a theoretical statement directly from an is either.

One implication of this insight is that both facts and values inform scientific knowledge. For example, Anderson (2004) has pointed out how feminist values contributed to an improved understanding of the consequences of a divorce. By including personal growth on the list of possible consequences of a dissolved marriage, the concept of a divorce changed. Similarly, by allowing narrative ethical voices to be heard in response to a moral dilemma, Gilligan broadened the scope of interpreting moral reasoning beyond the abstract and math-oriented tradition employed by Lawrence Kohlberg. Thus, an ethics grounded in care and identification with suffering people can provide different answers to a moral dilemma than an ethics of rule-based justice.

The analogical relevance for the humanistic theory of wellbeing is that a value-based approach to wellbeing may enhance our understanding of what the good life is. For example, if wellbeing is restricted to describe a particular experience, such as emotional happiness, it makes sense to say that "After a day spent killing his parents, Frank was happy" (Gilbert, 2006, p. 37). People would understand that we are referring to the feeling Frank had that day. But it does not make sense to say that Frank is performing his humanness well by killing his parents. A human life is not good if it violates basic humanistic values. Hence, equipped with the normative requirements of the HTW, Frank's assassination of his parents does not make his life go better for him. According to the theory, feelings and judgments are only constitutive of wellbeing if they are experienced for the right reasons. What we like in our lives is, in a way, only as good as the situation that creates it. This principle applies to all empirical observations employed in wellbeing research, which means that self-reported measures of what we like in life—such as being satisfied or feeling good—only can be taken as evidence for wellbeing when they are liked for the right reasons. For example, empirical studies show that both harming and hurting people can produce pleasure and positive affect (Chester, 2017; Sapolsky, 2017). However, if we accept that harming others is bad, it follows that it is better to feel good from comforting others than from hurting them. This value priority is made explicit in the HTW because the pleasure derived from comforting others is felt for the right reasons. In contrast, if mainstream wellbeing theories continue to insist on being value-free, they must accept that the pleasures we obtain from helping and the pleasure we get from harming are inseparable.

To Like One's Life

The HTW defines wellbeing as to like one's life for the right reasons. To like a life means that it both feels good and is thought of as good for the person living it. Thus, the term like is used broadly, somewhat akin to terms such as appreciate, approve, being in favor of, or being oriented toward something. Such a use of the word liking is not uncommon in the wellbeing literature. For instance, Diener has explained that a person has high subjective wellbeing when "both her cognitive and affective systems react favorably to what is happening in her life. She likes the life she is leading—it is desirable from her point of view" (Diener, 1998, p. 312). Veenhoven's conceptualization of wellbeing also comes close. He defines wellbeing, or happiness in his vocabulary, as "the degree to which an individual judges the overall quality of his or her life-as-a-whole favorably. In other words: how much he likes the life he leads" (Veenhoven, 1984, p. 22). Liking thus understood is not limited to fit the way it is used by neuropsychologists such as Berridge and Kringelbach (e.g., Berridge, 1996; Berridge & Kringelbach, 2011). In a strict, neuropsychological understanding, liking is basically a synonym for pleasure (see Chap. 5), but that meaning is not applied to the term in the HTW.

Good feelings come in many stripes, as do the thinking we make about our lives. The HTW organizes this multidimensionality according to the function these feelings and thinking serve in maintaining the three universal needs for stability, change, and care. Two overarching dimensions of wellbeing capture the ways in which the fulfillment of these needs are transformed into indicators of a good life. Stability is associated with hedonic wellbeing and reflects the wellness formed by successful maintenance of the stability need. Change is associated with eudaimonic wellbeing and reflects the wellness formed by successful facilitation of the stability need. Both stability and change are broadly conceptualized and relate to the biological, psychological, and social aspects of human living (e.g., Engel, 1977). The wellbeing indicators associated with the need to and for care straddle the hedonic-eudaimonic distinction and are integrated into both hedonic and eudaimonic elements of wellbeing. Figure 7.2 (Chap. 7) provides a graphical overview of the interaction between the three universal needs and hedonic and eudaimonic wellbeing.

Hedonic Wellbeing

Hedonic wellbeing (HWB) is about stability regulation and comprises two subcomponents: harmony feelings and spontaneous judgments. It is called hedonic because the primary function of HWB is to indicate how well we are performing in terms of need fulfillment and goal achievement, i.e., the constant task of rebalancing disequilibria throughout life. As will be detailed in subsequent chapters, what we often think of as hedonic seems to have evolved in our evolutionary past to serve such a stability-regulating function. For example, pleasure is involved in homeostasis and satisfaction is involved in goal achievement. The latent mechanism driving the indicators of HWB is spontaneous good-bad evaluations (SGBE) for which harmony feelings, including pleasure (Chap. 5), tranquility, contentment, happiness, and joy (Chap. 3), are prototypical indicators. The term harmony feelings is used interchangeably with hedonic feelings, and the category also include social feelings such as empathy and falling in love. The harmony feelings are generated according to the principles of basic emotions as described in the communicative theory of emotions (Chap. 3). The SGBE also regulates spontaneous judgments, which represents the thinking elements in HWB. The most important spontaneous judgment indicator is life satisfaction, but domain satisfaction and presence of meaning are also included in this dimension.

Eudaimonic Wellbeing

Eudaimonic wellbeing (EWB) is about change regulation and improvements, and it comprises three subcomponents: opportunity feelings, reflective judgments, and betterment orientations. EWB indicates how well we are performing in terms of managing the universal need for change, although it is limited to a restricted set of developments, such as our human potentials for wisdom, morality, and personal growth (Chap. 6). EWB can be accompanied by opportunity feelings such as interest, engagement, immersion, and wonder/awe. The term opportunity feelings is used interchangeably with the term eudaimonic feelings. Social feelings, such as compassion and romantic love, are also included in this category. In addition to a feeling dimension and a judgmental component, the EWB is also defined by a separate improvement indicator, referred to as betterment orientations. Personal growth, a search for meaning, and a will to be a good human being are important kinds of betterment orientations. Several mechanisms or operating modes are important for EWB. Major among them is an organismic drive to actualize one's human potential. The organismic idea will be more fully clarified in Chap. 6, and here I shall only say that it essentially suggests that biological organisms can build a structure of goals (including values) and plans to reach the goals and further execute these plans, without the influence of external rewards. This is not to say that organisms never are influenced by external rewards, only that they are able to operate without them. In a nutshell, EWB is about improvements that are regulated by a will to be a good human being.

References

't Hart, B., Struiksma, M. E., van Boxtel, A., & van Berkum, J. J. A. (2018). Emotion in stories: Facial EMG evidence for both mental simulation and moral evaluation [original research]. *Frontiers in Psychology, 9*(613). https://doi.org/10.3389/fpsyg.2018.00613

Adolphs, R., & Anderson, D. J. (2018). *The neuroscience of emotion: A new synthesis*. Princeton University Press.

Alexandrova, A., & Fabian, M. (2022). Democratising measurement: Or why thick concepts call for coproduction. *European Journal for Philosophy of Science, 12*(1), 7.
Allport, G. W. (1961). *Pattern and growth in personality*. Holt, Rinehart and Winston.
Ambady, N., & Rosenthal, R. (1993). Half a minute: Predicting teacher evaluations from thin slices of nonverbal behavior and physical attractiveness. *Journal of Personality and Social Psychology, 64*(3), 431–441. https://doi.org/10.1037/0022-3514.64.3.431
Anderson, E. (2002). Situated knowledge and the interplay of value judgments and evidence in scientific inquiry. In P. Gärdenfors, J. Woleński, & K. Kijania-Placek (Eds.), *In the scope of logic, methodology and philosophy of science: Volume two of the 11th international congress of logic, methodology and philosophy of science, Cracow, August 1999* (pp. 497–517). Springer Netherlands. https://doi.org/10.1007/978-94-017-0475-5_8
Anderson, E. (2004). Uses of value judgments in science: A general argument, with lessons from a case study of feminist research on divorce. *Hypatia, 19*(1), 1–24. https://doi.org/10.1111/j.1527-2001.2004.tb01266.x
Aristotle. (trans. 1908). *The Nicomachean ethics [Kindle]* (W. D. Ross, Trans.). Enhanced Media, 2017.
Arnold, M. (1960). *Emotion and personality*. Columbia University Press.
Baldwin, T. (2010). George Edward Moore. In E. N. Zalta (Ed.), *The Stanford encyclopedia of philosophy* (Summer 2010 Edition ed.). Available from http://plato.stanford.edu/archives/sum2010/entries/moore/.
Bargh, J. A. (1994). The four horsemen of automaticity: Awareness, intention, efficiency, and control in social cognition. In R. S. J. R. Wyer & T. K. Srull (Eds.), *Handbook of social cognition* (Vol. 1. Basic Processes, pp. 1–40). Lawrence Erlbaum.
Bargh, J. (1997). The automaticity of everyday life. In R. S. Wyer (Ed.), *The automaticity of everyday life* (Vol. X, pp. 1–61). Lawrence Erlbaum.
Bargh, J. A., Chaiken, S., Raymond, P., & Hymes, C. (1995). The automatic evaluation effect: Unconditional automatic attitude activation with a pronunciation task. *Journal of Experimental Social Psychology, 32*, 104–128.
Baron, J. (2024). *Thinking and deciding [Kindle]* (5th ed.). Cambridge University Press.
Barrett, L. F. (1995). Valence focus and arousal focus: Individual differences in the structure of affective experience. *Journal of Personality and Social Psychology, 69*(1), 153–166.
Barrett, L. F. (2006). Valence is a basic building block of emotional life. *Journal of Research in Personality, 40*(1), 35–55.
Baumeister, R. F. (1991). *Meanings of life*. Guilford Press.
Beauregard, E. M. (2022). We should all be marching: Why humanistic psychologists should take action toward social justice. *The Humanistic Psychologist, 50*(4), 594–606. https://doi.org/10.1037/hum0000269
Beebe-Center, J. G. (1932). The psychology of pleasantness and unpleasantness. .
Berridge, K. C. (1996). Food reward: Brain substrates of wanting and liking. *Neuroscience & Biobehavioral Reviews, 20*(1), 1–25. https://doi.org/10.1016/0149-7634(95)00033-B
Berridge, K. C., & Kringelbach, M. L. (2011). Building a neuroscience of pleasure and well-being. *Psychology of Well-Being, 1*(1), 1–26. https://doi.org/10.1186/2211-1522-1-3
Billman, G. E. (2020). Homeostasis: The underappreciated and far too often ignored central organizing principle of physiology. *Frontiers in Physiology, 11*, 200. https://doi.org/10.3389/fphys.2020.00200
Bjørndal, L. D., Nes, R. B., Czajkowski, N., & Røysamb, E. (2023). The structure of well-being: A single underlying factor with genetic and environmental influences. *Quality of Life Research, 32*(10), 2805–2816. https://doi.org/10.1007/s11136-023-03437-7
Blasi, A. (1976). Concept of development in personality theory. In J. Loevinger (Ed.), *Ego development* (pp. 29–53). Jossey–Bass.
Bornstein, R. F. (1989). Exposure and affect: Overview and meta-analysis of research, 1968–1987. *Psychological Bulletin, 106*(2), 265–289. https://doi.org/10.1037/0033-2909.106.2.265

Borsboom, D., van der Maas, H. L., Dalege, J., Kievit, R. A., & Haig, B. D. (2021). Theory construction methodology: A practical framework for building theories in psychology. *Perspectives on Psychological Science, 16*(4), 756–766.

Briggs, J. L. (1970). *Never in anger. Portrait of an eskimo family*. Harvard University Press.

Brinkmann, S. (2011a). Facts, values, and the naturalistic fallacy in psychology. In *Psychology as a moral science* (pp. 79–93). Springer. https://doi.org/10.1007/978-1-4419-7067-1_5

Brinkmann, S. (2011b). *Psychology as a moral science*. Springer. https://link.springer.com/book/10.1007/978-1-4419-7067-1

Brown, M. J. (2020). *Science and moral imagination. A new ideal for values in science*. University of Pittsburgh Press. https://doi.org/10.2307/j.ctv18b5d19

Bühler, C. (1928). Displeasure and pleasure in relation to activity. In M. L. Reymert (Ed.), *Feelings and emotions: The Wittenberg symposium* (pp. 195–199). Clark University Press.

Bühler, C. (1951). Maturation and motivation. *Dialectica, 5*(3–4), 312–361.

Butler, P. (2021). Humanism and the conceptualization of value and well-being. In A. B. Pinn (Ed.), *The Oxford handbook of humanism* (pp. 645–664). Oxford University Press.

Cannon, W. (1932). *The wisdom of the body*. Norton.

Carlquist, E., Ulleberg, P., Delle Fave, A., Nafstad, H. E., & Blakar, R. M. (2017). Everyday understandings of happiness, good life, and satisfaction: Three different facets of well-being. *Applied Research in Quality of Life, 12*, 481–505. https://doi.org/10.1007/s11482-016-9472-9

Casebeer, W. D. (2003). *Natural ethical facts: Evolution, connectionism, and moral cognition [Kindle]*. Cambridge University Press.

Chen, F. F., Jing, Y., Hayes, A., & Lee, J. (2013). Two concepts or two approaches? A bifactor analysis of psychological and subjective well-being. *Journal of Happiness Studies, 14*(3), 1033–1068. https://doi.org/10.1007/s10902-012-9367-x

Chester, D. S. (2017). The role of positive affect in aggression. *Current Directions in Psychological Science, 26*(4), 366–370. https://doi.org/10.1177/0963721417700457

ChoGlueck, C., & Lloyd, E. A. (2023). Values as heuristics: A contextual empiricist account of assessing values scientifically. *Synthese, 201*(6), 220. https://doi.org/10.1007/s11229-023-04198-z

Churchland, P. S. (2018). *Braintrust: What neuroscience tells us about morality [Kindle]*. Princeton Science Library.

Clore, G. L., & Schiller, A. J. (2016). New light on the affect–cognition connection. In L. F. Barrett, M. Lewis, & J. M. Haviland-Jones (Eds.), *Handbook of emotions* (pp. 532–546). Guilford Publications.

Crisp, R. (2006a). Hedonism reconsidered. *Philosophy and Phenomenological Research, 73*(3), 619–645. https://doi.org/10.1111/j.1933-1592.2006.tb00551.x

Crisp, R. (2006b). *Reasons and the good*. Clarendon Press.

Crisp, R. (2017). Well-being. In E. N. Zalta (Ed.), *The Stanford encyclopedia of philosophy*. Available from http://plato.stanford.edu/archives/fall2011/entries/well-being/.

Damasio, A. (1999). *The feeling of what happens: Body and emotion in the making of consciousness*. Avon Books.

Damasio, A. (2010). *Self comes to mind: Constructing the conscious brain [Kindle]*. Pantheon Books.

Damasio, A. (2018). *The strange order of things: Life, feeling, and the making of culture [Kindle]*. Pantheon Books.

Damasio, A. (2021). *Feeling & knowing: Making minds conscious [Kindle]*. Pantheon.

Darwall, S. (2002). *Welfare and rational care*. Princeton University Press.

Davies, S. E., Connelly, B. S., Ones, D. S., & Birkland, A. S. (2015). The general factor of personality: The "Big One," a self-evaluative trait, or a methodological gnat that won't go away? *Personality and Individual Differences, 81*, 13–22. https://doi.org/10.1016/j.paid.2015.01.006

De Waal, F. (2013). *The bonobo and the atheist: In search of humanism among the primates [Kindle]*. W.W. Norton.

Delle Fave, A., Brdar, I., Freire, T., Vella-Brodrick, D., & Wissing, M. (2011). The eudaimonic and hedonic components of happiness: Qualitative and quantitative findings. *Social Indicators Research, 100*(2), 185–207. https://doi.org/10.1007/s11205-010-9632-5
Denton, D. (2005). *The primordial emotions: The dawning of consciousness*. Oxford University Press.
Diener, E. (1984). Subjective well-being. *Psychological Bulletin, 95*(3), 542–575. https://doi.org/10.1037/0033-2909.95.3.542
Diener, E. (1998). Subjective well-being and personality. In D. F. Barone & M. Hersen (Eds.), *Advanced personality* (pp. 311–334). Plenum.
Disabato, D. J., Goodman, F. R., Kashdan, T. B., Short, J. L., & Jarden, A. (2016). Different types of well-being? A cross-cultural examination of hedonic and eudaimonic well-being. *Psychological Assessment, 28*(5), 471–482. https://doi.org/10.1037/pas0000209
Douglas, H. (2009). *Science, policy, and the value-free ideal [Kindle]*. University of Pittsburgh Press.
Ekman, P. (2003). *Emotions revealed: Recognizing faces and feelings to improve communication and emotional life*. Henry Holt.
Elliot, A., & Covington, M. (2001). Approach and avoidance motivation. *Educational Psychology Review, 13*(2), 73–92. https://doi.org/10.1023/a:1009009018235
Elliott, K. C. (2017). *A tapestry of values: an introduction to values in science [Kindle]*. Oxford University Press.
Engel, G. (1977). The need for a new medical model: A challenge for biomedicine. *Science, 196*(4286), 129–136. https://doi.org/10.1126/science.847460
Eregowda, N. I., Yadav, S., Parameshwarappa, P., & Basavraj, R. K. (2016). A girl with no pain: Congenital insensitivity to pain and anhidrosis (HSAN) type IV-A case report. *Journal of Clinical and Diagnostic Research: JCDR, 10*(2), ZL01.
Eronen, M. I., & Bringmann, L. F. (2021). The theory crisis in psychology: How to move forward. *Perspectives on Psychological Science, 16*(4), 779–788.
Feldman, F. (2010). *What is this thing called happiness?* Oxford University Press.
Festinger, L. (1954). A theory of social comparison processes. *Human Relations, 7*(2), 117–140.
Fishbach, A., & Ferguson, M. J. (2007). The goal construct in social psychology. In *Social psychology: Handbook of basic principles* (2nd ed., pp. 490–515). The Guilford Press.
Fiske, S. T., Cuddy, A. J. C., & Glick, P. (2007). Universal dimensions of social cognition: Warmth and competence. *Trends in Cognitive Science, 11*(2), 77–83.
Fodor, J. (2007). Why pigs don't have wings. *London Review of Books, 29*(20), 19–22.
Fox, A. S., Lapate, R. C., Shackman, A. J., & Davidson, R. J. (Eds.). (2018). *The nature of emotion: Fundamental questions*. Oxford University Press.
Fredman, S. (2008). *Human rights transformed: Positive rights and positive duties [Kindle]*. Oxford University Press.
Fredrickson, B. L. (2001). The role of positive emotions in positive psychology. The Broaden-and-build theory of positive emotions. *American Psychologist, 56*(3), 218–226.
Fredrickson, B. L. (2009). *Positivity: Groundbreaking research to release your inner optimism and thrive [Kindle]*. Crown Publishers.
Fredrickson, B. L. (2013). Positive emotions broaden and build. In D. Patricia & P. Ashby (Eds.), *Advances in experimental social psychology* (Vol. 47, pp. 1–53). Academic Press. https://doi.org/10.1016/B978-0-12-407236-7.00001-2
Freud, S. (1930). *Civilization and its discontents*. Norton.
Freud, S. (2012/1920). *Beyond the pleasure principle [Kindle]*. Liver.
Frijda, N. H. (1986). *The emotions*. Cambridge University Press.
Frijda, N. H. (2007). *The laws of emotions*. Lawrende Erlbaum Associates.
Frijda, N. H. (2010). On the nature and function of pleasure. In M. L. Kringelbach & K. C. Berridge (Eds.), *Pleasures of the brain* (pp. 99–112). Oxford University Press.
Geach, P. T. (1956). Good and evil. *Analysis, 17*(2), 33–42. https://doi.org/10.2307/3326442
Gilbert, D. (2006). *Stumbling on happiness*. Harper Press.

Gilligan, C. (1993). *In a different voice: Psychological theory and women's development*. Harvard University Press.
Gilligan, C. (2023). *In a human voice. The 40th anniversary edition [Kindle]*. Wiley.
Gilovich, T. D., Epley, N., & Hanko, K. (2005). Shallow thoughts about the self: The automatic components of self-assessment. In M. D. Alicke, D. Dunning, & J. Krueger (Eds.), *The self in social judgment* (5th ed., pp. 67–84). Psychology Press.
Goodman, F. R., Disabato, D. J., Kashdan, T. B., & Kauffman, S. B. (2018). Measuring well-being: A comparison of subjective well-being and PERMA. *The Journal of Positive Psychology, 13*(4), 321–332. https://doi.org/10.1080/17439760.2017.1388434
Griffin, J. (1986). *Well-being. Its meaning, measurement, and moral importance*. Clarendon Press.
Haidt, J. (2012). *The righteous mind: Why good people are divided by politics and religion [Kindle]*. Penguin Books.
Harmon-Jones, E., & Harmon-Jones, C. (2021). On defining positive affect (PA): Considering attitudes toward emotions, measures of PA, and approach motivation. *Current Opinion in Behavioral Sciences, 39*, 46–51. https://doi.org/10.1016/j.cobeha.2021.01.008
Hart, K. E., & Sasso, T. (2011). Mapping the contours of contemporary positive psychology. *Canadian Psychology/Psychologie Canadienne, 52*(2), 82–92. https://doi.org/10.1037/a0023118
Haybron, D. M. (2008). *The pursuit of unhappiness. The elusive psychology of well-being*. Oxford University Press.
Held, V. (2006). *The ethics of care: Personal, political, and global*. Oxford University Press.
Heyd, T. (1989). Mill and Comte on psychology. *Journal of the History of the Behavioral Sciences, 25*(2), 125–138. https://doi.org/10.1002/1520-6696(198904)25:2<125::AID-JHBS2300250203>3.0.CO;2-U
Hicks, D. J. (2014). A new direction for science and values. *Synthese, 191*(14), 3271–3295. https://doi.org/10.1007/s11229-014-0447-9
Hirata, J. (2011). *Happiness, ethics and economics*. Routledge.
Hogan, P. C. (2003). *The mind and its stories: Narrative universals and human emotion*. Cambridge University Press.
Hollander, B. (1901). Auguste Comte's positive psychology based on Gall's doctrine. In *The mental functions of the brain: An investigation into their localisation and their manifestation in health and disease* (pp. 447–464). Grant Richards. https://doi.org/10.1037/13814-011
Holman, B., & Wilholt, T. (2022). The new demarcation problem. *Studies in History and Philosophy of Science, 91*, 211–220. https://doi.org/10.1016/j.shpsa.2021.11.011
Huemer, M. (2021). *Knowledge, reality and value. A mostly common sense guide to philosophy [kindle]*. Samizdat.
Hume, D. (2006). *Enquiry concerning the principles of morals*. Cleardon Press.
Huppert, F. A., Marks, N., Clark, A., Siegrist, J., Stutzer, A., Vittersø, J., & Wahrendorf, M. (2009). Measuring well-being across Europe: Description of the ESS Well-being Module and preliminary findings. *Social Indicators Research, 91*(3), 301–315.
Hurka, T. (2015). Moore's moral philosophy. In E. N. Zalta (Ed.), *The Stanford encyclopedia of philosophy*. Available from http://plato.stanford.edu/archives/fall2015/entries/moore-moral/.
Izard, C. E. (1977). *Human emotions*. Plenum Press.
Jarvis, W. B. G., & Petty, R. E. (1996). The need to evaluate. *Journal of Personality and Social Psychology, 70*(1), 172–194.
Jensen, M. C. (2008). Foreword. In P. J. Zak (Ed.), *Moral markets: The critical role of values in the economy* (pp. ix–x). Princeton University Press.
Jousset, A., Eisenhauer, N., Materne, E., & Scheu, S. (2013). Evolutionary history predicts the stability of cooperation in microbial communities [Article]. *Nature Communications, 4*, 2573. https://doi.org/10.1038/ncomms3573
Kagan, J. (1998). *Three seductive ideas*. Harvard University Press.
Kagan, J. (2002). *Surprise, uncertainty, and mental structures*. Harvard University Press.

Kahneman, D. (1999). Objective happiness. In D. Kahneman, E. Diener, & N. Schwarz (Eds.), *Well-being: The foundations of hedonic psychology* (pp. 3–25). Russell Sage Foundation.
Kaiser, C., & Oswald, A. J. (2022). The scientific value of numerical measures of human feelings. *Proceedings of the National Academy of Sciences, 119*(42), e2210412119. https://www.pnas.org/doi/abs/10.1073/pnas.2210412119
Kazemi, S. A. (2023). Absolute goodness defended. *The Journal of Value Inquiry*. https://doi.org/10.1007/s10790-023-09947-4
Kendler, H. H. (2000). *Amoral thoughts about morality: The intersection of science, psychology, and ethics*. Charles C Thomas Publisher.
Kim, M. P., & Rosenberg, S. (1980). Comparison of two structural models of implicit personality theory. *Journal of Personality and Social Psychology, 38*, 375–389.
King, L., & Napa, C. K. (1998). What makes a life good? *Journal of Personality and Social Psychology, 75*(1), 156–165.
Kirchin, S. (2013a). Introduction: Thick and thin concepts. In S. Kirchin (Ed.), *Thick concepts* (p. 0). Oxford University Press. https://doi.org/10.1093/acprof:oso/9780199672349.003.0001
Kirchin, S. (2013b). *Thick concepts*. OUP Oxford.
Knobe, J., Prasada, S., & Newman, G. E. (2013). Dual character concepts and the normative dimension of conceptual representation. *Cognition, 127*(2), 242–257. https://doi.org/10.1016/j.cognition.2013.01.005
Kohlberg, L. (1975). The cognitive-developmental approach to moral education. *The Phi Delta Kappan, 56*(10), 670–677. http://www.jstor.org/stable/20298084
Kraut, R. (2012). *Against absolute goodness*. Oxford University Press. https://doi.org/10.1093/acprof:oso/9780199844463.001.0001
Kristjánsson, K. (2013). *Virtues and vices in positive psychology [Kindle]*. Cambridge University Press. https://doi.org/10.1017/cbo9781139177818
Krys, K., Capaldi, C. A., Zelenski, J. M., Park, J., Nader, M., Kocimska-Zych, A., Kwiatkowska, A., Michalski, P., & Uchida, Y. (2021). Family well-being is valued more than personal well-being: A four-country study. *Current Psychology, 40*(7), 3332–3343. https://doi.org/10.1007/s12144-019-00249-2
Kuhn, T. (2002). Objectivity, value judgment, and theory choice. In Balashov, Y., & Rosenberg, A. (Eds.), *Philosophy of science: Contemporary Readings* (pp. 421–437).
Lane, N. (2015). *The vital question: Energy, evolution, and the origins of complex life*. WW Norton & Company.
Lang, P. L. (1995). The emotion probe. Studies of motivation and attention. *American Psychologist, 50*(5), 372–385.
Lazarus, R. S. (1991). *Emotion and adaptation*. Oxford University Press.
Lazarus, R. S., & Folkman, S. (1984). *Stress, appraisal, and coping*. Springer.
Lercher, M. (2018). Homeostasis. In J. Brockman (Ed.), *This idea is brilliant. Lost overlooked and underappreciated scientific concepts everyone should know [Kindle]* (pp. 120–121). Harper Collins.
Leuthold, H., Kunkel, A., Mackenzie, I. G., & Filik, R. (2015). Online processing of moral transgressions: ERP evidence for spontaneous evaluation. *Social Cognitive and Affective Neuroscience, 10*(8), 1021–1029. https://doi.org/10.1093/scan/nsu151
Lewis, M. (2016). The emergence of human emotion. In L. F. Barrett, M. Lewis, & J. M. Haviland-Jones (Eds.), *Handbook of emotions* (pp. 272–292). Guilford Publications.
Longino, H. E. (1979). Evidence and hypothesis: An analysis of evidential relations. *Philosophy of Science, 46*(1), 35–56. http://www.jstor.org/stable/186801
Longino, H. E. (2002). *The fate of knowledge*. Princeton University Press.
Longino, H. E. (2008). Values, heuristics, and the politics of knowledge. In M. Carrier, D. Howard, & J. Kourany (Eds.), *The challenge of the social and the pressure of practice: Science and values revisited* (pp. 68–85). University of Pittsburgh Press. http://ebookcentral.proquest.com/lib/tromsoub-ebooks/detail.action?docID=2038168

Malle, B. F. (2021). Moral judgments. *Annual Review of Psychology, 72*(1), 293–318. https://doi.org/10.1146/annurev-psych-072220-104358
Marchetti, G., & Marchetti, S. (Eds.). (2016). *Facts and values: The ethics and metaphysics of normativity [Kindle]*. Taylor & Francis.
Maslow, A. (1954). *Motivation and personality*. Harper and Row.
Mayr, E. (1982). *The growth of biological thought. Diversity, evolution, and inheritance*. Harvard University Press.
Mayr, E. (2004). *What makes biology unique?: Considerations on the autonomy of a scientific discipline*. Cambridge University Press.
McGrath, R. E. (2015). Character strengths in 75 nations: An update. *The Journal of Positive Psychology, 10*(1), 41–52. https://doi.org/10.1080/17439760.2014.888580
Merton, R. K. (1938). Science and the social order. *Philosophy of Science, 5*(3), 321–337.
Mitchell, P., & Alexandrova, A. (2021). Well-being and pluralism. *Journal of Happiness Studies, 22*(6), 2411–2433. https://doi.org/10.1007/s10902-020-00323-8
Moen, O. M. (2012). *Because it feels good. A hedonistic theory of intrinsic value*. University of Oslo.
Montague, R. (2007). *Your brain is (almost) perfect: How we make decisions [Kindle]*. Dutton.
Murphy, G. L. (2002). *The big book of concepts*. The MIT Press.
Nafstad, H. E., Blakar, R. M., Botchway, A., & Rand-Hendriksen, K. (2009). Globalization, ideologies and well-being: a study of a West African and a North European society. *The Journal of Positive Psychology, 4*(4), 305–315. http://www.informaworld.com/10.1080/17439760902933773
Nesse, R. M. (2005). Natural selection and the elusiveness of happiness. In F. Huppert, N. Baylis, & B. Keverne (Eds.), *The science of well-being* (pp. 3–32). Oxford University Press.
Newell, A. (1973). You can't play 20 questions with nature and win: Projective comments on the papers of this symposium. In W. G. Chase (Ed.), *Visual information processing* (pp. 283–308). Academic Press.
Noddings, N. (2013). *Caring: A relational approach to ethics and moral education* (2nd ed.). University of California Press. http://www.jstor.org.ezproxy.uio.no/stable/10.1525/j.ctt7zw1nb
Nussbaum, M. C. (2001). *Upheavals of thought. The intelligence of emotions*. Cambridge University Press.
Nussbaum, M. C. (2008). Who is the happy warrior? Philosophy poses questions to psychology. *The Journal of Legal Studies, 37*(S2), s81–s113. https://doi.org/10.1086/587438
Oatley, K. (1992). *Best laid schemes. The psychology of emotions*. Cambridge University Press.
Oishi, S., Kushlev, K., & Schimmack, U. (2018). Progressive taxation, income inequality, and happiness. *American Psychologist, 73*(2), 157–168. https://doi.org/10.1037/amp0000166
Oishi, S., & Westgate, E. C. (2022). A psychologically rich life: Beyond happiness and meaning. *Psychological Review, 129*(4), 790–811. https://doi.org/10.1037/rev0000317
Oreskes, N. (2019). *Why trust science? [Kindle]*. Princeton University Press.
Osgood, C. E. (1969). On the whys and wherefores of E, P, and A. *Journal of Personality and Social Psychology, 12*(3), 194–199.
Osgood, C. E., May, W. H., & Miron, M. S. (1975). *Cross-cultural universals of affective meaning*. University of Illinois Press.
Osgood, C. E., Suci, G. J., & Tannenbaum, P. H. (1957). *The measurement of meaning*. University of Illinois Press.
Oveis, C., Horberg, E. J., & Keltner, D. (2010). Compassion, pride, and social intuitions of self-other similarity. *Journal of Personality and Social Psychology, 98*(4), 618–630. https://doi.org/10.1037/a0017628
Panksepp, J. (1998). *Affective neuroscience. The foundations of human and animal emotions*. Oxford University Press.
Pawelski, J. O. (2016a). Defining the 'positive' in positive psychology: Part I. A descriptive analysis. *The Journal of Positive Psychology, 11*(4), 339–356. https://doi.org/10.1080/17439760.2015.1137627

Pawelski, J. O. (2016b). Defining the 'positive' in positive psychology: Part II. A normative analysis. *The Journal of Positive Psychology, 11*(4), 357–365. https://doi.org/10.1080/17439760.2015.1137628
Perry, R. B. (1926). *General theory of value*. Harvard University Press.
Peterson, C., & Seligman, M. E. P. (2004). *Strengths and virtues: A handbook and classification*. American Psychological Association.
Phillips, J., De Freitas, J., Mott, C., Gruber, J., & Knobe, J. (2017). True happiness: The role of morality in the folk concept of happiness. *Journal of Experimental Psychology: General, 146*(2), 165–181. https://doi.org/10.1037/xge0000252
Phillips, J., Misenheimer, L., & Knobe, J. (2011). The ordinary concept of happiness (and others like It). *Emotion Review, 3*(3), 320–322. https://doi.org/10.1177/1754073911402385
Phillips, J., Nyholm, S., & Liao, S.-Y. (2014). The good in happiness. In T. Lombrozo, S. Nichols, & J. Knobe (Eds.), *Oxford studies in experimental philosophy* (Vol. 1, pp. 253–293). Oxford University Press.
Pinker, S. (2018). *Enlightenment now: The case for reason, science, humanism, and progress [Kindel]*. Penguin.
Plé, B. (2000). Auguste Comte on positivism and happiness. *Journal of Happiness Studies, 1*(4), 423–445.
Popper, K. R. (1963). Conjectures and refutations. The growth of scientific knowledge. .
Pratto, F. (1994). Consciousness and automatic evaluation. In P. M. Niedenthal & S. Kitayama (Eds.), *The heart's eye. Emotional influences in perception and attention* (pp. 115–143). Academic Press.
Primdahl, M. S. (2024). *The good, the bad, and the positive thinker: A qualitative study investigating positive thinking's influence on problem-solving* [Master thesis. Uit The Arctic University of Norway].
Prinzing, M. (2021). How to study well-being: A proposal for the integration of philosophy with science. *Review of General Psychology, 25*(2), 152–162. https://doi.org/10.1177/10892680211002443
Pross, A. (2016). *What is Life?: How chemistry becomes biology*. Oxford University Press.
Putnam, H. (1993). Objectivity and the science—Ethics distinction. In M. C. Nussbaum & A. Sen (Eds.), *The quality of life* (pp. 143–158). Clarendon Press.
Putnam, H. (2004). *The collapse of the fact/value dichotomy and other essays*. Harvard University Press.
Raatikainen, P. (2022). Gödel's incompleteness theorems. In E. N. Zalta (Ed.), *The Stanford encyclopedia of philosophy* (Spring 2022 ed.). Available from https://plato.stanford.edu/archives/spr2022/entries/goedel-incompleteness/.
Rawls, J. (1971). *A theory of justice*. Harvard University Press.
Reisenzein, R. (1992). A structuralist reconstruction of Wundt's three-dimensional theory of emotion. In H. Westmeyer (Ed.), *The structuralist program in psychology. Foundations and applications* (pp. 141–189). Hogrefe & Huber.
Rickless, S. (2012). Plato's parmenides. In E. N. Zalta (Ed.), *The Stanford encyclopedia of philosophy*. https://leibniz.stanford.edu/friends/members/preview/plato-parmenides/
Ridge, M. (2014). Moral non-naturalism. In E. N. Zalta (Ed.), *The Stanford encyclopedia of philosophy*. http://plato.stanford.edu/archives/fall2014/entries/moral-non-naturalism/
Robinson, F. (2011). *The ethics of care: A feminist approach to human security*. Temple University Press.
Rodolfo, K. (2000). *What is homeostasis?* Scientific American. https://www.scientificamerican.com/article/what-is-homeostasis/.
Rolls, E. T. (2005). *Emotions explained*. Oxford University Press.
Rooney, P. (1992). On values in science: Is the epistemic/non-epistemic distinction useful? *PSA: Proceedings of the Biennial Meeting of the Philosophy of Science Association, 1992*, 13–22. http://www.jstor.org.mime.uit.no/stable/192740
Ross, D., & Ross, W. D. (2002). *The right and the good*. Oxford University Press.

Ruckmick, C. A. (1925). The psychology of pleasantness. *Psychological Review, 32*(5), 362–383.
Russell, J. A. (1980). A circumplex model of affect. *Journal of Personality and Social Psychology, 39*(6), 1161–1178. https://doi.org/10.1037/h0077714
Russell, J. A. (2003). Core affect and the psychological construction of emotion. *Psychological Review, 110*(1), 145–172.
Russell, J. A., & Barrett, L. F. (1999). Core affect, prototypical emotional episodes, and other things called emotion: Dissecting the elephant. *Journal of Personality and Social Psychology, 76*(5), 805–819.
Sapolsky, R. M. (2017). *Behave. The biology of humans at our best and worst [Kindle]*. Penguin Press.
Sauer, H. (2017). Between facts and norms: Ethics and empirical moral psychology. In B. G. Voyer & T. Tarantola (Eds.), *Moral psychology: A multidisciplinary guide* (pp. 5–27). Springer. https://doi.org/10.1007/978-3-319-61849-4_2
Sayer, A. (2011). *Why things matter to people: Social science, values and ethical life [Kindle]*. Cambridge University Press.
Scherer, K. R., Schorr, A., & Johnstone, T. (Eds.). (2001). *Appraisal processes in emotion. Theory, methods, research*. Oxford University Press.
Schlosberg, H. (1954). Three dimensions of emotion. *Psychological Review, 61*, 81–88.
Schneirla, T. C. (1959). An evolutionary and developmental theory of biphasic processes underlying approach and withdrawal. In *Nebraska symposium on motivation, 1959* (pp. 1–42). University of Nebraska Press.
Schrödinger, E. (2010/1946). What is life? (selections). In C. E. Cleland, & M. A. Bedau (Eds.), *The nature of life: Classical and contemporary perspectives from philosophy and science* (pp. 50–69). Cambridge University Press. (Original work published in 1946). https://doi.org/10.1017/CBO9780511730191.007.
Searle, J. R. (1995). *The construction of social reality*. Pinguin.
Seligman, M. E. P. (1998). *What is the 'good life'? Editorial*. APA Monitor.
Seligman, M. E. P. (1999). The president address. *American Psychologist, 54*(8), 559–562.
Seligman, M. E. P. (2002). *Authentic happiness. Using the new positive psychology to realize your potential for deep fulfillment*. Nicholas Brealey Publishing.
Seligman, M. E. P., & Csikszentmihalyi, M. (2000). Positive psychology: An introduction. *American Psychologist, 55*(1), 5–14. https://doi.org/10.1037/0003-066X.55.1.5
Sheldon, K. M. (2011). What's positive about positive psychology? Reducing value-bias and enhancing integration within the field. In K. Sheldon, T. Kashdan, & M. Steger (Eds.), *Designing positive psychology: Taking stock and moving forward* (pp. 421–429). Oxford University Press.
Sheldon, K. M., Fredrickson, B., Rathunde, K., Csikszentmihalyi, M., & Haidt, J. (2000). *A positive psychology manifesto*. https://ppc.sas.upenn.edu/sites/default/files/Positive%20Psychology%20Manifesto.docx.
Shue, H. (2020). *Basic rights: Subsistence, affluence, and US foreign policy [Kindle]*. Princeton University Press.
Slote, M. (2007). *The ethics of care and empathy*. Routledge.
Smith, C. A., Tong, E. M. W., & Ellsworth, P. C. (2014). The differentiation of positive emotional experience as viewed through the lens of appraisal theory. In M. M. Tugade, M. N. Shiota, & K. N. Kirby (Eds.), *Handbook of positive emotions* (pp. 11–27). Guilford.
Springer, K. W., & Hauser, R. M. (2006). An assessment of the construct validity of Ryff's scales of psychological well-being: Method, mode, and measurement effects. *Social Science Research, 35*(4), 1080–1102.
Springer, K. W., Hauser, R. M., & Freese, J. (2006). Bad news indeed for Ryff's six-factor model of well-being. *Social Science Research, 35*(4), 1120–1131.
Stanford, K. (2021). Underdetermination of scientific theory. In E. N. Zalta (Ed.), *The Stanford encyclopedia of philosophy*.
Steyl, S. (2019). *Towards an Aristotelian Theory of care: A comparison of Neo-Aristotelian virtue ethics with feminist ethics of care, and the fundaments of a virtue ethical theory of care*. (Doctor

of Philosophy (College of Philosophy and Theology)). University of Notre Dame Australia. https://researchonline.nd.edu.au/theses/246
Sumner, L. W. (1996). *Welfare, happiness, and ethics*. Clarendon Press.
Suppe, F. (1977). *The structure of scientific theories*. University of Illinois Press.
Taylor, S. E. (2002). *The tending instinct. Women, men, and the biology of our relationships*. Times Books.
Taylor, S. E. (2006). Tend and befriend: Biobehavioral bases of affiliation under stress. *Current Directions in Psychological Science, 15*(6), 273–277. https://doi.org/10.1111/j.1467-8721.2006.00451.x
Taylor, J. B. (2008). *My stroke of insight [Kindle]*. Hodder & Stoughton.
Tesser, A., & Martin, L. (1996). The psychology of evaluation. In E. T. Higgins & A. W. Kruglanski (Eds.), *Social psychology. Handbook of basic principles* (pp. 400–431). The Guildford Press.
Thagard, P. (1992). *Conceptual revolutions*. Princeton University Press.
Thagard, P. (2010). *The brain and the meaning of life [Kindle]*. Princeton University Press.
Thagard, P. (2012). *The cognitive science of science*. The MIT Press.
Thorndike, E. L. (1920). A constant error in psychological ratings. *Journal of Applied Psychology, 4*(1), 25–29. https://doi.org/10.1037/h0071663
Thorndike, E. L. (1927). The law of effect. *The American Journal of Psychology, 39*(1/4), 212–222. https://doi.org/10.2307/1415413
Tiberius, V. (2013a). Recipes for a good life: Eudaimonism and the contribution of philosophy. In A. Waterman (Ed.), *The best within us. Positive psychology perspectives on eudaimonia* (pp. 19–38). American Psychological Association. https://doi.org/10.1037/14092-002
Tiberius, V. (2013b). Theorizing: On the division of labor between moral philosophy and positive psychology. In S. Kirchin (Ed.), *Thick concepts* (pp. 217–234). Oxford University Press.
Tiberius, V. (2015). *Moral psychology: A contemporary introduction*. Routledge.
Tiberius, V. (2017a). Does virtue make us happy? A new theory for an old question. In W. Sinnott-Armstrong & C. B. Miller (Eds.), *Moral psychology: Virtue and character [Kindle]* (pp. 547–578). Mit Press. http://www.jstor.org/stable/j.ctt1n2tvzm.41
Tiberius, V. (2017b). On the division of labor between philosophers and psychologists: a "Goldilocksian" reply to comments from Saucedo & Gruber and Kristjánsson. In W. Sinnott-Armstrong & C. B. Miller (Eds.), *Moral psychology: Virtue and character [Kindle]* (pp. 597–604). Mit Press. http://www.jstor.org/stable/j.ctt1n2tvzm.41
Tomasello, M. (2016). *A natural history of human morality [Kindle]*. Harvard University Press.
Tomasello, M. (2018). The origins of morality. *Scientific American, 319*(3), 70–75. https://doi.org/10.1038/scientificamerican0918-70
Tomasello, M. (2019). *Becoming human: A theory of ontogeny [Kindle]*. Belknap Press.
Tomkins, S. S. (1962). *Affect, imagery, consciousness. Vol 1. The positive affects*. Springer.
Tranel, D., & Damasio, A. (1993). The covert learning of affective valence does not require structures in hippocampal system or amygdala. *Journal of Cognitive Neuroscience, 5*, 79–88.
Turp, M.-J. (2016). Goodness: Attributive and predicative. *Les ateliers de l'éthique/The Ethics Forum, 11*(2–3), 70–87. https://doi.org/10.7202/1041767ar
UN. (1948). *The United Nations General Assembly's Universal Declaration of Human Rights*. http://www.un.org/en/universal-declaration-human-rights/index.html
Van Berkum, J. J. A., Holleman, B., Nieuwland, M., Otten, M., & Murre, J. (2009). Right or wrong?:The Brain's fast response to morally objectionable statements. *Psychological Science, 20*(9), 1092–1099. https://doi.org/10.1111/j.1467-9280.2009.02411.x
Veenhoven, R. (1984). *Conditions of happiness*. Kluwer Academic.
Vittersø, J. (2016). The feeling of excellent functioning: Hedonic and eudaimonic emotions. In J. Vittersø (Ed.), *Handbook of eudaimonic well-being* (pp. 253–276). Springer International Publishing. https://doi.org/10.1007/978-3-319-42445-3_17
Weijers, D. (2021). Hedonism. *Internet Encyclopedia of Philosophy*. https://iep.utm.edu/hedonism/
Wessman, A. E., & Ricks, D. F. (1966). *Mood and personality*. Holt, Reinehart & Winston.

Wierzbicka, A. (1999). *Emotions across languages and cultures: Diversity and universals*. Cambridge University Press.
Williams, B. (2011/1985). *Ethics and the limits of philosophy*. Taylor & Francis. (Original work published 1985).
Willis, J., & Todorov, A. (2006). First impressions. Making up your mind after a 100 ms exposure to a face. *Psychological Science, 17*(7), 592–598.
Winkielman, P., Schwarz, N., Fazendeiro, T. A., & Reber, R. (2003). The hedonic marking of processing fluency: Implications for evaluative judgment. In J. Musch & K. C. Klauer (Eds.), *The psychology of evaluation. Affective processes in cognition and emotion* (pp. 189–217). Lawrence Erlbaum.
Wong, P. T. P. (2011). Positive psychology 2.0: Towards a balanced interactive model of the good life. *Canadian Psychology/Psychologie Canadienne, 52*(2), 69–81. https://doi.org/10.1037/a0022511
Young, P. T. (1961). *Motivation and emotion: A survey of the determinants of human and animal activity*. Wiley.
Zajonc, R. B. (1968). Attitudinal effects of mere exposure. *Journal of Personality and Social Psychology (Monograph Supplement), 9*(part 2, no.2), 2–27.
Zajonc, R. B. (1980). Feelings and thinking: Preferences need no inferences. *American Psychologist, 35*(2), 151–175. https://doi.org/10.1037/0003-066X.35.2.151
Zimmerman, M. J. (2015). Value and normativity. In I. Hirose & J. Olson (Eds.), *The Oxford handbook of value theory* (pp. 13–28). Oxford University Press.

Chapter 2
Happiness and Wellbeing

Introduction

> "When I went to school, they asked me what
> I wanted to be when I grow up. I wrote down 'happy.'
> They told me I didn't understand the assignment,
> and I told them they didn't understand life."
> John Lennon (cited in Lieberman, 2013)[1]

Humans have wrangled over the notion of happiness for ages, but two decades ago, the British psychologist Michael Argyle boldly declared that "most people know very well what [happiness] is" (Argyle, 2001, p. 1). Could Argyle be right? Had a common understanding of happiness finally been carved out, or was Argyle just overly optimistic on behalf of the new discipline of happiness research? According to the cartoonist Matt Groening, the latter must be the case. Reflecting on the well-known wish for a "Happy New Year," Groening commented, "I understand the 'New Year' part, but what do they mean by 'Happy'?" (Haybron, 2008, p. 29). Beyond anecdotes and cartoons, the bewildering about the meaning of happiness is present in practically every approach to the study of happiness, being it historical (McMahon, 2006), cultural (Lomas, 2018), linguistic (Wierzbicka, 2004), philosophic (Fletcher, 2015), scientific (Kahneman et al., 1999b; Veenhoven, 1984), or folk theory (Carlquist et al., 2016). Happiness is what Flanagan (2007, p. 162) refers to as a polysemic term; it has many different meanings. Indeed, everybody seems to have obtained their own definition of it (Haybron, 2008, p. 3). These circumstances have, unfortunately, led the study of happiness into dire conceptual straits, and we must accept that happiness belongs to the group of ideas that evade themselves from a clear definition.

[1] Lieberman doubts that Lennon ever wrote this and suggests that it might just be an internet meme (p. 224).

J. Vittersø, *Humanistic Wellbeing*, https://doi.org/10.1007/978-3-031-69292-5_2

One reason for the confusion about happiness is the jingle fallacy (Thorndike, 1913), i.e., that a single term (such as happiness) means diverse things to different people. Another confusion is the jangle fallacy (Kelley, 1927), i.e., that different words (such as happiness and wellbeing) are used to refer to the same concept. Much of the writing on happiness suffers from these fallacies (see, Vittersø, 2016b). One recent example is a book entitled *The Origins of Happiness: The Science of Well-Being Over the Life Course,* authored by the world's leading happiness economists (Clark et al., 2018). The book uses happiness and wellbeing as synonyms in the title, whereas all the empirical analyses are about life satisfaction.

The practice of using happiness, wellbeing, and sometimes even life satisfaction indiscriminately is traceable at least back to Bentham (Sumner, 1996). Among psychologists we find, again, that Argyle (2001) has a particularly clear opinion on the matter as he simply claims that happiness "has come to be called subjective well-being, SWB for short, which means *exactly* (italics added) the same thing" (p. 2). Other authorities, such as Kahneman (1999, p. 5), Seligman (2003, p. 127), Diener and Tov (2012, p. 137), Veenhoven (2012, p. 66), and very many others are also explicit about their use of happiness and wellbeing as synonyms.

But Bentham, Kahneman, Seligman, Diener, Veenhoven, and many others do not consider happiness and wellbeing to be *exactly* the same. Bentham, for example, made at times "a distinction between wellbeing as the net balance of pleasure over pain, and happiness to describe pleasures of unusual intensity" (Sumner, 1996, p. 85). Most modern researchers are similarly less vigorous than Argyle and follow the tradition of using happiness and wellbeing *loosely* as synonyms (e.g., Easterlin, 2001; Martin, 2008; Van Praag & Ferrer-i-Carbonell, 2004; Vella-Brodrick, 2014). As for the terminology of the current chapter, I use the term wellbeing and think of it as a loose synonym for happiness. Subsequent chapters will be more particular about differences between the two concepts.

The problems with the jingle and jangle fallacies are, to some extent, acknowledged in the field. In a recent review, Diener and his colleagues expressed their concern for how the term happiness "can be confusing, because it means different things in different contexts and to different people. It may mean positive feelings at the moment, long-term life satisfaction, all forms of well-being, or even the causes of subjective well-being" (Diener, Lucas, & Oishi, 2018, p. 3). Algoe et al. (2011) are even more critical of the plethora of meanings that have been applied to the term happiness and seriously suggest that the word should be banned: "even in the unlikely event that scientists were to agree on its meaning, such understanding could hardly compete with all multiple meanings of the word 'happy' within common usage" (p. 116). The authors list a range of ways in which happiness can be used, with examples such as a momentary feeling state, an overarching emotional term, a personality trait, as the ultimate goal of life, or in the sense of conveying simple acceptance—as in the phrase "I'll be happy to help."

Philosophical Approaches

The essential objective in the philosophy of wellbeing is to identify the ultimate human goodness, i.e., determining the things that "make someone's life go better for them" (Crisp, 2006, p. 622) or what "the good for a person [is] in the broadest sense"[2] (Tiberius, 2015, p. 158). Haybron describes wellbeing as "a normative or evaluative concept that concerns what *benefits* a person, is in her *interest*, is *good for* her, or *makes her life go well* for her" (Haybron, 2008, p. 29, italics in original). Other terms used to express the idea of wellbeing include advantage, prudential value, welfare, happiness, flourishing, eudaimonia, and utility (Moore & Crisp, 1996, p. 599). Alexandrova explains that these concepts aim to deliver "a maximally general account of goods non-instrumentally valuable to the agent" (Alexandrova, 2017, p. 28). She also points out that mainstream theories about wellbeing are concerned with "the most general evaluation of the value of a state to a person and not anything else."

Philosophical theories of wellbeing are normative. They use value-laden terms, such as better, good, advantage, interest, flourishing, etc., to describe wellbeing as an inherently valuable state that we have reason to think of as favorable for any individual. In Chap. 1, the distinction between prudential and deontological values was introduced, and I pointed out that most philosophers argue that wellbeing is about prudential and not deontological values. Philosophical theories of wellbeing further try to answer both substantive and formal questions about such prudential goodness. Chapter 1 pointed out that substantive questions concern the nature of wellbeing, and they ask what constitutes a good life. Formal questions ask what it is about the ingredients of wellbeing that make them good. These questions pertain to the methodologies or principles used to understand why something is good.

Endless Lists of Human Goods

There is no lack of suggestions as to what constitute a human good. For example, when Agustine, in the year 426, published *The City of God*, he complained about the high number of theories of happiness that ancient philosophers had produced. Augustine counted 288 competing theories, although Hudson (1996) suspected that this number was an exaggeration. A more reliable account of early attempts at list making is found in MacIntyre (2007), who discusses disagreements over various records of character traits circulating in ancient Athens. The heroes in Homer's *Iliad* had, for instance, only one concern or item on their list: to beat the enemy and keep the fruits of victory for himself. MacIntyre further tells us that Socrates also had a

[2] This is confusing, because the phrase "broadest sense" can hardly mean only in a prudential sense. A life that is good for me in a broad sense can arguably include the notion that my life is good for me if it is good for others.

single item on his list of things worth pursuing, and that was knowledge. Plato includes wisdom, justice, courage, temperance, and sometimes piety on his list, whereas Aristotle offers 13 moral virtues and several intellectual virtues, although he "does not seem to be claiming that his list is complete" (Curzer, 2018, p. 114). The 13 virtues are courage, temperance, liberality, magnificence, proper pride, right ambition, good temper, wit, truthfulness, friendliness, shame, poetic justice, and justice. The most comprehensive list of virtues I have heard of comes from Pincoffs (1986), who operates with no less than 221 personal qualities that can be considered as virtues (cited in Held, 2006, p. 55).

Moral theology has often focused on the dark part of human nature and is known for the seven deadly sins, each with an opposite virtue (humility, charity, chastity, gratitude, temperance, patience, and diligence). A selected group of values lists four cardinal virtues (prudence, temperance, fortitude, and justice). Following Churchland (2018), other historical lists of vises and virtues include the "three poisons" (hatred, craving, and delusion) from the Buddhist Abhidharma. This Buddhist approach also operates with the "Four Noble Truths" (loving kindness, compassion, appreciative joy, and equanimity). A list from the Chinese philosopher Mencius (fourth c. BCE) contains four overarching virtues: benevolence, righteousness, propriety, and wisdom. Benjamin Franklin (2005) held 13 virtues to be of particular importance (temperance, silence, order, resolution, frugality, industry, sincerity, justice, moderation, cleanliness, tranquility, chastity, and humidity), whereas Bennett (1993) operates with 10 virtues (self-discipline, compassion, responsibility, friendship, work, coercion, perseverance, honesty, loyalty, and faith).

Modern philosophers have also contributed to list making about wellbeing, and a review by Fletcher (2015) mentions four examples. The first comes from John Finnis and contains life itself, knowledge and aesthetic experience, some degree of excellence in work and play, friendship, self-integration, self-expression, and religion. List 2 comes from Guy Fletcher and contains achievement, friendship, happiness, pleasure, self-respect, and virtue. List 3 comes from Mark Murphy and contains life, knowledge, aesthetic experience, excellence in play and work, excellence in agency, inner peace, friendship and community, religion, and happiness. Finally, List 4 comes from Derek Parfit and contains moral goodness, rational activity, development of abilities, having children and being a good parent, knowledge, and awareness of true beauty.

The problem of list making has elegantly and ironically been demonstrated by the Argentine short story writer Jorge Luis Borges. His book *The Analytical Language of John Wilkins* famously ridicules the seventeenth-century philosopher and bishop John Wilkins for his ambitious attempt at making a classification scheme of a "natural language." Borges polemically mocked all kinds of quasi-scientific classifications, and about Wilkins' taxonomy in particular, he claimed that it resembles "a certain Chinese encyclopedia" which divided animals "into (a) those that belong to the Emperor, (b) embalmed ones, (c) those that are trained, (d) suckling pigs, (e) mermaids, (f) fabulous ones, (g) stray dogs, (h) those that are included in this classification, (i) those that tremble as if they were mad, (j) innumerable ones, (k) those drawn with a very fine camel's hair brush, (I) others, (m) those that have just broken a flower vase, (n) those that resemble flies from a distance" (Borges, 1964, p. 103).[3]

Classifying Philosophical Theories of Wellbeing

There is an obvious need to clean up and systematize the many candidates that compete to define the human good, and in current philosophical literature, three main categories of philosophical wellbeing theories seem to have been identified. An early taxonomy was offered by von Wright (1963). In the book, *Varieties of Goodness*, von Wright referred to the first of his three major classes of wellbeing theories as "Epicurean ideals," because the valuable attribute of wellbeing (or "true happiness" as von Wright calls it) comes "above all from having things which please" (p. 92). He went on to name a second category of wellbeing theories for "Utilitarian happiness," because they suggest that wellbeing depends upon the satisfaction of desires. The third and final category in von Wright's scheme was "Aristotelian happiness," in which wellbeing is thought to come from the pleasure that one takes in certain doings or activities—especially those that involve capacities that one has made an effort to develop. The three major categories proposed by von Wright were later relabeled and slightly changed 20 years later, when Parfit (1984, pp. 493–502) sorted wellbeing theories into (1) hedonistic theories (what would be best for someone is what would make his life happiest), 2) desire-fulfillment theories (what would be best for someone is what, throughout his life, would best fulfill his desires), or (3) objective list theories (certain things are good or bad for us, whether or not we want to have the good things, or to avoid the bad things). A brief survey of the main arguments from these three wellbeing theories follows next.

Hedonism, Satisfactionism, and Objective Lists

Theories of hedonism come in many stripes. A prototypical one is from Bentham, who famously proclaimed that "Nature has placed mankind under the governance of two sovereign masters, pain and pleasure. It is for them alone to point out what we ought to do, as well as to determine what we shall do" (Bentham, 1789/1948, p. 1). Based on this verdict and subsequent explanations, hedonism can be separated into a moral version and a prudential version. Prudential hedonism, according to Weijers (2021), is a monist theory holding that "only pleasure intrinsically makes people's lives go better *for them* (italics in original) and all and only pain intrinsically makes their lives go worse *for them*" (italics in original). In other words, pleasure (net of

[3] Needless to say, the Chinese encyclopedia is a fiction made up by Borges.

pain) is the only thing in life that is truly valuable, both individually (prudential hedonism) and morally (value hedonism). More relaxed versions of hedonism exist, some of them replace pleasure with enjoyment, while others replace pleasure with the much broader concept of positive experiences. But the basic structure remains—pleasure/enjoyment/positive experiences are the only thing desirable as an end, and pain/suffering/negative experiences are the only thing not desirable as our ultimate end (Gregory, 2015). We will look more closely into the pros and cons of hedonism in Chap. 5.

Desire-fulfillment theories, which are sometimes referred to as satisfactionism, is another group of monist theories about prudential goodness (Crisp, 2017; Heathwood, 2015). Briefly, it says that getting what you want is good for you and not getting what you want is bad for you (Fletcher, 2016, p. 27). Another way of formulating the essence of desire-fulfillment theories is to say that your life is going well to the extent that you are succeeding in getting what you want (Sumner, 1996, p. 113) or that the good of the person is synonymous with the satisfaction of subjective material preferences (Annett, 2022, p. 131). Hence, it is not pleasure or any other feeling that constitutes the good; the only thing that matters is to get what you desire, since the fulfillment of a strong desire counts directly as your interest (Parfit, 1984, p. 465). The subjective sovereignty inherent in the desire-fulfillment approaches seems to make these theories infallible. If the idea that a person cannot be wrong about their own wellbeing is taken on face value, the desire-fulfillment theories cannot be falsified beyond the individual's own claim. Nevertheless, the desire-fulfillment theories are popular and often regarded as the dominant account of wellbeing in philosophy, welfare economics, and political theory (e.g., Fabian & Pykett, 2021; Tiberius, 2013b).

The last category in the philosophical tripartite taxonomy of wellbeing is often called objective list theories (e.g., Parfit, 1984, pp. 493–502). Sumner (1996) mentions four theories within this category: (1) private ownership theory (goodness means to own something that is good), (2) need theories (goodness is to get ones' basic needs satisfied), (3) capability theories (goodness is the opportunity to do and be what you have reason to value), and (4) teleological theories (goodness defined as Aristotelian eudaimonism). Objective list theories have a dubious reputation in many philosophical circles, and Sumner argues that their objective nature makes them unable to account for prudential wellbeing. Toward the end of the present chapter, however, and again in Chaps. 6 and 7, objective list theories will be discussed in a slightly more favorable light. First, we refer to Searle's taxonomy of ontologies and epistemologies (this chapter), then we draw on Aristotelian eudaimonism (Chap. 6), and finally we benefit from social epistemology (Chap. 7).

Competing Taxonomies

Although Parfit's catalog of wellbeing theories is popular (e.g., Angner, 2010; Crisp, 2017), many competing taxonomies exist. Sumner (1996) has, for instance, argued that a reasonable conceptualization of wellbeing can be established by restricting happiness to be a subjective phenomenon, i.e., by removing the objective accounts from Parfit's classification scheme. As briefly mentioned in Chap. 1, Sumner's theory defines wellbeing as authentic happiness, which is the happiness of an informed and autonomous subject (Sumner, 1996, p. 171). His arguments against objectivity will be reviewed in more details in the "Subjective Versus Objective Wellbeing" section, which suffice it here to say that Sumner's minimalistic taxonomy is one in which hedonic theories and desire-fulfillment theories are the only overarching approaches to the philosophical study of wellbeing.

Others have expanded rather than reduced the number of classes of wellbeing theories suggested by von Wright and Parfit. Fletcher (2016) has, for instance, suggested that four main categories are reasonable: hedonism, desire-fulfillment theory, objective list theory, and perfectionism. Haybron (2008) has presented a list that comprises five classes: hedonic theories, desire-fulfillment theories, authentic theories, eudaimonic (or "nature fulfillment") theories, and list theories. Tiberius (2013a) operates with a slightly different fivefold taxonomy: hedonic theories, desire-fulfillment theories, life satisfaction theories, nature fulfillment theories, and objective list theories about wellbeing. As a final example, *The Routledge Handbook of Philosophy of Well-Being* (Fletcher, 2015) suggests that seven major categories of wellbeing theories are needed to provide a decent overview: hedonism, perfectionism, desire-fulfillment theory, objective list theories, hybrid theories, wellbeing and subjective dependence, and eudaimonism.

The list of proposed wellbeing taxonomies is much longer, but this brief review illustrates that philosophers disagree about "what we have when our lives go well for us." Beyond the overarching disagreements about taxonomies, there is also much debate among philosophers about the specific content within each theory.

Philosophical approaches also suffer from jingle and jangle fallacies. Chapter 1 mentioned that Haybron (2008) uses the word *happiness* as a referent for a psychological state approach to a good life and the word *wellbeing* as a referent for a philosophical approach to a good life. Happiness is purely descriptive, Haybron says, and has two components: pleasure, which is defined as "a mental state that contains pleasure" (p. 289) and life satisfaction, which is defined as "an attitude of being satisfied with your life as a whole" (p. 30). Such a conceptualization comes close to popular definitions of SWB. Thus, for Haybron, subjective wellbeing is used interchangeably with happiness but is distinct from the term wellbeing. By contrast, eudaimonia is an evaluative,[4] not psychological, term corresponding roughly to

[4] The philosophical use of evaluative as an exclusively normative—and not psychological—term is another example of a jingle fallacy in the wellbeing literature. As demonstrated in Chap. 1, evaluation is a concept frequently studied in psychology and other scientific disciplines.

Haybron's term "wellbeing" (Haybron, 2008, p. 9). This is why Haybron maintains that Aristotle did not articulate a theory of happiness, but rather a theory of wellbeing (Haybron, 2008, p. 32).

As the above review shows, the philosophy of wellbeing is no better off than the science of wellbeing when it comes to conceptual confusion and a lack of theoretical agreements. Sumner observes, for instance, that "no simple theory about the nature of happiness enjoys much support among philosophers; there is not even agreement that such a theory is possible" (Sumner, 1996, p. 139). This may not come as a surprise. According to van Inwagen and Sullivan (2020), there is almost no thesis in philosophy overall about which scholars agree, and there is barely any collective convergence for the major questions in the discipline (Chalmers, 2015). For example, Bourget and Chalmers (2014) asked a sample of university philosophers ($N = 931$), about their opinions about 30 central philosophical issues. Only one issue reached a level of consensus of 80% agreement (the issue was about non-skeptical realism about the external world). In addition, the participants were remarkably unaware of the wide discrepancies regarding the 30 issues. The situation is radically different in science, at least the natural sciences, because empirical observations have "the power to compel agreement on the answers to the big question" (Chalmers, 2015, p. 16). Moreover and in contrast to philosophers, scientists agree more frequently on the premises for their methodological reasoning and are thus more able to resolve opposing arguments and consent on conclusions. Central elements in philosophical reasoning, such as articulating thesis and developing arguments in their favor, seldom contribute consensus. To the contrary, Chalmers (2015, p. 19) finds that "philosophical arguments typically lead not to agreement but to sophisticated disagreement." A new theory by Mercier and Sperber (2017) even suggests that reasoning did not evolve as a mechanism to help us in finding truths and understand the universe. The main function of human reasoning is rather to support and protect our own biases in debates with others.

Scientific Approaches

When scientists began to study wellbeing, the focus was not on identifying the highest or most valuable of all states. The emphasis was rather directed toward "understanding the antecedents and consequences of subjective well-being, assuming that it was good regardless of whether it was the highest good" (Diener, 2009b, p. 1). This strategy has been foundational to the empirical study of wellbeing. Critical issues are now reasonably well understood, and many questions asked 50 years ago have been settled or rephrased to become more understandable and relevant. A review of the literature overwhelmingly reveals that empirical advancements have been made and that a long list of correlates and causes of indicators of wellbeing have reliably been established. In one excellent overview, Diener, Oishi, and Tay (2018) reported that the fulfillment of basic and psychological needs is positively associated with SWB, that richer countries and richer individuals and families are better off than their poorer counterparts, that people who achieve their valued goals are more satisfied than those who do not, that wellbeing is beneficial for health and longevity, and that happy people are more likely to marry, have more friends, have a better work life, and so on. The understanding of how income relates to wellbeing has also grown remarkably well since Easterlin (1974) and other pioneers of happiness economics first formulated testable hypotheses about it (e.g., Killingsworth et al., 2023). A recent Science publication similarly points out that optimism leads to hope which again provides investments by individuals in work, health, and education and that these positive consequences are particularly important in developing countries (Graham et al., 2018). Indeed, a study including approximately 700,000 participants showed that a single life satisfaction item is a more powerful predictor than a combined set of economic indicators for a bundle of outcome variables related to housing, partner separation, job, and hospitalization (Kaiser & Oswald, 2022). The list of evidence and putative facts regarding wellbeing has become unmanageably large—and it continues to grow (e.g., Diener, Lucas, & Oishi, 2018; Diener et al., 1999; Helliwell et al., 2022; Lyubomirsky et al., 2005; Michalos, 2021; Pressman & Cohen, 2005; Sirgy, 2021).

The scientific study of happiness spans four centuries and includes work by Sinclair (1791), Kirwan (1810), and Spencer (1850), although the conception of happiness applied in this early research was radically different from ours. For instance, Sinclair kept detailed scores of the living conditions in Scotland in the eighteenth century and referred to the purpose of his statistical inquiry as "ascertaining the quantum of happiness enjoyed by its inhabitants, and the means of its future improvement" (Thin, 2012, pp. 4–5). What Sinclair basically measured, however, was agricultural products. Nevertheless, empirical studies based on self-reported happiness and wellbeing have been published regularly over the last 100 years (e.g., Beckham, 1929; Flügel, 1925; Hartmann, 1934; Ruckmick, 1925; Watson, 1930), although the role of happiness studies was limited before World War II (Jones, 1953).

As long as wellbeing has been investigated empirically, debates have been raised about the quality and relevance of the measures that have been used (e.g., Alexandrova, 2016; Angner, 2013; Deaton & Stone, 2016; Diener, 2009a; Goldings, 1954; Graham et al., 2018; Layard, 2010; McMahan & Estes, 2011; Oswald & Wu, 2010; Weinberg et al., 2018; Wilson, 1967). In psychometrics, the quality and relevance of a measurement are often evaluated in terms of reliability (numerical precision) and validity (conceptual precision). For the core instruments used in wellbeing studies, acceptable reliability has regularly been reported since the 1930s. For instance, Watson (1930) reported a Spearman-Brown reliability of 0.83 for a self-reported happiness scale. A few years later, Hartmann (1934) found a test-retest correlation of 0.70 for his happiness instrument, measured 1 month apart. Thus, Wilson (1967) announced more than 50 years ago that "It is already established that avowed happiness can be determined reliably" (p. 294). Since Wilson's review, empirical analyses of the psychometric quality of happiness and wellbeing scales has basically confirmed Watson's conclusion, and it is currently fair to say that wellbeing can be reliably measured (Diener et al., 2013; Lucas, 2018). But when it comes to validity, things are different. Although empirical studies typically report their wellbeing measures to be both reliable and valid, the validity part of that phrase is uncertain. This is because the techniques utilized to estimate validity are questionable.

If validity is taken to be a test's ability to measure a particular concept—"what it intends to measure"—then the evidence for validity should come from showing how variation in a relevant attribute of that concept causes the variation observed in the test scores (Bringmann & Eronen, 2016). Such procedures are rare, however, which means that the validity of wellbeing measures is largely unknown (Eronen & Bringmann, 2021). Note that from this perspective, Cronbach and Meehl's (1955) popular notion of construct validity is not a factual question of whether a test measures a real attribute. Their construct validity regards "the complexe question of whether test score interpretations are consistent with a nomological network involving theoretical and observational terms" (Borsboom et al., 2004, p. 1061). Thus, the problem of validity cannot be solved by psychometrics or models alone, which implies that a popular technique such as a multitrait multimethod correlation table will not, on its own, determine the validity of a test. Moderately high correlations between self-reports and informant reports of wellbeing (e.g., Sandvik et al., 1993; Schneider & Schimmack, 2009) indicate criteria-based validity, which is helpful, although it cannot solve the crucial validity question. To test validity properly, Borsboom et al. argue, one must identify how variation in a concept, or an attribute of a concept, produces variance in a measurement outcome. A test is "valid for measuring an attribute if (a) the attribute exists and (b) variations in the attribute causally produce variation in the measurement outcomes" (p. 1061). Therefore, before something can be measured, precise knowledge about the concept must be established, which is to say that only substantial theoretical work can solve the problem of validity. It is not the psychometrics that is difficult about validation, the true challenge is to determine what one intends to measure (Borsboom et al., 2004, p. 67).

Therefore, solving the issue of validity in wellbeing research depends on the development of better theories and more precise concepts. If conceptual clarity is the place to start to determine the question of validity, more attention should be devoted to those areas of wellbeing studies. And that is precisely where we are heading next, beginning with the historical development of the concept of wellbeing.

Subjective Wellbeing

The term subjective wellbeing (SWB) was introduced to the social sciences by Burger (1964), an ergonomist. Burger's concern was jobholders who worked too hard, and he defined SWB in relation to an optimal level of workload, specified to be 1/3 of the maximal workload. This perspective of SWB never entered the framework of happiness research, however, and the term had to wait 20 years to gain popularity.

A handful of books published in the 1960s and 1970s were instrumental for making the term subjective wellbeing a lead concept in the empirical study of wellbeing. These pioneers did not use the term SWB explicitly, but they voiced the idea that a scientific study of wellbeing can be established on the basis of survey responses to items adapted from the philosophical traditions of hedonism and desire-fulfillment theories. Gurin et al. (1960) is an early example of a hedonic-inspired approach to wellbeing, although the main inspiration behind this publication was grounded in the study of mental health. Bradburn's (1969) hedonistic orientation was also important in establishing an empirical tradition of measuring positive and negative affect. Twenty years before Ryff's (1989) more well-known use of the term, Bradburn dubbed his study field psychological wellbeing.[5] Happiness, as he also called it, could be studied by measuring "subjective feeling states that individuals experience in their daily lives" (Bradburn, 1969, p. 225). He classified these feelings into two kinds, positive affect and negative affect, which in many respects, Bradburn noted, "is similar to older pleasure-pain or utility models that view an individual's happiness or wellbeing in terms of the degree to which pleasure predominates over pain in his life experiences" (p. 9).

At about the same time and theoretically located somewhere between the hedonic and desire-fulfillment approaches, Wessman and Ricks (1966) offered a remarkably modern perspective on wellbeing. The authors developed, for instance, an early version of the Day Reconstruction Method, a data collection procedure typically attributed to Kahneman (e.g., Kahneman et al., 2004).[6] Other books that prepared the groundwork for today's default conceptualization of SWB were Bauer (1966) who took a social indicator perspective on wellbeing and Brickman and Campbell (1971) who had a hedonic orientation. Some journal articles, such as Wilson (1967), Neugarten et al. (1961), Davies (1962), Parducci (1968), Locke (1969), Allard (1973), and Easterlin (1974), were also instrumental in establishing a science of wellbeing in the 1970s and early 1980s.

Two early steppingstones came with Campbell et al. (1976) and Andrews and Withey (1976). These authors did not refer to their own work in terms of subjective wellbeing, although Andrews and Withey (1976, p. 19) referred to the work of Campbell and coworkers as studies of "subjective well-being." In their own writings, however, Campbell, Converse, and Rogers used the phrase "perceived well-being." The Campbell et al. book was primarily about satisfaction, specified as both life satisfaction and domain satisfaction, but it contributed important insights into other areas of wellbeing as well, such as happiness, affects, and the development of competence. Andrews and Withey had a particular interest in the affective components of wellbeing, although they also included satisfaction in their framework. The main ideas in the two classic books from 1976 have been adopted in popular definitions of subjective wellbeing, as shown in Table 2.1.

---

[5] Others who operate with the concept of psychological wellbeing includes Su et al. (2014), Vallerand (2016), and Harms et al. (2018).

[6] This might be a version of *misonomy*, i. e., a tendency for misattributing effects in science to persons other than those who truly discovered them (see Salsburg, 2002, p. 16).

Table 2.1 Some definitions of subjective wellbeing

Definitions	Sources
1. SWB consists of three components: life satisfaction, the presence of positive mood, and the absence of negative mood, together often summarized as happiness	Ryan and Deci (2001, p. 144)
2. Subjective wellbeing—i.e., how people think about and experience their lives. (…) This definition of subjective wellbeing hence encompasses three elements: (1) life evaluation, (2) affect, and (3) eudaimonia	OECD (2013, p. 3 and 10)
3. Subjective wellbeing (SWB) represents individuals' evaluations of the quality of their lives and functioning in life. The nature of SWB has been divided into two streams of research. The first equates wellbeing with feeling good; the second equates wellbeing with functioning well in life	Keyes et al. (2015, p. 656)
4. We consider SWB as an aspect of an individual's overall utility function	Adler et al. (2017, p. 1)
5. Subjective wellbeing is conceptualized as the general feelings that people have about the quality and course of their lives	Oropesa (1995, p. 224)
6. Subjective wellbeing refers to all of the various types of evaluations, both positive and negative, that people make of their lives	Diener (2006, pp. 399–400)
7. Although pleasure is included as one aspect of subjective wellbeing, the concept is much broader in that it includes purpose, meaning, and feelings of fulfillment	Diener and Tov (2012, p. 139)
8. Subjective wellbeing is defined as people's evaluations of their lives—the degree to which their thoughtful appraisals and affective reactions indicate that their lives are desirable and proceeding well	Diener et al. (2015, p. 234)
9. SWB refers to the extent to which a person believes or feels that his or her life is going well	Diener et al. (2018, p. 1)
10. Subjective wellbeing (SWB) reflects an overall evaluation of the quality of a person's life from her or his own perspective	Diener et al. (2018, p. 1)

Until the early 1980s, the literature on wellbeing included fewer than 1000 references, yet, in his comprehensive and influential book *Conditions of Happiness,* Veenhoven reported more than 100 different meanings of the phrase wellbeing (Veenhoven, 1984, p. 33). At this stage in his career, Veenhoven preferred the term happiness rather than SWB, and he defined it as "the degree to which an individual judges the overall quality of his or her life-as-a-whole favorably. In other words, how much he likes the life he leads" (p. 22). In Veenhoven's work, happiness has two main components: hedonic level (defined as pleasant experiences) and contentment (defined as the degree to which an individual perceives that his aspirations are being met). To some degree, the dimensions of pleasant experiences and contentment in Veenhoven's theory correspond to the hedonic and desire-fulfillment theories in philosophy. Contrary to strict hedonism, however, there are no monist claims in Veenhoven's texts; other things than pleasure, or contentment, can be valuable (e.g., Vittersø, 2021).

"Dienerology"

It was Ed Diener more than anyone else who made SWB important. In his path-breaking 1984 article, Diener came to use subjective wellbeing, happiness, and wellbeing interchangeably. But the paper was entitled "Subjective Well-Being," and SWB, together with happiness, evolved to become the preferred term for scientific studies of wellbeing (cf. Fig. 1.1). Until he passed away in 2021, Diener spear-headed a movement of SWB research with astonishing scientific merits, and his footprints are visible in practically all the current wellbeing literature. He has published over 400 papers in his career and is currently cited approximately 300,000 times (see also Biswas-Diener & Oishi, 2021). Thus, Haybron has half-jokingly referred to SWB research as "Dienerology" (Haybron, 2008, p. xi).

Some of Diener's work is nicely summarized in Diener, 2009, Vol I–III and (Eid & Larsen, 2008), but his contributions continue to accumulate, and a full account is beyond the practical limits of any summary (see Biswas-Diener & Kashdan, 2021). In comparison, my review is rather brief and covers only a fraction of Diener's impressive empirical work. Given that the present chapter is a review of theories and conceptualizations of happiness and wellbeing, the following comments focus on Diener's conceptualizations of SWB.

In an important paper published in 2006, the following formulation of SWB was agreed upon by more than 50 signatories:

> Subjective well-being refers to all of the various types of evaluations, both positive and negative, that people make of their lives. It includes reflective cognitive evaluations, such as life satisfaction and work satisfaction, interest and engagement, and affective reactions to life events, such as joy and sadness. Thus, subjective well-being is an umbrella term for the different valuations people make regarding their lives, the events happening to them, their bodies and minds, and the circumstances in which they live. Although well-being and ill-being are "subjective" in the sense that they occur within a person's experience, manifestations of subjective well-being and ill-being can be observed objectively in verbal and nonverbal behavior, actions, biology, attention, and memory. The term well-being is often used instead of subjective well-being because it avoids any suggestion that there is something arbitrary or unknowable about the concepts involved. (Diener, 2006, pp. 399–400)

The first sentence declares that SWB refers to *all* the various types of evaluations people make of their lives. The "all-inclusiveness" nature of SWB is reiterated when SWB is described as an umbrella term for the different valuations people make regarding their lives. It also appears in many of Diener's texts, such as when SWB is assumed to "include a global assessment of all aspects of a person's life" (Diener, 1984, p. 544) or as a "general term referring to the various types of subjective evaluations of one's life, including both cognitive evaluations and affective feelings" (Diener, Lucas, & Oishi, 2018, p. 3). However, the common opinion among wellbeing researchers is that SWB is limited to three kinds of evaluations: life satisfaction (LS), positive affect (PA), and negative affect (NA). Describing SWB, Phillips et al. (2017) claim that "One key advantage within this field has been the convergence on a conception of happiness that involves three elements: *high positive affect, low negative affect, and high life satisfaction*" (p. 165).[7] In other words, only to the extent that LS, PA, and NA can capture *all various kinds of evaluations and valuation* a person can make about their life is what Phillips et al. refer to as the common view of SWB consistent with Diener's definition of the concept.

One element that is explicitly excluded from the popular tripartite operationalization of SWB is domain satisfaction (DS). This component was frequently included as a fourth dimension of SWB in the early days of Diener's writing (e.g., Diener et al., 1999). The unique role of DS as an explicit component of SWB, on equal footing with LS, PA, and NA, is, for instance, articulated in a paper entitled "The evolving concept of subjective well-being" (Diener et al., 2009). Central to that paper is a model introduced as "A model of happiness," which is depicted in Fig. 2.1.

The model has three levels, the first—or highest in the hierarchy—is named SWB. Below it, four second-level components are located: pleasant emotion, unpleasant emotions, global life judgments, and domain satisfaction. There are in other words clear differences between the model presented in Fig. 2.1 and the mainstream conceptualization of SWB as life satisfaction (LS), positive affect (PA), and negative affect (NA), which can be formulated as SWB = LS + PA – NA. Another irregularity is the inclusion of fulfillment and meaning as kinds of global life judgments on conceptual pairs with life satisfaction. This contrasts with other taxonomies, which suggest that meaning and fulfillment belong to a eudaimonic dimension of wellbeing and not to a global life judgment dimension that includes life satisfaction. For example, Diener, Oishi, and Tay (2018) write about eudaimonic wellbeing, which, in contrast to SWB, "refers to well-being defined as desirable psychological characteristics such as meaning and purpose, positive social relationships, mastery,

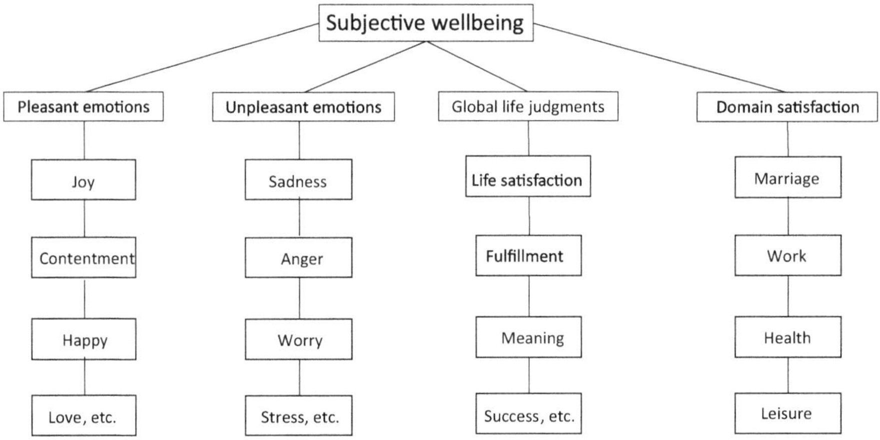

Fig. 2.1 A hierarchical model of subjective wellbeing presented in by Diener and colleagues in 2009. Reprinted with permission from Springer Nature

[7] Phillips and coworkers use the term happiness, but their reference for the definition is to papers by the "Diener camp," and in the original literature, the term SWB is used.

autonomy, virtues, and so forth" (p. 3). This issue will be discussed in more depth in Chaps. 4, 6, and 7.

A different taxonomy has also been suggested by Diener and his colleagues, first presented in Su et al. (2014). Here, the authors propose a model of what they call psychological wellbeing, comprising 18 components nested within 7 theoretical wellbeing dimensions: (1) relationship, (2) engagement, (3) mastery, (4) autonomy, (5) meaning, (6) optimism, and (7) subjective wellbeing. Again, meaning is not considered a part of SWB but rather constitutes an independent dimension of psychological wellbeing. SWB is further presented as a subcategory of psychological wellbeing. If this conceptualization is correct, SWB can no longer be defined as *all* the various types of evaluations and valuation people make of their lives, since all the remaining dimensions reflect something evaluable or valuable in people's lives. A competing taxonomy has been suggested in Bjørndal et al. (2023), which was introduced in Chap. 1. This paper identified six first-order wellbeing factors: (1) absence of negative affect, (2) social, (3) well-functioning, (4) positive activation, (5) autonomy, and (6) life satisfaction.

Another area of disagreement concerns the definitions of LS, PA, and NA. As will be detailed in Chaps. 3 and 4, the literature offers a variety of theoretical opinions and empirical practices regarding these core wellbeing concepts. One issue addresses how LS, PA, and NA are related to each other. Busseri (e.g., 2011, 2015) has noted that multiple conflicting conceptualizations about the structure of SWB exist, but few researchers have systematically debated this topic. For example, PA, NA, and LS can be treated as three separate components. Alternatively, they can be treated as hierarchical concepts, as in a reflective model in which a latent SWB variable causes variance in the observed manifest variables of PA, NA, and LS. They can also constitute a formative model, in which PA, NA, and LS are added to create an SWB composite variable. Finally, SWB can be treated as a causal system, in which PA and NA are the causes of LS. However, in a recent meta-analysis (Busseri, 2018), the hierarchical structure of SWB, in which PA, NA, and LS[8] load on a latent SWB factor, was reported to be very robust. But finding that PA, NA, and LS can be accounted for by a common factor does not prove anything other than such a structure is empirically possible. Busseri's results cannot be interpreted as conceptual evidence for a particular way of defining the causal relationships among the three major components of SWB.

These examples illustrate that we still have a way to go before a conceptual consensus about SWB has been reached. Until then and as plainly stated by Tiberius (2016), SWB researchers should stop pretending that such an agreement has been established.

---

[8] In these studies, PA and NA were measured with SPANE (Diener et al., 2010), a 12-item measure of the frequency of positive (six items, e.g., joyful, happy, contented) and negative (six items, e.g., sad, angry, afraid) affective experiences. LS was measured with the Satisfaction with Life Scale (SWLS; Diener et al., 1985). The average correlations across 40 samples ($N = 34{,}298$) were PA-NA, −0.49; PA-LS, 0.53; and NA-LS, −0.37.

Kahneman and Objective Happiness

Coming from studies of judgment and decision-making, Daniel Kahneman introduced a refreshing perspective on happiness in the 1990s (e.g., Kahneman, 1999; Kahneman & Snell, 1992; Kahneman & Verey, 1991; Kahneman et al., 1997). With Peter Wakker and Rakesh Sarin, he reinterpreted Benthamian hedonism and introduced the distinction between "experienced utility" and "decision utility" (Kahneman et al., 1997). Experienced utility means hedonic quality as in Bentham's usage, i.e., degrees of felt pleasure or displeasure. These pleasures can be either instant (the pleasure of the moment) or remembered (the retrospective evaluation of the total pleasure associated with past outcomes). Decision utility is the weight of an outcome in a decision and has to do with choices and preferences.

Total utility is suggested to be a third important concept. Briefly, it reflects an aggregate of instant pleasures as summarized according to a set of axiomatic proofs and normative rules of substantial symbolic complexity. For example, for the proposed logic to stick, the report of a person's momentary pleasures must contain all the information relevant for a person's wellbeing at that moment. It must further have a functional zero point that makes all experiences above the zero-point positive and all those below negative. This feature makes the experience interpersonally comparable. The intensity of the experiences must also satisfy the conditions of ordinal measurement. The logical and symbolic nomenclature used by Kahneman and colleagues to construct their normative theorems are amazingly complicated, and to be honest, I have trouble understanding what their six-page-long appendix of formal analysis and proofs means.

Fortunately, an extended and less formal version of Kahneman's notion of a good life is presented in a text entitled "Objective Happiness." It was published as the opening chapter of a volume with the ambitious aim of establishing a new scientific field: Hedonic psychology (Kahneman et al., 1999b). In the chapter, Kahneman (1999) follows up on the ideas from the 1997 paper and articulates a theory in which happiness is defined as an aggregate of instant experienced utility. Kahneman operates with two kinds of happiness. Subjective happiness refers to the overall happiness that is traditionally measured by self-reports. Objective happiness is the total utility as explained above. Despite its name, the core element in objective happiness is purely subjective since it is nothing more than an aggregation of experienced pleasures. It is labeled objective because the procedure that takes us from subjective pleasure to objective happiness is governed by a logical rule and could, in principle, be performed by an observer with access to a continuous score of an individual's online feelings of pleasure, or the temporal profile of instant utility, as Kahneman calls it (Kahneman, 1999, p. 5).

Memory and thinking are important elements in Kahneman's theory. Clearly, the affects we remember from a certain episode are no blueprints of the real-time feelings that occurred during the episode, and Kahneman has identified several mechanisms that explain how the memory of a feeling is altered with time. The peak-end rule is one such mechanism and duration neglect is another The peak-end rule suggests that maximum feeling intensity (peak) and the feeling at the end of the episode are key features in the process of remembering the experience of an episode. Duration neglect is a cognitive trap that contributes to downplaying the time dimension of an episode. The duration is basically ignored when an experience is transformed into a memory. A famous example that illustrates how the two effects work is a study that asked patients who underwent an unpleasant colonoscopy to report on the intensity of their pain every 60 seconds during the procedure (Redelmeier & Kahneman, 1996). After the procedure, the patients also indicated their "total amount of pain" for the whole episode. The peak-end average correlated with this total pain report at $r = 0.67$, whereas duration (which varied from 4 to 67 min) correlated with total pain at $r = 0.03$. In an experimental follow-up study (reported in Kahneman et al., 1997), a randomized group of patients had the procedure extended by leaving the colonoscope in place but at rest, for approximately 1 min after the clinical examination was completed. Despite the extra time spent in this slightly uncomfortable state, the experimental group reported less total pain than did the controls, who had a briefer pain episode.

According to Kahneman's theory, the subjective feeling of objective happiness is identified as an evaluation. It is sometimes referred to as a "hedonic commentary" and is conceived of as automatized and nonreflective. Kahneman also calls this evaluative process the good-bad dimension (GBD) and explains that the term GBD is preferred to avoid an "overly intellectual connotation" that comes with the word evaluation (Kahneman, 1999, p. 3). The GBD is a favorable state of being that includes experiences such as enjoyment and having fun but also broader concepts such as being satisfied and happy. The GBD rests on two assumptions: The first is that the hedonic commentary is continuously constructed by the brain. The second is that the commentary is adequately summarizing the goodness and badness as one experiential dimension and that such a summation can be captured by a single value. This value reflects what Kahneman refers to as instant utility. If it is continuously measured according to the procedures laid out in Kahneman et al. (1997), the resulting temporal integral[9] is the objective happiness for the reference period.

The quantifiable and unidimensional nature of the GBD is the centerpiece of objective happiness and signifies the strengths and weaknesses of Kahneman's theory. By defining happiness as the sum of momentary pleasures accumulated over a lifetime, Kahneman accommodates to Occam's ideal of simplicity. "All of us prefer unitary definitions to definitions that are all over the place," Kahneman argues (cited in Winerman, 2012).

Kahneman's simplicity ambition fails, however, and for the same reasons that Bentham's reductionism failed (see Chap. 5). In contrast to Bentham, however, Kahneman realizes the perils of crafting theories that are too simple and came to change his mind about one-dimensional wellbeing models: "the quality of life cannot be reduced to the balance of pleasure and pain" (Kahneman et al., 1999a, p. x).

---

[9] Kahneman's temporal integral is a two-dimensional space, with the intensity of pleasant feelings plotted vertically and time plotted horizontally. The area under the plotted line can be calculated as the integral.

In an interview with the APA Monitor, he explains that for wellbeing "a unitary definition doesn't work because you cannot ignore life satisfaction as a measure of well-being" (Winerman, 2012).

Kahneman has therefore abandoned his one-dimensional thinking about the good life (Kahneman, 2009). One adjustment came with the concepts of an experiencing self and a remembering self (Kahneman & Riis, 2005). Briefly, the experiencing self is about being happy IN your life, whereas the remembering self is about being happy WITH your life. With this move, Kahneman came closer to mainstream SWB, and the experiencing self was no longer constrained to reflect a single pleasure component. By including a remembering self in his theory, the concept of life satisfaction also became important to Kahneman. Somewhat later, he even showed signs of approving a third, independent dimension of wellbeing. In a foreword to Paul Dolan's *Happiness by Design* (Dolan, 2015), Kahneman praised the inclusion of the experience of meaning as an important component of happiness (Kahneman, 2015). Studies of meaning in life, and the notion of personal growth and self-fulfillment more generally, have gradually become a popular extension or alternative to mainstream happiness and subjective wellbeing approaches, often referred to as eudaimonic wellbeing (Vittersø, 2016a). The eudaimonic turn in wellbeing research will be discussed in Chap. 6.

Subjective Versus Objective Wellbeing

Subjectivity is roughly speaking something that "relates to or characterizes a subject" (Merriam-Webster Dictionary), whereas objectivity is something that "is not influenced by personal feelings or opinions" (Oxford Dictionary of English). Clarifying the distinction between subjectivity and objectivity is arguably the most critical issue in the study of wellbeing (e.g., Sumner, 1996), because it addresses definitional ownership. Who can decide if a person's life goes well or badly? Is it the person who lives it, is it a cultural group such as a scientific community, or is it a combination of subjective and objective perspectives? Sumner argues in favor of the person and claims that "The great advantage of a subjective theory is that it makes well-being responsive to an individual's own schedule of concerns" (Sumner, 1996, p. 93).

Sumner spends much of his book explaining why wellbeing must be a subjective, or subjective-relative, rather than an objective concept. Wellbeing is *subject-relative*, Sumner argues, because it has a subjective-perspective character. Recall that for most modern philosophers, wellbeing is not a relational but a rational concept. It is supposed to apply to informed, independent, and rational actors. Wellbeing is also prudential, having "to do with how people's lives are going for them, rather than with how their lives are going from the moral point of view" (Hall & Tiberius, 2015, p. 174). Sumner therefore stipulates that wellbeing "stands out by virtue of incorporating an internal reference to its bearer" (Sumner, 1996, p. 42). He further explains that "the defining feature of all subjective theories is that they make your well-being depend on your own concerns: the things you care about, attach importance to, regard as mattering, and so on" (p. 42). This reasoning leads Sumner to conclude that something counts as good for a person only if that person has the right attitude toward it, i.e., is in favor of it. Sumner drives home the point that wellbeing depends logically on such a subjective attitude and believes that objective theories "denies this dependency." Objective theories hold that something can be good for a person even if that person does not favor it. Objectively speaking, therefore, "my life can be going well despite my failing to have any positive attitude toward it" (Sumner, 1996, p. 38). According to objective theory, attitudes are therefore not a *sufficient* constituent of wellbeing. As mentioned in Chap. 1, however, it is difficult to see how Sumner's distrust in the happiness of uninformed and dependent individuals conforms to his own ideal of subjectivity.

But is a favorable attitude *necessary* for objective wellbeing? Not at all, Sumner tells us, because subjective and objective approaches to wellbeing are "both mutually exclusive and jointly exhaustive" (p. 39). Sumner therefore concludes that none of the objective theories can respond to his challenge, not even Aristotelian eudaimonism (see Chap. 6).[10] With the demise of eudaimonism, he argues, objectivists must realize that they are unable to construct "a descriptively adequate objective theory of welfare"[11] (Sumner, 1996, p. 80).

Another philosophical approach to the issue of subjectivity and objectivity is provided by Hall and Tiberius (2015). These authors mention that Haybron defends a subjective theory that "defines well-being in terms of a feature of the individual, namely, the person's emotional state. This theory allows that different people, due to differing emotional and physical makeups, will be happy in different circumstances, but it does not make well-being dependent on our attitudes" (Hall & Tiberius, 2015, p. 182). Another subjective approach can be found in Tiberius's value fulfillment theory (e.g., DeYoung & Tiberius, 2022; Tiberius, 2018). Here, wellbeing is defined in terms of individuals' values rather than their desires. According to the value fulfillment theory, "a person's life goes well to the extent that she pursues and fulfills or realizes a subjectively appropriate system of values together over time" (Hall & Tiberius, 2015, p. 180).

Hall and Tiberius also operate with a category of subjectivity theories referred to as subject-transcending. These theories "ground well-being in factors that transcend the particular individual, such as species-level traits or objectively valuable goods" (p. 176). One example is the rational care theory developed by Stephen Darwall (2002). His writing is tough going for nonphilosophers, but a book review described the idea of rational care as follows: "What is best for you is not simply what you happen to want for yourself, or what I, who care for you, want for you. It is what I and others should rationally want for you" (Campbell, 2015, p. 44). Darwall's

[10]An important element in Sumner's argument is that Aristotelian eudaimonism (or teleological theory as he calls it) depends critically on the functioning argument, which Sumner takes to be is a subjectivist concept. Sumner also criticizes Aristotelian eudaimonism for being perfectionist and not prudential. Hence, with regard to wellbeing, the theory "answers the wrong question."

[11]Recall that welfare is Sumner's word for wellbeing.

reasoning is hard to follow, and even an ethics authority such as Joseph Raz (2006, p. 401) admits that he finds it difficult to make out what Darwall is up to.[12]

Another objection against Sumner's strict subjectivism comes from MacLeod (2015). MacLeod considers all wellbeing theories to be *sobjective*, by which term he means a mixture of subjectivity and objectivity. Thus, wellbeing theories can be located along a continuum that runs from extremely subjective to extremely objective. MacLeod calls this continuum "a dimension of wellbeing constraints." A low constraint reads subjective since a lack of constraints means that people are allowed to define wellbeing themselves. The more objective factors a model includes, the more constrained it is. MacLeod considers life satisfaction to be the least constrained theory of wellbeing, since it only requires that to be well all a person needs to do is to say so. Broad hedonism is more constrained, since it specifies that a person must feel good to be well. Strict hedonism is even more constrained because the only feeling it considers relevant for wellbeing is pleasure. The most constrained theory in MacLeod's continuum is Aristotelian eudaimonism, which claims that to be well we have no choice but to act rationally and virtuously.

John Searle

Reflections on subjectivity and objectivity about wellbeing can be inspired by the writings of John Searle, who over the last 20 years have been concerned with ontological and epistemological dimensions of subjectivity and objectivity (e.g., Searle, 1992, 1995, 1998, 2011). Searle's reasoning starts with two distinctions, one regarding ontology and epistemology (existence versus statements) and the other regarding objectivity and subjectivity. This taxonomy makes for a two-by-two table, in which the two columns represent ontological existence (objective or subjective) and the two rows represent epistemological statements (objective or subjective). For example, a mountain such as Mt. Everest is *ontologically objective* because it exists independently of a perceiving subject. In contrast, a conscious state such as pain is *ontologically subjective* because its existence depends on a perceiving subject.

However, the sentence "I have pain in my toe" is *epistemically objective* because it is stating a matter of fact. The statement "is made true by the existence of an actual fact that is not dependent on any stance, attitude, or opinions of observers. However, the phenomenon itself, the actual pain, has a subjective mode of existence" (Searle, 1995, p. 9).

[12] Here are some of Darwall's theses that Raz finds particularly difficult: (1) *the necessary equivalence thesis,* "What is for someone's good or welfare is what one ought to desire and promote in so far as one cares for him"; (2) *the rational care thesis*, "a person's good is constituted… by what one (perhaps she) should want in so far as one cares about her"; and (3) *the identity version*, "What it is for something to be good for someone just is for it to be something one should desire for him for his sake" (Raz, 2006, pp. 401–402).

A valuation of the pain, however, such as saying that "the pain in the toe is bad for me" is an *epistemically subjective* statement, an opinion that cannot be verified as a matter of fact. Similarly, the statement "Bill Clinton was President in the USA" is *epistemically objective* because it expresses a matter of fact. But to say that "Bill Clinton was a good President for the USA" is *epistemically subjective* because it depends on a subjective opinion. A visualization of this idea is shown in Table 2.2.

The statements in Table 2.2 are relevant for the study of wellbeing. For example, in most studies of subjective wellbeing, statement 3 ("I feel pleasure") is taken to indicate a person's wellbeing because statement 4a ("My pleasure is good for me") is presupposed. An alternative position would be to say that statement 3 is a mere description of a psychological state; thus, none of the statements in cell 4 are relevant for the scientific study of wellbeing. As discussed in Chap. 1, however, such a value-free approach is problematic. For example, both the statement "I feel pleasure" and the statement "I see a red square" are epistemically objective, but only the former is considered an indicator of wellbeing. To suggest that a psychological state is a kind of wellbeing therefore requires a normative claim, for instance, one of the statements in cell 4. In other words, it takes a value statement to claim that pleasure is a component of wellbeing, and it makes little sense to say that pleasure is indicative of wellbeing unless one also assumes that pleasure is good for the person experiencing it. But is this value claim by necessity epistemically subjective? No, the humanistic theory of wellbeing argues, some value statements are epistemologically objective. This idea will be more fully developed in Chap. 7, but with regard to Table 2.2, the following reasoning will hopefully suffice.

Searle's scheme implies that statements 4a to 4d in Table 2.2 are epistemologically subjective. Yet, there is a significant difference between statements 4a and 4b, which are subjective, and statements 4c and 4d, which are objective. Furthermore, statements 4b and 4d are arguments against hedonism because they do not take pleasure to be an unconditional and ultimate good. The goodness of pleasure must be evaluated against the context in which it is felt. An eccentric example in case comes from the clinical neurologist Harold Klawans, who diagnosed one of his patients as suffering from "complex partial epilepsy." This woman tended to be overwhelmed by orgasms, but they occurred in awkward situations such as when

Table 2.2 Searle's taxonomy of ontologies and epistemologies presented as a two-by-two table

	Ontologically objective	Ontologically subjective
Epistemically objective	1. Bill Clinton was President in the USA	3. I feel pleasure
Epistemically subjective	2. Bill Clinton was a good president for the USA	4. (a) My pleasure is good for me (b) My pleasure is not necessarily good for me (c) Your pleasure is good for you (d) Your pleasure is not necessarily good for you

she took her child to the dentist or paid for her groceries. Isolated speaking, she experienced the orgasms as warm, pleasant, and intense. It was not that these moments were unpleasant, but rather that they were inconvenient. Thus, regardless of how pleasurable the incidents were, the woman did not want them (cited in Bergsma, 2000). It seems fair to say that an unwanted orgasm is an example of a pleasure that is "not necessarily good for me."

The concept of eudaimonism brings this principle into the moral domain by claiming that pleasure experienced during acts of immoral behavior is not good for you (statement 4d). Relatedly, statement 4b includes a subjective uptake of the eudaimonic idea, coming from a person who has realized that the prudential value of their pleasures cannot be completely detached from its sources. Statement 4d also counterargues Sumner's insistence about subjective and objective approaches to wellbeing being "mutually exclusive and jointly exhaustive" (Sumner, 1996, p. 39). Adopting the objective of statement 4d, the humanistic theory of wellbeing argues against Sumner's subjectivism by claiming that only if a life is liked for the right reasons will the liking indicates a good life. However, the "right reason" argument is not subjective in the sense that it belongs to a particular perceiving subject. It is a third-person perspective and must be agreed upon by a moral community (see Chap. 7).

Somewhat analogically, the statement that Bill Clinton was a good president is not entirely subjective in the sense that it merely reflects a first-person opinion. Some evaluative criteria about a presidency can be established by means of social perspective taking, i.e., the give-and take process elaborated in feminist epistemology and discussed in Chap. 1. Searle is open to categorizing some value statements as epistemological objective, given that they are grounded in common cultural ground. For example, the statement that "earthquakes are bad for real estate values" is epistemologically objective (Searle, 1995, p. 12). However, I am not sure that Searle would allow for the values expressed in statements 2 and 4c and 4d to be epistemically objective. Lin (2016) maintains, for instance, that Searle would not. Lin therefore criticizes Searle for excluding statements about relational goodness or axiological subjectivity from the taxonomy (p. 919). In the example of Bill Clinton, Lin argues that it is possible to set up criteria or standards for good and bad presidency and then judge Clinton according to these standards. The criteria are not subjective in the sense Searle defines it, i.e., "as grounded in attitudes, feelings, and points of views of the maker" (Searle, 1995, p. 8). The critique against Searle's subjectivity arguments does not imply, however, that established criteria for good presidency will cover every thinkable judgment about a president's conduct. Some parts of the evaluation expressed in statement 2 may remain subjective in the sense that they are not commonly agreed upon.

Certain weaknesses in Sumner's theory are revealed when confronted with Searle's system of subjectivity-objectivity classifications. Sumner's position, as laid out in Chap. 6 of his *Welfare, Happiness, and Ethics*, holds that feelings are causes of wellbeing, not their ingredients (Sumner, 1996, pp. 108–109). Feelings such as the one in statement 3 are in themselves not good for you; they only become so if you are (1) fully informed about their circumstances, (2) your feelings are not manipulated, and (3) you have a positive attitude toward them. Sumner seems here to disregard his own definition of subjectivity, which requires that individuals should themselves decide what their own wellbeing consists of. By introducing the theory of authentic happiness, Sumner has imposed some rather strict constraints on a person's freedom to decide what their wellbeing is about (Chap. 1).

References

Adler, M. D., Dolan, P., & Kavetsos, G. (2017). Would you choose to be happy? Tradeoffs between happiness and the other dimensions of life in a large population survey. *Journal of Economic Behavior & Organization, 139*, 60–73. https://doi.org/10.1016/j.jebo.2017.05.006

Alexandrova, A. (2016). Is well-being measurable after all? *Public Health Ethics*. https://doi.org/10.1093/phe/phw015

Alexandrova, A. (2017). *A philosophy for the science of well-being*. Oxford University Press.

Algoe, S. B., Fredrickson, B. L., & Chow, S.-M. (2011). The future of emotions research within positive psychology. In K. M. Sheldon, T. B. Kashdan, & M. F. Steger (Eds.), *Designing positive psychology: Taking stock and moving forward* (pp. 115–132). Oxford University Press. https://doi.org/10.1093/acprof:oso/9780195373585.003.0008

Allard, E. (1973). *About dimensions of welfare, and exploratory analysis of a comparative Scandinavian survey* [Research Report](No 1).

Andrews, F. M., & Withey, S. B. (1976). *Social indicators of well-being*. Plenum Press.

Angner, E. (2010). Subjective well-being. *The Journal of Socio-Economics, 39*(3), 361–368. https://doi.org/10.1016/j.socec.2009.12.001

Angner, E. (2013). Is it possible to measure happiness? *European Journal for Philosophy of Science, 3*(2), 221–240.

Annett, A. M. (2022). *Cathonomics: How catholic tradition can create a more just economy [Kindle]*. Georgetown University Press.

Argyle, M. (2001). *The psychology of happiness* (2nd ed.). Routledge.

Augustine, S. (2009/426). *The city of God*. Hendrickson Publishers. (Original work published 426).

Bauer, R. A. (Ed.). (1966). *Social indicators*. MIT Press.

Beckham, A. S. (1929). Is the negro happy? *Journal of Abnormal and Social Psychology, 24*, 186–190.

Bennett, W. J. (1993). *Book of virtues: A treasury of great moral stories*. Simon and Schuster.

Bentham, J. (1789/1948). *An introduction to the principles of moral and legislation [Kindle]*. Hafner (Available from http://www.econlib.org/library/Bentham/bnthPML1.html).

Bergsma, A. (2000). Transhumanism and the wisdom of old genes: Is neurotechnology a source of future happiness. *Journal of Happiness Studies, 1*(3), 401–417.

Biswas-Diener, R., & Kashdan, T. B. (2021). Three lessons from Ed Diener. *International Journal of Wellbeing, 11*(2), 73–76. https://doi.org/10.5502/ijw.v11i2.1705

Biswas-Diener, R., & Oishi, S. (2021). Ed Diener (1946–2021). *American Psychologist*. https://doi.org/10.1037/amp0000900

Bjørndal, L. D., Nes, R. B., Czajkowski, N., & Røysamb, E. (2023). The structure of well-being: A single underlying factor with genetic and environmental influences. *Quality of Life Research*. https://doi.org/10.1007/s11136-023-03437-7.

Borges, J. L. (1964). The analytical language of John Wilkins. In J. L. Borges (Ed.), *Other inquisitions, 1937–1952*. University of Texas Press. https://en.wikipedia.org/wiki/The_Analytical_Language_of_John_Wilkins

Borsboom, D., Mellenbergh, G. J., & van Heerden, J. (2004). The concept of validity. *Psychological Review, 111*(4), 1061–1071. https://doi.org/10.1037/0033-295X.111.4.1061

Bourget, D., & Chalmers, D. J. (2014). What do philosophers believe? [journal article]. *Philosophical Studies, 170*(3), 465–500. https://doi.org/10.1007/s11098-013-0259-7
Bradburn, N. M. (1969). *The structure of psychological well-being*. Aldine.
Brickman, P., & Campbell, D. T. (1971). Hedonic relativism and planning the good society. In I. H. Appley (Ed.), *Adaption level theory*. Academic Press.
Bringmann, L. F., & Eronen, M. I. (2016). Heating up the measurement debate: What psychologists can learn from the history of physics. *Theory & Psychology, 26*(1), 27–43. https://doi.org/10.1177/0959354315617253
Burger, G. C. E. (1964). Permissible load and optimal adaptation. *Ergonomics, 7*(4), 397–417.
Busseri, M. A. (2015). Toward a resolution of the tripartite structure of subjective well-being. *Journal of Personality, 83*(4), 413–428. https://doi.org/10.1111/jopy.12116
Busseri, M. A. (2018). Examining the structure of subjective well-being through meta-analysis of the associations among positive affect, negative affect, and life satisfaction. *Personality and Individual Differences, 122*, 68–71. https://doi.org/10.1016/j.paid.2017.10.003
Busseri, M. A., & Sadava, S. W. (2011). A review of the tripartite structure of subjective well-being: Implications for conceptualization, operationalization, analysis, and synthesis. *Personality and Social Psychology Review, 15*(3), 290–314.
Campbell, S. M. (2015). The concept of well-being. In G. Fletcher (Ed.), *The Routledge handbook of philosophy of well-being* (pp. 402–414). Routledge.
Campbell, A., Converse, P. E., & Rodgers, W. L. (1976). *The quality of American life*. Sage.
Carlquist, E., Ulleberg, P., Delle Fave, A., Nafstad, H. E., & Blakar, R. M. (2016). Everyday understandings of happiness, good life, and satisfaction: three different facets of well-being [journal article]. *Applied Research in Quality of Life*, 1–25. https://doi.org/10.1007/s11482-016-9472-9
Chalmers, D. J. (2015). Why isn't there more progress in philosophy? *Philosophy, 90*(1), 3–31. https://doi.org/10.1017/S0031819114000436
Churchland, P. S. (2018). *Braintrust: What neuroscience tells us about morality [Kindle]*. Princeton Science Library.
Clark, A. E., Flèche, S., Layard, R., Powdthavee, N., & Ward, G. (2018). *The origins of happiness: The science of well-being over the life course [Kindle]*. Princeton University Press.
Crisp, R. (2006). Hedonism reconsidered. *Philosophy and Phenomenological Research, 73*(3), 619–645. https://doi.org/10.1111/j.1933-1592.2006.tb00551.x
Crisp, R. (2017). Well-being. In E. N. Zalta (Ed.), *The Stanford encyclopedia of philosophy*. Available from http://plato.stanford.edu/archives/fall2011/entries/well-being/
Cronbach, L. J., & Meehl, P. E. (1955). Construct validity in psychological tests. *Psychological Bulletin, 52*(4), 281–302.
Curzer, H. (2018). Aristotle and moral virtue. In N. E. Snow (Ed.), *The Oxford handbook of virtue* (p. 0). Oxford University Press. https://doi.org/10.1093/oxfordhb/9780199385195.013.14
Darwall, S. (2002). *Welfare and rational care*. Princeton University Press.
Davies, J. C. (1962). Toward a theory of revolution. *American Sociological Review, 27*(1), 5–19.
Deaton, A., & Stone, A. A. (2016). Understanding context effects for a measure of life evaluation: How responses matter. *Oxford Economic Papers, 68*(4), 861–870. https://doi.org/10.1093/oep/gpw022
DeYoung, C. G., & Tiberius, V. (2022). Value fulfillment from a cybernetic perspective: A new psychological theory of well-being. *Personality and Social Psychology Review, 27*(1), 3–27. https://doi.org/10.1177/10888683221083777
Diener, E. (1984). Subjective well-being. *Psychological Bulletin, 95*(3), 542–575. https://doi.org/10.1037/0033-2909.95.3.542
Diener, E. (2006). Guidelines for national indicators of subjective well-being and ill-being. *Journal of Happiness Studies, 7*(4), 397–404. https://doi.org/10.1007/s10902-006-9000-y
Diener, E. (Ed.). (2009a). *Assessing well-being. The collected works of Ed Diener* (Vol. III). Springer. https://doi.org/10.1007/978-90-481-2350-6_2

Diener, E. (2009b). Introduction—The science of well-being: Reviews and theoretical articles by Ed Diener. In E. Diener (Ed.), *The science of well-being: The collected works of Ed Diener* (Vol. I, pp. 1–10). Springer. https://doi.org/10.1007/978-90-481-2350-6_1

Diener, E., Emmons, R. A., Larsen, R. J., & Griffin, S. (1985). The satisfaction with life scale. *Journal of Personality Assessment, 49*, 71–75. https://doi.org/10.1207/s15327752jpa4901_13

Diener, E., Inglehart, R., & Tay, L. (2013). Theory and validity of life satisfaction scales. *Social Indicators Research, 112*(3), 497–527. https://doi.org/10.1007/s11205-012-0076-y

Diener, E., Lucas, R. E., & Oishi, S. (2018). Advances and open questions in the science of subjective well-being. *Collabra: Psychology, 4*(1).

Diener, E., Oishi, S., & Lucas, R. E. (2015). National accounts of subjective well-being. *American Psychologist, 70*(3), 234–242. https://doi.org/10.1037/a0038899

Diener, E., Oishi, S., & Tay, L. (2018). Advances in subjective well-being research. *Nature Human Behaviour, 2*(4), 253–260. https://doi.org/10.1038/s41562-018-0307-6

Diener, E., Scollon, C. N., & Lucas, R. E. (2009). The evolving concept of subjective well-being. The multifaceted nature of happiness. In E. Diener (Ed.), *Assessing well-being. The collected works of Ed Diener* (pp. 67–100). Springer.

Diener, E., Suh, E. M., Lucas, R. E., & Smith, H. L. (1999). Subjective well-being: Three decades of progress. *Psychological Bulletin, 125*(2), 276–302. https://doi.org/10.1037/0033-2909.125.2.276

Diener, E., & Tov, W. (2012). National accounts of well-being. In K. C. Land, A. C. Michalos, & M. J. Sirgy (Eds.), *Handbook of social indicators and quality of life research* (pp. 137–157). Springer Netherlands. https://doi.org/10.1007/978-94-007-2421-1_7

Diener, E., Wirtz, D., Tov, W., Kim-Prieto, C., Coi, D.-W., Oishi, S., & Biswas-Diener, R. (2010). New well-being measures: Short scales to assess flourishing and positive and negative feelings. *Social Indicators Research, 97*, 143–156.

Dolan, P. (2015). *Happiness by design: Finding pleasure and purpose in everyday life [Kindle]*. Penguin.

Easterlin, R. A. (1974). Does economic growth improve the human lot? In P. A. David & M. W. Reder (Eds.), *Nations and households in economic growth* (pp. 89–125). Academic Press. http://graphics8.nytimes.com/images/2008/04/16/business/Easterlin1974.pdf

Easterlin, R. A. (2001). Income and happiness: Towards a unified theory. *The Economic Journal, 111*, 465–484.

Eid, M., & Larsen, R. J. (Eds.). (2008). *The science of subjective well-being*. Guilford Press.

Ekman, P. (2003). *Emotions revealed: Recognizing faces and feelings to improve communication and emotional life*. Henry Holt.

Eronen, M. I., & Bringmann, L. F. (2021). The theory crisis in psychology: How to move forward. *Perspectives on Psychological Science, 16*(4), 779–788.

Fabian, M., & Pykett, J. (2021). Be happy: Navigating normative issues in behavioral and well-being public policy. *Perspectives on Psychological Science, 0*(0), 1745691620984395. https://doi.org/10.1177/1745691620984395

Flanagan, O. (2007). *The really hard problem. Meaning in a material world*. The MIT Press.

Fletcher, G. (Ed.). (2015). *The Routledge handbook of philosophy of well-being [Kindle]*. Routledge.

Fletcher, G. (2016). *The philosophy of well-being: An introduction*. Routledge.

Flügel, J. C. (1925). A quantitative study of feeling and emotion in everyday life. *British Journal of Psychology, 15*, 318–355.

Franklin, B. (2005). *The autobiography of Benjamin Franklin*. Digireads.com Publishing.

Goldings, H. J. (1954). On the avowal and projection of happiness. *Journal of Personality, 23*, 30–47.

Graham, C., Laffan, K., & Pinto, S. (2018). Well-being in metrics and policy. *Science, 362*(6412), 287–288. https://doi.org/10.1126/science.aau5234

Gregory, A. (2015). Hedonism. In G. Fletcher (Ed.), *The Routledge handbook of philosophy of well-being* (pp. 113–123). Routledge.

Gurin, G., Veroff, J., & Feld, S. (1960). *Americans view their mental health*. Basic Books.
Hall, A., & Tiberius, V. (2015). Well-being and subjective dependence. In G. Fletcher (Ed.), *The Routledge handbook of philosophy of well-being* (pp. 175–186). Routledge.
Harms, P. D., Brady, L., Wood, D., & Silard, A. (2018). Resilience and well-being. In E. Diener, S. Oishi, & L. Tay (Eds.), *Handbook of subjective well-being*. DEF Publishers. https://doi.org/nobascholar.com
Hartmann, G. W. (1934). Personality traits associated with variations in happiness. *Journal of Abnormal and Social Psychology, 29*, 202–212.
Haybron, D. M. (2008). *The pursuit of unhappiness. The elusive psychology of well-being*. Oxford University Press.
Heathwood, C. (2015). Desire-fulfilment theory. In G. Fletcher (Ed.), *The Routledge handbook of philosophy of well-being* (pp. 161–174). Routledge.
Held, V. (2006). *The ethics of care: Personal, political, and global*. Oxford University Press.
Helliwell, J. F., Layard, R., Sachs, J. D., De Neve, J.-E., Aknin, L. B., & Wang, S. (Eds.). (2022). *World happiness report 2022*. https://worldhappiness.report/.
Hudson, D. W. (1996). *Happiness and the limits of satisfaction*. Rowman & Littlefield Publishers.
van Inwagen, P., & Sullivan, M. (2020). Metaphysics. In E. N. Zalta (Ed.), *The Stanford encyclopedia of philosophy*. Available from https://plato.stanford.edu/archives/spr2020/entries/metaphysics/.
Jones, H. M. (1953). *The pursuit of happiness*. Harvard University Press.
Kahneman, D. (1999). Objective happiness. In D. Kahneman, E. Diener, & N. Schwarz (Eds.), *Well-being: The foundations of hedonic psychology* (pp. 3–25). Russell Sage Foundation.
Kahneman, D. (2009). What constitutes life satisfaction? In J. E. Brockman (Ed.), *What have you changed your mind about?: Today's leading minds rethink everything*. HarperPerennial.
Kahneman, D. (2015). Foreword. In P. Dolan (Ed.), *Happiness by design: Finding pleasure and purpose in everyday life* (pp. 1–2). Penguin.
Kahneman, D., Diener, E., & Schwarz, N. (1999a). Preface. In D. Kahneman, E. Diener, & N. Schwarz (Eds.), *Well-being: The foundations of hedonic psychology*. Russel-Sage.
Kahneman, D., Diener, E., & Schwarz, N. (Eds.). (1999b). *Well-being: The foundations of hedonic psychology*. Russel-Sage.
Kahneman, D., Krueger, A. B., Schkade, D., Schwarz, N., & Stone, A. (2004). A survey method for characterizing daily life experience: The Day Reconstruction Method. *Science, 305*(5702), 1776–1780. https://doi.org/10.1126/science.1103572
Kahneman, D., & Riis, J. (2005). Living, and thinking about it: Two perspectives on life. In F. Huppert, N. Baylis, & B. Keverne (Eds.), *The science of well-being* (pp. 285–304). Oxford University Press.
Kahneman, D., & Snell, J. (1992). Predicting a changing taste: Do people know what they will like? *Journal of Behavioral Decision Making, 5*(3), 187–200. https://doi.org/10.1002/bdm.3960050304
Kahneman, D., & Verey, C. (1991). Notes on the psychology of utility. In J. Elster & J. E. Roemer (Eds.), *Interpersonal comparison of well-being* (pp. 127–159). Cambridge University Press.
Kahneman, D., Wakker, P. P., & Sarin, R. (1997). Back to Bentham? Explorations of experienced utility. *Quarterly Journal of Economics, 112*(2), 375–405.
Kaiser, C., & Oswald, A. J. (2022). The scientific value of numerical measures of human feelings. *Proceedings of the National Academy of Sciences, 119*(42), e2210412119. https://www.pnas.org/doi/abs/10.1073/pnas.2210412119
Kelley, T. L. (1927). *Interpretation of educational measurements*. World Book.
Keyes, C. M., Kendler, K. S., Myers, J. M., & Martin, C. C. (2015). The genetic overlap and distinctiveness of flourishing and the big five personality traits. *Journal of Happiness Studies, 16*(3), 655–668. https://doi.org/10.1007/s10902-014-9527-2
Killingsworth, M. A., Kahneman, D., & Mellers, B. (2023). Income and emotional well-being: A conflict resolved. *Proceedings of the National Academy of Sciences, 120*(10), e2208661120. https://doi.org/10.1073/pnas.2208661120

Kirwan, R. (1810). Of happiness. *The Transactions of the Royal Irish Academy, 11*, 1–190.

Layard, R. (2010). Measuring subjective well-being. *Science, 327*(29 January), 534–535. https://doi.org/10.1126/science.1186315

Lieberman, M. D. (2013). *Social: Why our brains are wired to connect [Kindle]*. Oxford University Press.

Lin, C.-T. (2016). A critique of epistemic subjectivity. *Philosophia, 44*(3), 915–920. https://doi.org/10.1007/s11406-016-9724-9

Locke, E. A. (1969). What is job satisfaction? *Organizational Behavior and Human Performance, 4*(4), 309–336. https://doi.org/10.1016/0030-5073(69)90013-0

Lomas, T. (2018). *Translating happiness: A cross-cultural lexicon of well-being [Kindle]*. MIT Press.

Lucas, R. E. (2018). Reevaluating the strengths and weaknesses of self-report measures of subjective well-being. In E. Diener, S. Oishi, & L. Tay (Eds.), *Handbook of subjective well-being. Noba Scholar Handbook series: Subjective well-being*. DEF Publishers. https://doi.org/nobascholar.com

Lyubomirsky, S., King, L., & Diener, E. (2005). The benefits of frequent positive affect: Does happiness lead to success? *Psychological Bulletin, 131*(6), 803–855.

MacIntyre, A. (2007). *After virtue [Kindle]* (3rd ed.). University of Notre Dame Press.

MacLeod, A. (2015). Well-being: Objectivism, subjectivism or sobjectivism? *Journal of Happiness Studies, 16*(4), 1073–1089. https://doi.org/10.1007/s10902-014-9561-0

Martin, M. W. (2008). Paradoxes of happiness. *Journal of Happiness Studies, 9*(2), 171–184.

McMahan, E. A., & Estes, D. (2011). Measuring lay conceptions of well-being: The beliefs about well-being scale [journal article]. *Journal of Happiness Studies, 12*(2), 267–287. https://doi.org/10.1007/s10902-010-9194-x

McMahon, D. (2006). *The pursuit of happiness. A history from the Greeks to the present*. Allen Lane.

Mercier, H., & Sperber, D. (2017). *The enigma of reason. A new theory of understanding [Kindle]*. Pinguin.

Michalos, A. C. (Ed.). (2021). *The pope of happiness. A Festschrift for Ruut Veenhoven*. Springer Nature. https://doi.org/10.1007/978-3-030-53779-1_27

Moore, A., & Crisp, R. (1996). Welfarism in moral theory. *Australasian Journal of Philosophy, 74*(4), 598–613. https://doi.org/10.1080/00048409612347551

Neugarten, B. L., Havighurst, R. J., & Tobin, S. S. (1961). The measurement of life satisfaction. *Journal of Gerontology, 16*, 134–143.

OECD. (2013). *OECD Guidelines on measuring subjective well-being*. https://doi.org/10.1787/9789264191655-en

Oropesa, R. S. (1995). Consumer possessions, consumer passions, and subjective well-being. *Sociological Forum, 10*(2), 215–244.

Oswald, A. J., & Wu, S. (2010). Objective confirmation of subjective measures of human well-being: Evidence from the U.S.A. *Science, 327*, 576–579. https://doi.org/10.1126/science.1180606

Parducci, A. (1968). The relativism of absolute judgments. *Scientific American, 219*, 84–90.

Parfit, D. (1984). *Reasons and persons*. Oxford University Press.

Phillips, J., De Freitas, J., Mott, C., Gruber, J., & Knobe, J. (2017). True happiness: The role of morality in the folk concept of happiness. *Journal of Experimental Psychology: General, 146*(2), 165–181. https://doi.org/10.1037/xge0000252

Pincoffs, E. L. (1986). *Quandaries and virtues: Against reductivism in ethics*. University Press of Kansas.

Pressman, S. D., & Cohen, S. (2005). Does positive affect influence health? *Psychological Bulletin, 131*(6), 925–971.

Raz, J. (2006). Darwall on rational care. *Utilitas, 18*(4), 400–414. https://doi.org/10.1017/S0953820806002184

Redelmeier, D. A., & Kahneman, D. (1996). Patients' memories of painful medical treatments: Real-time and retrospective evaluations of two minimally invasive procedures. *Pain, 66*(1), 3–8. https://doi.org/10.1016/0304-3959(96)02994-6
Ruckmick, C. A. (1925). Thc psychology of pleasantness. *Psychological Review, 32*(5), 362–383.
Ryan, R. M. M., & Deci, E. L. D. (2001). On happiness and human potentials: A review of research on hedonic and eudaimonic well-being. *Annual Review of Psychology, 52*, 141–166. http://psych.AnnualReviews.org/cgi/reprint/52/1/141.pdf
Ryff, C. D. (1989). Happiness is everything, or is it? Explorations on the meaning of psychological well-being. *Journal of Personality and Social Psychology, 57*, 1069–1081. https://doi.org/10.1037/0022-3514.57.6.1069
Salsburg, D. (2002). *The lady tasting tea*. Holt Paperback.
Sandvik, E., Diener, E., & Seidlitz, L. (1993). Subjective well-being: The convergence and stability of self-report and non-self-report measures. *Journal of Personality, 61*(3), 317–342.
Schneider, L., & Schimmack, U. (2009). Self-informant agreement in well-being ratings: A meta-analysis. *Social Indicators Research, 94*(3), 363. https://doi.org/10.1007/s11205-009-9440-y
Searle, J. R. (1992). *The rediscovery of the mind*. MIT Press.
Searle, J. R. (1995). *The construction of social reality*. Pinguin.
Searle, J. R. (1998). *Mind, language and society. Philosophy in the real world*. Basic Books.
Searle, J. (2011). The mystery of consciousness continues. *The New York Review of Books, June*, 50–52.
Seligman, M. P. E. (2003). Psychology. Fundamental assumptions. *The Psychologist, 16*(3), 127.
Sinclair, J. (1791). *The statistical account of Scotland*.
Sirgy, M. J. (2021). *The psychology of quality of life: Wellbeing and positive mental health*. Springer. https://doi.org/10.1007/978-3-030-71888-6_2
Spencer, H. (1850). *Social statistics, the conditions essential to human happiness specified and the first of them developed*. Routledge & Keagan.
Su, R., Tay, L., & Diener, E. (2014). The development and validation of the Comprehensive Inventory of Thriving (CIT) and the Brief Inventory of Thriving (BIT). *Applied Psychology: Health and Well-Being, 6*(3), 251–279. https://doi.org/10.1111/aphw.12027
Sumner, L. W. (1996). *Welfare, happiness, and ethics*. Clarendon Press.
Thin, N. (2012). *Social happiness. Theory into policy and practice*. The Policy Press.
Thorndike, E. L. (1913). *An introduction to the theory of mental and social measurements* (2nd ed.). Teachers College Press. (Original work published 1904). https://doi.org/10.1037/10866-002.
Tiberius, V. (2013a). Recipes for a good life: Eudaimonism and the contribution of philosophy. In A. Waterman (Ed.), *The best within us. Positive psychology perspectives on eudaimonia* (pp. 19–38). American Psychological Association. https://doi.org/10.1037/14092-002
Tiberius, V. (2013b). Theorizing: On the division of labor between moral philosophy and positive psychology. In S. Kirchin (Ed.), *Thick concepts* (pp. 217–234). Oxford University Press.
Tiberius, V. (2015). Prudential value. In I. Hirose & J. Olson (Eds.), *The Oxford handbook of value theory* (pp. 158–174). Oxford University Press.
Tiberius, V. (2016). The future of eudaimonic well-being: Subjectivism, objectivism and the lump under the carpet. In J. Vittersø (Ed.), *Handbook of eudaimonic well-being* (pp. 565–569). Springer. https://doi.org/10.1007/978-3-319-42445-3_38
Tiberius, V. (2018). *Well-being as value fulfillment: How we can help each other to live well [Kindle]*. Oxford University Press.
Vallerand, R. J. (2016). On the synergy between hedonia and eudaimonia: The role of passion. In J. Vittersø (Ed.), *Handbook of eudaimonic well-being* (pp. 191–204). Springer. https://doi.org/10.1007/978-3-319-42445-3_13
Van Praag, B. M. S., & Ferrer-i-Carbonell, A. (2004). *Happiness quantified. A satisfaction calculus approach*. Oxford University Press.
Veenhoven, R. (1984). *Conditions of happiness*. Kluwer Academic.

Veenhoven, R. (2012). Happiness: Also known as "life satisfaction" and "subjective well-being". In K. C. Land, A. C. Michalos, & M. J. Sirgy (Eds.), *Handbook of social indicators and quality of life research* (pp. 63–77). Springer Netherlands. https://doi.org/10.1007/978-94-007-2421-1_3

Vella-Brodrick, D. (2014). Pleasure, engagement, meaning, and happiness. In A. Michalos (Ed.), *Encyclopedia of quality of life and well-being research*. Springer.

Vittersø, J. (Ed.). (2016a). *Handbook of eudaimonic well-being*. Springer.

Vittersø, J. (2016b). The most important idea in the world: An introduction. In J. Vittersø (Ed.), *Handbook of eudaimonic well-being* (pp. 1–24). Springer. https://doi.org/10.1007/978-3-319-42445-3_1

Vittersø, J. (2021). A passion for happiness: Ruut Veenhoven, eudaimonia and the good life. In A. C. Michalos (Ed.), *The pope of happiness: A Festschrift for Ruut Veenhoven* (pp. 261–275). Springer. https://doi.org/10.1007/978-3-030-53779-1_27

Watson, G. (1930). Happiness among adult students of education. *The Journal of Educational Psychology, 21*, 79–109.

Weijers, D. (2021). Hedonism. *Internet Encyclopedia of Philosophy*. https://iep.utm.edu/hedonism/.

Weinberg, M. K., Seton, C., & Cameron, N. (2018). The measurement of subjective wellbeing: Item-order effects in the personal wellbeing index—adult [journal article]. *Journal of Happiness Studies, 19*(1), 315–332. https://doi.org/10.1007/s10902-016-9822-1

Wessman, A. E., & Ricks, D. F. (1966). *Mood and personality*. Holt, Reinehart & Winston.

Wierzbicka, A. (2004). "Happiness" in cross-linguistic and cross-cultural perspective. *Daedalus, 34*(2), 34–43.

Wilson, W. (1967). Correlates of avowed happiness. *Psychological Bulletin, 67*(4), 294–306.

Winerman, L. (2012). A machine for jumping to conclusions. *APA Monitor*, 24–27. http://www.apa.org/monitor/2012/02/conclusions.aspx.

von Wright, G. H. (1963). *The varieties of goodness*. Routledge.

Chapter 3
Affect

Introduction

> Our good depends on the quality and breadth of our emotions.
> George Eliot, Middlemarch

Affect is a fundamental part of human experience and has always been central to philosophy and psychology. The concept was for long considered to be the opposite of intellectual, and in the history of thinking, there has often been a conflict between the idea of affect and the idea of reason (e.g., Hilgard, 1980; Oatley, 2004). Immanuel Kant, for instance, regarded affect as "sickness of the mind" (Frijda, 1999) and saw it as short-term eruptions of strong and immediate desire (Frevert, 2016). Miron (1969, p. 189) explains that although it is "intuitively satisfying to take the theoretical position that whatever it is we mean by affect, it is orthogonal to something we might call cognitive," such a view is misguided. Thus, a renewed perspective on the distinction between affect and reasoning—or emotion and thinking—emerged with the cognitive revolution in the late 1950s. Since then and particularly since 1980, a rapid growth in knowledge about affect has occurred (Clore & Schnall, 2005; Damasio, 1994; Salovey & Mayer, 1990; Zajonc, 1980). Neo-Aristotelians might object to this timeline, though, and rather claim that the modern perspective has reemerged from Aristotelian and ancient Roman views (Nussbaum, 2001). Regardless, the current understanding of affect and cognition is more integrative than previous perspectives were, even if the two concepts still are treated as distinct phenomena (e.g., Adolphs & Anderson, 2018; Dukes et al., 2021; Fox et al., 2018; Keltner et al., 2019).

Terminologically, it has been customary to use affect as a synonym for emotion (e.g., Russell & Barrett, 1999, p. 805). Psychologists such as Murray, Maslow, and Piaget investigated what they referred to as affects in this way. However, the interest in affective/emotional studies in the early phase of psychology was not very intense, as testified by the few studies that were published about it. According to Schimmack and Crites (2005), the term affect only appeared in 175 publication titles before

J. Vittersø, *Humanistic Wellbeing*, https://doi.org/10.1007/978-3-031-69292-5_3

1960. Tomkins' influential work in the early 1960s marked a change in the tide. His work was highly respected and contributed to establishing the tradition of using the term affect in ways that resemble how we talk about emotions today (Tomkins, 1962, 1963). This practice was also adopted when the field of affective neuroscience was introduced (Adolphs & Anderson, 2018; Panksepp, 1998a), and many neuroscientists still use affect and emotions interchangeably. But the word affect has also been given other meanings, two of which will be reviewed below: the top-down approach and the bottom-up approach. For the record, it can also be mentioned that the word affect can mean something that produces change, and Barrett and Bliss-Moreau (2009) point out that affect in the "emotional" sense also bears connotation to the idea of being mentally influenced or affected by something.

When affect is used to denote an overarching top-down concept, it stands as the superordinate concept in a hierarchical IS—A KIND OF taxonomy. The structure of such taxonomies will be further elaborated in Chap. 7, but briefly, they locate superordinate categories high in the taxonomy and subordinate categories further down. Emotion is therefore a *kind of* affect in this nomenclature, not a synonym. As an umbrella term, affect embraces many other subcategories beyond emotions, such as temperament (personality), moods, and feelings. A clear example of this conceptualization is from Matsumoti and Ekman (2009), who claim that "We consider the universe of affective phenomena to include emotions, moods, affect related personality traits, some psychopathologies, and wellbeing; emotion, therefore, is one class of affective phenomena" (p. 69). In some schemes, preferences and evaluations are also added as subcategories of affect (Huntsinger et al., 2014; Keltner et al., 2014).

In contrast, some scientists use affect as a bottom-up concept. Moods, emotions, feelings, and so on are considered not as different kinds of affects, but rather as the product of an affective component. Such conceived, affect is an omnipresent "building block" that constitutes one of the elements that always are included in all kinds of emotional or affective experiences. An early articulation of this perspective was formulated by Floyd Allport. In his monumental work on social psychology, Allport referred to affect as a pleasure-displeasure dimension and argued that it is included in all emotions: "Every emotion has an *affective element* (italics in original); that is, it may be classified as either pleasant or unpleasant" (Allport, 1924, p. 85). More recently, Batson et al. (1992) have supported this idea and argued that the concept of affect is more phylogenetically and ontogenetically primitive than the concept of emotion. The authors explain that affect is present in everything from "the yelp of a dog and in the coo or cry in an infant" (p. 298). Batson and coauthors argue that the functional element of affects is to signal valence, i.e., positivity and negativity. It is the valence part that makes affect functional because it informs an organism about what they should value.

Similarly, Frijda (1999) supports the idea that affect is a one-dimensional feeling element that runs from pleasant to unpleasant. He defines affect as "hedonic experience, the experiences of pleasure or pain" (p. 194). The most popular use of affect as a building block concept comes, however, from theories of core affect (Russell, 2003; Russell & Barrett, 1999). Here, affect is described as simple features of valence (varying from pleasure to displeasure) and arousal (varying from energization to lassitude) "which are part of every waking moment of consciousness, including but not limited to, emotional episodes" (Barrett, 2018, p. 37).

I will return to the notion of core affect below but shall first mention a third usage of the term affect. This is the synonym approach, in which affect is used interchangeably with mood, emotion, or feeling or some combination of these three elements (see Ekkekakis, 2013, for similar examples). Scholars such as Watson, Clark, and Tellegen use affect as a synonym for mood and feeling, but not for emotion. According to David Watson (2000), emotions are more organized and specific than moods. In contrast to moods, emotions are also shorter in duration, have a noncyclical pattern, and are experienced as stronger and less attenuated. Moods, by contrast, can be defined as "transient episode of feeling or affect" (p. 4). Thus, when the influential Positive and Negative Affect Schedule (PANAS) was first introduced, it was used as a mood scale (Watson et al., 1988, p. 1069). Later, it was recategorized into a measure of arousal, with PA and NA relabeled as positive activation and negative activation, respectively (Watson et al., 1999).

To add a few more examples of how affect is defined according to the three different categories of approaches to the study of affect, a small sample of definitions of the word is provided in Table 3.1.

The first three definitions are based on the top-down approach, with the first two being more specific than the third. The next four examples are bottom-up definitions in the sense that affect is the building block of "anything emotional." Definition 5 describes affect as a "conglomerate of phenomenon," which could indicate a top-down perspective. However, Damasio and Damasio explain elsewhere that all affective phenomena are valenced in the sense that they are "good, bad, or somewhere in between" (Damasio & Damasio, 2018, p. 3), which is why I consider it consistent with the bottom-up approach. The remaining definitions are synonym perspectives, using affect as another word for emotion, feeling, and the like. The last definition, by Frijda, uses affect as another word for hedonia, which is often used to label the experience of pleasure and pain.

The variety and idiosyncratic ways in which affect is conceptualized reminds us about the difficulties of reaching conceptual agreements in science. This unfortunate situation poses a problem for wellbeing research, because it is difficult to generate common knowledge about affective wellbeing until we agree about what we are to study when investigating affect. For example, when positive and negative affect are included as core elements in the definition of subjective wellbeing, should these concepts then refer to pleasure and pain (definition 12), to what we feel more generally (definition 9), to core affect (definition 4), or to a combination of feelings, emotions, moods, and temperaments (definition 1)?

In the Diener camp, terms such as affect, emotions, mood, and feelings are often used without discriminating sharply between them (e.g., Diener & Lucas, 2000; Diener et al., 1999). But these terms refer to different concepts (e.g., Dukes et al., 2021; Ellsworth, 1994). A feeling refers to a continuous experience and is always present in consciousness (e.g., Damasio, 1999). Emotions, by contrast, are infrequent, brief, intense, and typically persist for seconds or perhaps minutes before disappearing. If the affective element of wellbeing is restricted to the brief periods

Table 3.1 Some definitions of affect

Definition	Source
1. We consider the universe of affective phenomena to include emotions, moods, affect-related personality traits, some psychopathologies, and wellbeing; emotion, therefore, is one class of affective phenomena	Matsumoti and Ekman (2009, p. 69)
2. A general term that we use to refer to any evaluative reaction. Such reactions are representations of value; they are about the goodness-badness of something. Thus, there are affective feelings, affective thoughts, affective expressions, and so on. Common terms referring to different kinds of affective conditions include emotion, mood, attitude, and temperament	Huntsinger et al. (2014, p. 600)
3. Affect is an umbrella term for psychological states that involve valuation or a "good-for-me" versus "bad-for-me" judgment	Inzlicht et al. (2015, p. 126)
4. Affect is described as simple features of valence and arousal which are part of every waking moment of consciousness, including, but not limited to, emotional episodes	Barrett (2018, p. 37)
5. The conglomerate of phenomena designated by such terms as drives, motivations, emotions, and the feelings that correspond to them	Damasio and Damasio (2018, p. 6)
6. Affect is the manner in which emotional events influence behavior and subjective feelings, often operationalized in terms of valence and arousal	Kragel and LaBar (2016, p. 445)
7. Small flashes of positive or negative feeling that prepare us to approach or avoid something. Every emotion (such as happiness or disgust) includes an affective reaction, but most of our affective reactions are too fleeting to be called emotions	Haidt (2012, p. 65)
8. A synonym for emotion	Cabanac (2009, p. 49)
9. What the organism feels	Ortony et al. (2005, p. 173)
10. Sometimes (affect) refer to values, sometimes to emotional states	Mandler (1984, p. 191)
11. A sense of purely physical, prelinguistic, unconscious emotion	Plamper (2015, p. 11)
12. A hedonic experience, the experience of pleasure and pain	Frijda (1999, p. 194)

in which we are experiencing an emotion (see the "Emotions" section), how should the experiences of the remaining time of our conscious life be counted? Even moods, which last longer than emotions and often extend into hours and days, are not ubiquitously present when feelings are experienced (Ekkekakis, 2013; Fox et al., 2018; Keltner et al., 2014). However, in the formative years of SWB research, these differences were seldom articulated, resulting in a "jingle-jangle" practice with unfortunate consequences. To better see why this is so, a brief review of the distinct subcategories of affect, understood from the overarching, i.e., top-down, perspective is helpful. Starting with the broadest elements in the taxonomy of affects, the next sections will review the concepts of temperament, mood emotions, feelings, and evaluations. The last two sections will look more closely into emotional happiness and emotional interest. Note that pleasure, which arguably is the most important concept in the family of affects, will be discussed loosely throughout the chapter but will be treated more systematically in Chap. 5.

Temperament and Mood

Temperament

The most abstract category in the affect taxonomy is temperament, which comes from the Latin *temperare:* "to mix." The Greeks and Romans believed that a mix of bodily fluids, or humors, created our mental states of rationality and emotionality, and the temperamental types proposed by the second-century physician Galen are the most well-known of the ancient theories today (e.g., Kagan, 1998). Galen's idea was that the balance between the four humors blood, phlegm, yellow bile, and black bile determines an individual's temperament and personality. For example, a sanguine person is cheerful and optimistic because of an excess of blood in the body, leading to a warm and moist mix of humors. The choleric personality has an excess of yellow bile, the melancholic personality has too much black bile, and the phlegmatic person has a surplus of phlegm. Galen's typology inspired personality psychologists such as Gustav Jung and Hans Eysenck. Jung invented the terms introversion and extroversion to mirror melancholic and sanguine temperaments, whereas Eysenck grounded his personality theory on the two bipolar dimensions of extroversion vs. introversion and neuroticism vs. stability. These dimensions have striking similarities to the axes of sanguine vs. melancholic and choleric vs. phlegmatic.

We often think of temperament as a general tendency to feel or act in certain ways, such as being fearful or cheerful. Thus, one conventional definition describes temperaments as "stable behavioral and emotional reactions that appear early and are influenced in part by genetic constitution" (Kagan, 1998, p. 264). In another definition, temperament refers to "a set of biologically rooted, early appearing, and relatively stable individual differences in reactivity to stimuli and self-regulation of that reactivity" (Bates, 2000, p. 384).

Several basic temperamental types exist. One commonly observed propensity relates to the experience of pleasure and can, according to Shiner (2018), be observed very early in human development. It includes children's tendencies to smile and laugh, experience excitement, and take pleasure in interactions with others. Another temperamental propensity is a fear/inhibition disposition that includes withdrawal from novel and stressful situations. A third kind relates to irritability/anger/frustration, whereas a fourth type is referred to as activity level. This disposition "involves the vigor and frequency of motor movements and seems to be related to both positive emotions/extraversion and poor self-control, depending on how it is measured" (Shiner, 2018, p. 62).

Kagan (2018) has spent a lifetime studying temperament and has become convinced that two traits stand out as particularly important. They are referred to as "high reactive" and "low reactive." Already at 4 months, Kagan has found, 20% of babies can be classified as high reactive and 40% can be classified as low reactive. High-reactive infants are born with a characteristic neurochemistry and are avoidant and distressed by unfamiliar events, a tendency that tends to persist into youth and adulthood for many of these toddlers. The high-reactive disposition can later be observed as a vulnerability to anxiety and depression and as a high score for the personality trait of introversion. The low-reactive infants are born with a different neurochemistries and show signs of sociability and fearlessness, a temperament that tends to follow them throughout their life span. As adults, they are typically described as extraverts.

Despite the distinctive traits observed by Shiner, Kagan, and others, researchers disagree about the underlying structure of temperament typology. Some, such as Cloninger (1987), believe that "avoidance of danger, seeking of novelty, and dependence on social rewards constitute the primary temperamental types" (cited in Kagan, 1998, p. 43). Others posit emotionality, activity, and sociability as the three major temperaments (e.g., Buss & Plomin, 1975). A yet different take is offered by Richard Davidson, who thinks of temperament as a kind of emotional style (e.g., Davidson, 1998, 2018; Davidson & Begley, 2012). In contrast to personality, Davidson claims that emotional style can be traced to specific, neural circuits that can be classified into six basic dimensions (resilience, outlook, social intuition, self-awareness, sensitivity to context, and attention). Davidson's taxonomy appears more emotional than temperamental, so it is at least a borderline case of a temperamental typology.

Temperament and personality share some similarities but are also separable. For example, cognitive style is more prominent in personality than in temperament. Personality traits further tend to encompass emotions that emerge slightly later in childhood, such as empathy, guilt, and shame (Shiner, 2018). Among the parallels between temperaments and personality, we find the resemblances that Eysenck pointed out between the extroversion-introversion and neuroticism-stability dimensions of personality and how they reflect the notion of sanguine vs. melancholic and choleric vs. phlegmatic. Similarly, extraversion, as conceptualized in the five-factor model of personality, shares some qualities with modern conceptualization of temperament, such as the tendencies to experience pleasure and sociability, and with activity level (De Pauw et al., 2009). Overlaps also exist between neuroticism and temperamental inhibition and between the trait conscientiousness and temperaments such as impulse control, persistence, orderliness, and striving for high standards. According to Shiner and DeYoung (2013), agreeableness has a less direct temperamental counterpart, although it shares some similarities with empathy and soothability at its high end, similar to anger and irritability at its low end. Interestingly, the trait openness to experience seems to lack a clear temperamental counterpart. Openness involves tendencies to be perceptive, curious, artistic, and quick to learn. It further encompasses the engagement that arises from opportunity emotions such as interest and curiosity (DeYoung, 2015). The temperamental content representing openness is almost completely ignored, although there seems to be some kinship between openness and perceptual sensitivity (De Pauw et al., 2009).

Few studies on SWB and temperament exist, but Diener spent some time discussing Galen's theory and how his temperamental types relate to affective wellbeing in a book chapter from 1998 (Diener, 1998). In it, Diener basically argued that Galen's typology could be accounted for in a two-dimensional space of affect and intensity. Choleric then becomes a combination of high (intense) positive affect and high negative affect. Phlegmatic is the opposite of melancholic and is characterized by low positive affect and low negative affect. Melancholic covers the span from low to high negative affect, whereas sanguine is located between high positive and low negative affect. More recently, a few studies have examined more modern operationalizations of temperament and correlated these with indicators of wellbeing. Bojanowska and Piotrowski (2021) reported, for instance, negligible effect sizes for measures of life satisfaction and temperament traits such as briskness and perseveration. Using a different temperament questionnaire, Viñas et al. (2014) found some associations between personal wellbeing and traits such as affiliation and (lack of) shyness.

Overall, SWB researchers are much more interested in personality traits than in temperaments (Diener & Lucas, 1999, 2018; Lucas & Diener, 2015). For example, numerous studies have shown that neuroticism is the trait that explains the most SWB variance, followed by extraversion. Agreeableness and conspicuousness also correlate positively with SWB, whereas openness to experience seems almost unrelated to subjective wellbeing (Anglim et al., 2020; Steel et al., 2008; Vittersø & Nilsen, 2002).

Mood

At least two opposing views about mood can be identified. One regards moods as "little emotions," which is the idea that mood is merely an attenuated form of emotion. The other perspective sees mood as a distinctive construct that is structurally, phenomenologically, and functionally different from emotion (Morris, 1999). When considered "little emotions," mood is typically described as diffuse affective states that are not directed toward a specific object. The difference attributed to moods and emotions within this paradigm is that moods last longer and are less intense. My impression is that Diener and his colleagues subscribe to the "moods as little emotions" perspective. For example, their texts often define affective wellbeing by referring to moods and emotions in a single phrase, without specifying similarities and differences between them and without articulating how the two concepts might relate to wellbeing in distinct ways (e.g., Diener, 1998, pp. 311–312; Diener et al., 2009, p. 191; Diener et al., 1999, p. 277; Kesebir & Diener, 2008, p. 118).

The alternative approach considers moods fundamentally different from emotions. Here, mood is conceptualized as more of an overall kind of evaluation, an experience related to one's current state of being more globally. In this view and in contrast to emotions, moods can last for hours, or days, and sometimes longer, and it is often unclear when they start and stop (Keltner et al., 2014). Moods are often considered objectless and free floating, and they vary in a cyclic pattern with diurnal changes and, to some extent, follow seasonal changes over a yearly cycle (Watson, 2000). According to Morris (1999), moods inform us of temporary fluctuations in the likelihood of occurrence of future pleasurable and painful events, whereas emotions are the result of present hedonically relevant events. He sees the mood system as a homeostatic mechanism that serves us by assessing the adequacy of our current resources and producing feelings that are capable of influencing goal-directed activity. More concretely, mood solves a problem for us by continuously monitoring the availability of resources necessary for meeting current demands: "they constitute a feeling-based prediction about the likelihood of success of goal-directed behavior in the near term" (Morris, 1999, p. 169). This suggests that an intimate connection between mood and subjective wellbeing exists. For instance, Diener and his colleagues described SWB "as an internal barometer of 'how life is going'—it is a gauge of the extent to which other aspects of psychological well-being or needs are fulfilled" (Su et al., 2014, p. 254).

When mood is conceived as an overall kind of evaluation, it is not functionally oriented toward particular life goals like emotions are. Moods do not acutely change the physiology, cognition, or action of the experiencing person (Kagan, 1994; Stein & Hernandez, 2007). Thus, whereas emotions tend to be directed toward specific goals, moods are barometers that evaluate a person's general situation in life (Morris, 1999, p. 170). Mood has been described as a monitor that informs us about our long-term relationship with the environment and as the "products of appraisals of the existential background of our lives" (Lazarus, 1994, p. 84).

Batson et al. (1992) give the following description of the functional role moods play in our everyday lives. "Good moods signal that we are passing through a land of milk and honey and should reach out, pluck the fruit, and enjoy. Bad moods signal that we should pull our cloak tight and trudge stolidly ahead, or stop and reassess out itinerary, or hunk down, conserve resources, and wait for the storm to pass" (p. 299). In other words, positive moods motivate us to take advantage of our favorable current circumstances. Negative moods convey more varied meanings, including an urge to push on or, in other circumstances, to stop and/or prepare for the worst. To determine how the function and experience of moods differ from those of emotions, a survey of the most important literature on emotions will be provided next.

Emotions

The word emotion came from French to English during the seventeenth and eighteenth centuries but did not refer to anything mental until the mid-nineteenth century (Scarantino, 2016). Then and initiated by important work by Darwin (1872),

James (1884), Freud and Breuer (1895), and others, a busy period of emotion research was initiated before the black box ideology of behaviorism sat the study on halt.[1] In the late 1950s, a new generation of scientists again took the study of emotion seriously, and in the early 1980s, interest in and knowledge about emotion escalated. By then and after a hundred years of scientific investigation, the number of different understandings and definitions had accumulated. For example, Plutchik and Kellerman (1980) identified 28 definitions of emotion, and Kleinginna and Kleinginna (1981) noted 92 definitions in their literature review. It has frequently been remarked that no singular or even preferred definition of emotion exists (e.g., Cabanac, 2009, p. 215), and the plethora of different meanings has led the field into "a glaring need for conceptual clarity" (Berscheid, 1990). Although such clarity remains to be achieved, recent decades have witnessed important progress in knowledge and insights. The disagreements have become more focused and, as we will see below, more directed toward a restricted and better articulated set of puzzles. Comprehensive investigations and research programs have begun to provide a fair understanding of at least some basic properties of emotions and not at least some answers to important questions such as what an emotion is and why emotions exist.

Current scholars seem to agree that an emotion is a multidimensional state of readiness to act in a certain way when an event is appraised as affecting a concern that we have (Oatley, 2018). A recent review by Moors (2012) identified five key features of an emotion: (1) a cognitive component, referring to the processing or appraisal of a stimulus; (2) a motivational component, referring to action tendencies; (3) a somatic component, referring to central and peripheral physiological activity; (4) a motor component, referring to behavior (e.g., facial and vocal expressions, gross actions); and (5) an experiential component,[2] referring to the phenomenological or feeling part of an emotion.

According to Oatley (1992), emotions are "a part of the biological solution to the problem of how to plan and to carry out actions aimed at satisfying multiple goals in environments which are not perfectly predicable" (p. 35). In its broadest sense, an emotion brings together cognitions, evaluations, neurophysiological processes, somatic changes, subjective feelings, facial expressions, and behaviors (Johnson-Laird & Oatley, 2000, p. 459). Moreover, emotions are short-lived and "defined by distinct feelings, expressive behavior, and physiological patterning in the central and peripheral nervous systems" (Keltner & Oatley, 2022). As an approximation to define them, Keltner et al. (2014) suggest that "one may treat emotions, at least to start with, as *multicomponent responses to challenges or opportunities that are important to the individual's goals, particularly social ones*" (p. 27, italics in original). Somewhat simpler, Lambie and Marcel (2002) tentatively define an emotion state as what is common to a certain set of evaluative representations, attitudinal behaviors, and physical states.

[1] Skinner never though highly about emotions and basically considered them as an irrelevant epiphenomenon (Smith & Lazarus, 1990).

[2] Moors uses the term subjective, but I believe the term experiential is more precise.

An emotion is thus a state of action readiness that relates events to what is important for a person, a state "that prompt plans and provide outline structures for relations with others" (Oatley & Jenkins, 1996, p. 130). This insight was well articulated by Simon (1967), who realized that, in a critical situation, it is impossible to search one's repertoire of knowledge for all possible solutions before a decision is made. Simon proposed that emotions are part of the solution to this problem and argued that emotions are integrated parts of an information processing system with multiple goals and needs.

One crucial feature of emotions is their ability to interrupt one's current interaction with the environment. If a more urgent goal suddenly is at stake, it is critical to change the current plan and undertake the behavior immediately required to manage the challenges that appear in one's proximal circumstances. With respect to specific emotions, Simon maintained that they reprioritize goals, feelings, and actions according to challenges in the environment. Here is an example of how the process may proceed. Suppose you are deeply involved in a conversation as you start crossing a street. Then, you suddenly hear the screeching brakes from a car: "You stop your conversation, jump back onto the sidewalk. You find your head pounding, thinking you could have been hurt, and you determine to be more careful, not to become so deeply involved in conversations. The event is evaluated as important, and priorities are changed, interrupting your previous actions. You are shaken bodily, and you make plans about what to do" (Oatley & Johnson-Laird, 1996, p. 96).

There is a general agreement among emotion researchers about the features just described. For other elements, however, controversies are heatedly discussed, and common ground has not been reached. An example is the disagreement about whether emotions should be considered discrete or dimensional. It is "The great emotions debate," as Barrett et al. (2007) call it. According to the discrete approach, a set of basic emotions represents specific and partly innate bundles of central characteristics, such as feelings, expressions, and physiological patterns. The central idea about basic emotions is that this set of characteristics must be *unique* for each emotion—other emotions or mental states cannot have them (e.g., Celeghin et al., 2017). In contrast, the continuous approach rejects this idea and argues instead that emotions derive from a construction process. This process can be explained by a system of biological and psychological structures, as proposed by appraisal theories of emotion (e.g., Ortony et al., 2022). However, they can also be created less systematically by social and linguistic factors. This is the perspective proposed by constructed emotion theories (e.g., Barrett, 2017a).

Discrete (Basic) Emotions

The notion of basic emotions is old. Sophocles of the fifth century BCA, known for his ancient Greek tragedies, wrote about the "delineation of the great primitive emotions" (cited in Oatley, 1992, p. 55). Closer in time, Descartes had ideas about basic emotions or fundamental passions in his vocabulary. Using his well-known discourse method, Descartes concluded that six passions were more fundamental than others: wonder, joy, sadness, love, hatred, and desire (Power & Dalgleish, 2015, p. 28). Later, philosophers developed more elaborate theories about emotions, but Darwin introduced the first scientific theory of basic emotions. Unlike Skinner and the behaviorists, Darwin realized that emotions existed for a reason; they must somehow be relevant for survival. As explained by Oatley and Jenkins (1996), Darwin's ideas about emotions were not very sophisticatedly articulated in *On the Origin of Species* (Darwin, 1859), but his book *The Expression of the Emotions in Man and Animals* Darwin (1872) was far more detailed. For example, Darwin issued questionnaires to English-speaking individuals worldwide and thus collected information about emotional expressions cross-culturally. Darwin's idea was that these expressions had a core of universality, which again suggested that emotions had been a useful communicative tool in our evolutionary past.

Building on Darwin's ideas, scholars such as Tomkins, Ekman, Izard, Levenson, Panksepp, and Oatley developed theories that account for the adaptiveness of basic emotions and how their "basicness" functions by improving our ability to interact successfully with the environment. One important feature of basic emotions is the assumption that they comprise an unanalyzable feeling element, a unique phenomenology that cannot be decomposed to simpler parts. This element is also adopted as a core premise of the humanistic theory of wellbeing, which relies heavily on Oatley's idea that biology equips humans with a variety of feeling quality as a means of communication. Feelings communicate messages to ourselves and to others about how we are doing in terms of reaching our goals and fulfilling basic needs (Oatley, 1992).

The Ekman Six

Ekman (e.g., Ekman, 1980, 1992; Ekman & Cordaro, 2011) took a clear position in "The great emotions debate," by insisting that each of a limited set of basic emotions must have unique features, such as what they signalize, how they are physiologically organized, and what their antecedent events are. Ekman (1992) detailed nine criteria to guide the scientific study of emotion and summarized that these patterns "should be specific to these emotions and not found in other mental activity" (Ekman, 1994, p. 18). He held that six emotions were universally expressed and recognized: anger, disgust, fear, sadness, surprise, and happiness. For these six emotions, Ekman argues, "there is robust, consistent evidence of a distinctive, universal facial expression" (Ekman, 1992, p. 175).

A more recent version of Ekman's theory comes from a group of researchers led by Dacher Keltner. This theory is called "social functional theory" and suggests that the dimensionality of human emotion is much richer than what was proposed by Ekman. The social functional approach also advocates that the boundaries between emotions are not discrete but rather fuzzy and that emotion categories such as amusement, awe, and fear are more important drivers of emotional experiences than valence and arousal. In several studies, Keltner and his coworkers reported that 18 emotional states can be identified with distinct facial expressions, vocalizations, and prosody (Cowen & Keltner, 2020; Cowen et al., 2021; Keltner & Oatley, 2022).

Keith Oatley and Communicative Theory

The communicative theory of emotions was introduced by Oatley and Johnson-Laird in 1987 and is rooted in the Aristotelian idea that emotions are feelings that change our judgments (Oatley & Johnson-Laird, 2011, p. 424). Emotions are evaluations of events that are important for goals and plans, and the initial argument for the communicative theory was that "a small number of basic emotions are linked to a small number of junctures of plans and that are recognizable and that reoccur" (Oatley, 1992, pp. 55–56). Emotions are therefore heuristics that organize action in a world that is always imperfectly known.

> Each goal and plan has a monitoring mechanism that evaluates events relevant to it. When a substantial change of probability occurs of achieving an important goal or subgoal, the monitoring mechanism broadcasts to the whole cognitive system a signal that can set it into readiness to respond to this change. Humans experience these signals and the states of readiness they induce as emotions. (Oatley, 1992, p. 50)

More concretely, each basic emotion is linked to a specific pattern of juncture plans and action tendencies. For example, happiness occurs when a subgoal is achieved, whereas sadness occurs when a major plan fails or a valuable goal is lost. In terms of communication, our feelings of happiness, sadness, or other basic emotions are evaluative signals that are broadcasted throughout our minds to set the mental architecture in a certain state of action readiness.

Basic emotions are psychological primitives and irreducible in the sense that they "cannot be decomposed into lower-level states or processes that are not themselves emotions" (Oatley & Johnson-Laird, 2011, p. 426). For example, the feeling of happiness is not a composite of pleasure, arousal, or other more basic units. What we feel when we are happy is something genuine for happiness and cannot be further decomposed. More technically, basic emotions are grounded in nonpropositional signals that have no semantic meaning, which is to say that emotional feelings cannot be articulated as verbalized statements.

Basic feelings operate automatically by switching emotional modules on or off. The message sets the brain into a mode adapted to deal with a recurrent situation—a kind of action tendency template. For happiness, the template is to continue with the ongoing plan and progress toward the overarching goal. For sadness, the template is to do nothing or search for a new plan. The signal for fear, which is another basic emotion, is about a threatened self-preservation goal or goals that are in conflict. The recurring action tendency is an urge to stop the current plan and attend vigilantly to the environment, alternatively to freeze and/or escape. Anger occurs when an active plan is frustrated, inciting a tendency to try harder and/or aggress (Oatley & Johnson-Laird, 1987).

Hence, emotions coordinate our plans and goals, and they do so under constraints of time and other limited resources. In this regard, the feeling element is important because it creates an immediate valuation of a particular outcome of a situation. This is in line with the argument made by Simon (1967) above, about emotions as a mechanism that reprioritizes goals and actions to meet a sudden and interruptive challenge that occurs in the environment.

A central implication embedded in the communicative theory is that emotions are not about evaluating events per se. Rather, they are about evaluating goals and plans related to these events. This is important, given the variety of emotional responses that can be observed to relatively similar circumstances, and vice versa, when a variety of circumstances give rise to comparable emotional responses. Darwin gives a recognizable example from an encounter with a native of Tierra del Fuego. The man touched Darwin's meal with a finger, which made Darwin somewhat disgusted. The native, on the other hand, was disgusted from the soft consistency of Darwin's food. For both, however, the goal of not eating contaminated food was violated (cited in Oatley, 1992, p. 57).

Originally, the communicative theory suggested five basic emotions: happiness, sadness, fear, anger, and disgust. In a revised version, disgust was reclassified into a category of basic emotion that necessarily has objects (Oatley & Johnson-Laird, 1996, 2011). Oatley and Johnson-Laird also expanded the category of basic emotions to include hate, sexual love, parental love, and love for caregivers. These five emotions are basic in the sense of being founded on innate biological substrates. However, since they always have objects, these emotions can only be experienced in relation to someone or something, which is why they constitute a subcategory of basic emotions (Oatley & Johnson-Laird, 1996, p. 374).

The exact number of basic emotions is not the most important aspect of the theory and may change without altering the basic structure of the theory. Altering the number of basic emotions will therefore not falsify the theory. But if it can be established that a culture lacks a particular basic emotion or that individuals can immediately experience a basic emotion at will, then the theory will be in trouble (Oatley & Johnson-Laird, 2011).

Jaak Panksepp and Affective Neuroscience

Jaak Panksepp was a pioneer in affective neuroscience, and even though his theory of basic emotions is based largely on older animal studies, it still inspires affective neuroscientists (Adolphs & Anderson, 2018). Panksepp (1998a, 2000) separates affect concepts into three levels of categories: The first contains pleasure, pain, and the startle reflex (among others) and is organized low in the brain stem. The second category is that of basic emotions, including those corresponding roughly to the English terms interest, joy, fear, sadness, anger, joy, and affection, but for which, as we will see below, Panksepp uses a more idiosyncratic vocabulary. There is also a higher, third layer in his theory, which organizes more subtle emotions such as shame, guilt, envy, and humor.

Like Ekman and Oatley, Panksepp assumes that specific modules corresponding to specific and basic emotions exist. Panksepp refers to these modules as "intrinsic psychobehavioral systems in the brain" (Panksepp, 1998a, p. 3). Unlike Ekman and Oatley, however, Panksepp operates with seven basic emotional systems, four of which mature soon after birth: SEEKING[3] (expectancy), RAGE (anger), FEAR (anxiety), and PANIC/GRIEF (sadness). Three additional systems develop somewhat later: LUST (sexual excitement), CARE (nurturance), and PLAY (social joy).

Panksepp organizes four basic emotions under the umbrella concept he refers to as a "higher-order construct of positive affect" (1988, p. 46). These are LUST, CARE, PLAY, and SEEKING. The LUST system is associated with sexual urges, is regulated by hormones such as oxytocin, and includes a special set of sexual feelings. The CARE system involves some of the same neurological physiology and anatomy as the LUST system but is devoted to a much broader area of social bonding. The PLAY system is interesting because of its role in regulating pleasure. The PLAY system occurs in familiar circumstances, and most young mammals play. What Panksepp calls rough-and-rumble play takes the form of pouncing on each other, chasing, and wrestling. PLAY is not an aggressive behavior; rather, it is an intense social joy that occurs in familiar circumstances and is accompanied by positive affect. In contrast, the SEEKING system is activated when novel territories are explored (Panksepp & Biven, 2012).

The SEEKING system is a general-purpose appetitive motivational system that holds a special place in Panksepp's emotional system. It developed in the mammalian brain as a foraging/exploration/investigation/curiosity/interest/expectancy system that leads organisms to eagerly pursue all kinds of resources that exist in their environments (Panksepp & Biven, 2012, p. 103). He considers the system to represent a basic emotion for several reasons. One is that SEEKING has distinct similarities with the concept of interest as accounted for in other basic emotion theories, such as the one developed by Izard (1977) and the one proposed by Plutchik (1980). Another reason is that the underlying circuits of SEEKING are genetically prewired and designed to respond to stimuli arising from major life-challenging circumstances, that SEEKING allows the performance of a large number of goal-seeking behaviors, and that the system has emotive circuits that interact with brain mechanisms that elaborate higher decision-making processes (Panksepp, 1998a, p. 150). SEEKING overlaps strongly with the concept of interest as a feeling and will therefore be further elaborated in the section "Interest as an Emotion" toward the end of the chapter.

[3] In accordance with his idiosyncratic terminology, I use capital letters to name Panksepp's affective concepts.

Wrapping Up Basic Emotions

More theories on basic emotions than the ones presented above exist (see Power & Dalgleish, 2015, for a nice review). At the same time, the notion of emotional basicness continues to attract criticism. Consider, for instance, the two editions of the very useful handbook *The Nature of Emotion: Fundamental Questions*. Both are organized by a set of fundamental questions about the nature and origin of emotions. The first edition was spearheaded by Paul Ekman and Richard Davidson (Ekman & Davidson, 1994), and its first question was about basic emotions. Two chapters supported this notion (Ekman, 1994; Panksepp, 1994), and two chapters contradicted it (Scherer, 1994; Schweder, 1994). It was easy for the editors to conclude that more and better data were needed to settle the issue. However, after 25 years, the disagreements have not been resolved (Fox et al., 2018). Ekman and Panksepp still defended their positions, and Keltner and coauthors presented new arguments in favor of the basic emotion approach. Scherer and Schweder did not contribute to the new volume, but others, such as Barrett and Clore, keep the counterarguments alive. However, the gap between basic and nonbasic emotion theorists is shrinking in the sense that the discussion is more focused and that the basic emotion camp has abandoned their more simplistic models.

Much has been written about basic emotion between the two editions of *The Nature of Emotion*, and it is beyond the scope of this book to cover the debate in any detail. But useful milestones along the way can be found in Moors (2009), the special edition of *Emotion Review* in October 2011 (Russell, 2011) and an edited volume by Zachar (2012). Several meta-studies have also contributed to this discussion (Barrett et al., 2019; Cowen et al., 2019; Elfenbein & Ambady, 2002; Kirby & Robinson, 2017; Lench et al., 2011; Lindquist et al., 2012; Siegel et al., 2018; Vytal & Hamann, 2010; Wager et al., 2015).

The results presented in these meta-studies differ. Sometimes, the same findings are used to reach opposing conclusions, such as in the studies by Vytal and Hamann (2010) and Lindquist et al. (2012). Vytal and Hamman argue that "the current meta-analysis results indicate that the key elements of basic emotion views are reflected in neural correlates identified by neuroimaging studies" (p. 2864), whereas Lindquist et al. "found little evidence that discrete emotion categories can be consistently and specifically localized to distinct brain regions. Instead, we found evidence that is consistent with a psychological constructionist approach to the mind" (p. 121). More recent meta-studies have reported evidence in favor of the basic emotion approach. For example, Kranzbühler et al. (2020) concluded that within the domain of firm-customer encounters, their study clearly showed that discrete emotion models outperform models of core affect. Celeghin et al. (2017) further argue that "recent meta-analyses do not seem to us to provide enough solid ground for rejecting the existence basic emotion at the neurobiological level" (p. 4).

To move forward, Celeghin et al. suggested that basic emotion theorists need to update and reformulate too rigid definitional criteria with respect to what the basic emotions are. They must let go of the notion of a one-to-one relationship between individual brain areas and specific emotions. Celeghin and collaborators concluded that "the bulk of evidence lends support to the existence of relatively segregated neural networks for the processing of different basic emotions" (Celeghin et al., 2017, p. 8).

Continuous (Dimensional) Emotions

All emotion theories reduce emotions either to a set of irreducible states that are themselves emotions or to a set of irreducible states that are not emotions. Whereas basic emotion theories support the first kind of reduction, the continuous approach favors the latter. According to continuous theories, all emotions vary along a few common dimensions. These dimensions can be affective or cognitive. The affective component approach harks back to Wundt and the first versions of his monumental *Outlines of Physiological Psychology.* Here, Wundt argued that three dimensions, namely, pleasure-displeasure, excitement-inhibition, and tension-relaxation, were the fundamental building blocks of a feeing state. However, Wundt came to change his mind, and in the fourth edition of the book, he claimed that the only irreducible qualia are the feelings of pleasure and pain (Reisenzein, 1992). Later developments in the affective approach to continuous emotions have, however, operated with two constitutive dimensions of emotions: valence and arousal.

The cognitive-oriented approaches to continuous emotions are typically referred to as appraisal theories. Historically, they owe much to Aristotle and to the thinking of Hume, Spinoza, and Sartre (Moors et al., 2013). In a review by Gendron and Feldman Barrett (2009), scholars such as Spencer, Irons, Dewey, Titchener, and Young were also included as early appraisal theorists. However, the scientific origin of appraisal theories is typically attributed to Arnold (1954, 1960), Lazarus (1966), and, to some extent, Schachter and Singer (1962).

Appraisal Theories

An appraisal is basically a process that detects and assesses the significance of the environment for our wellbeing (Moors et al., 2013). Cognitive appraisals ask how individuals ascribe personal meaning to their circumstances and how these individualized evaluations create emotions. For example, the sadness felt when a romantic relationship ends may be elicited by the appraisal that something desired has been lost (Roseman & Smith, 2001). Some appraisal theories defend the idea of basic emotions (e.g., Lazarus, 1991b; Oatley & Johnson-Laird, 1987), but others are dimensional theories (e.g., Ortony et al., 1988; Roseman, 1984; Scherer, 1988; Smith & Ellsworth, 1985). Hence, the structure of this part of the chapter is slightly misleading since some appraisal theories belong to the category of basic emotion theories, whereas appraisal theories in general are presented as theories of continuous emotions.

According to the appraisal perspective, emotions are processes rather than states, and they unfold in phases. Organisms constantly scan their environments to detect and reevaluate changes; thus, an appraisal is often followed by "reappraisal" (Scherer et al., 2001). Moreover, a central element in the emotional process is situation-person appraisals, and the dimensions along which appraisals are construed are explicitly specified. The number of dimensions involved varies across theories, but an initial goodness and badness evaluation, judgment about goal relevance, certainty, agency, and coping potential are included in most appraisal theories.

For example, in his pioneering theory, Lazarus (1966) proposed that emotions unfold in two major phases, following the mechanisms of two categories of appraisals. During the first, called primary appraisals, we evaluate what our relationship to the environment implies for our wellbeing: is the situation or stimulus we encounter good or bad? The emotional outcome is positive if the circumstances are appraised as beneficial. It is negative if the circumstances are appraised as harmful (Smith & Lazarus, 1993). In the next phase, called secondary appraisals, one's coping resources are evaluated by an assessment of the ability available to manage the consequences of the event. In collaboration with colleagues such as Folkman, Lazarus later revised his theory to make it more about emotions and less about stress (Lazarus, 1991a, 1991b). The new theory was named "cognitive-motivational-relational," and the primary appraisals were now specified for three kinds of goal evaluations: goal relevance, goal congruence, and ego-involvement. Secondary appraisals were described as problem-focused and emotion-focused coping strategies.

Other phases and appraisal dimensions have been proposed. For instance, Scherer (1984) developed a multilevel sequential check model that considers emotions to involve "a rapidly occurring sequence of hierarchically organized stimulus processing steps" (p. 306), where each step is a stimulus evaluation check. The first check is for novelty, the second for pleasantness, the third for goal conduciveness, the fourth for coping potential, and the fifth for compatibility with norms. Emotions unfold successively along these dimensions over milliseconds to seconds, and the involved information processing becomes increasingly elaborate. Moreover, the sequential nature of Scherer's evaluation checks combines three main components of the emotion system (the sensory-motor level, the schematic level, and the conceptual level) and four appraisal objectives (relevance, implications, coping potential, and normative significance). Scherer's theory is very detailed and somewhat complicated. For example, one tabulated presentation of the core ideas of the model spans four full pages (Scherer, 2009, pp. 1310–1313). Admittedly, this scheme is quite complex and formal, and empirical work remains to fully support it.

A final combination of appraisals worth mentioning is that of Smith and Ellsworth (1985). They suggest that eight dimensions are involved in determining an emotional process: (1) pleasantness, (2) anticipated effort/activation, (3) attentional activity/novelty, (4) control agency/coping potential, (5) certainty, (6) goal-path obstacle/goal relevance, (7) legitimacy, and (8) responsibility. Various blends of these dimensions can account for similarities and differences between emotions.

For example, Smith and Ellsworth found that both happiness and pride were rated very high on pleasantness and very low on effort. Happiness was also found to differ from pride due to the high standard of personal achievements associated with pride. High personal achievement standards were not emphasized for happiness.

The Theory of Constructed Emotion

The constructive theory of emotions (sometimes referred to as "the conceptual act theory") was developed by Lisa Feldman Barrett, a prolific researcher and neuropsychologist also known for her work on core affect (a blend of pleasure and activation to be discussed below). This theory was partly developed in collaboration with James Russell (e.g., Barrett, 2013, 2016a, 2017a; Barrett & Russell, 2014). The theory of constructed emotion is an ambitious, comprehensive, and holistic attempt to integrate insights from psychological, philosophical, social, and biological knowledge. It incorporates a rich corpus of modern neuroscience and is strongly focused on emotional feelings. The central idea of Barrett's theory is, as the name indicates, that emotions are constructions of the world, not reactions to it. Emotions are built up in the brain and occur when core affect is categorized with knowledge from the conceptual system, and these culture-based interpretations give emotional experiences their specificity (Barrett, 2006). One implication of this view is that emotions are not different from any other concepts, such as colors, trees, or money (Barrett, 2017a, p. 134). In other words, no distinct emotional categories exist, and no prewired neural structures or "biological fingerprints" have evolved to create our emotions. Rather, they are conceptual inventions. "You need an emotion concept in order to experience or perceive the associated emotion. It's a requirement. Without a concept for 'Fear,' you cannot experience fear" (Barrett, 2017a, p. 141).

Barrett argues that fear is absent from the emotional repertoire of some cultures, such as the !Kung people of the Kalahari Desert (Barrett, 2017a, p. 145). But her argument for the claim is surprisingly thin and factually wrong. Barrett's reasoning boils down to a word the !Kung uses to describe a particular feeling associated with ritual events. This word, "kua," is variably translated as awe, fear, or respect (Shostak, 1981, p. 388). Since this kind of fear is different from fear more universally understood, Barrett suggests that !Kung does not feel fear. However, the fact that a word exists in a language to describe a mixed feeling involving fear does not mean that fear cannot occur as a basic emotion among the users of that language. For example, the Norwegian word "ærefrykt" means awe and is composed of two parts: ære (honor/respect) and frykt (fear). This does of course not exclude Norwegians from being able to experience fear as a universal, basic emotion. Neither does the existence of the word "kua" by necessity prevent !Kung from experiencing fear as a basic emotion. In "*Nisa,*" Marjorie Shostak's brilliant !Kung monography, a handful of women tell stories from their lives as gatherers and hunters in the Kalahari desert during the first half of the twentieth century. Reports of experienced fear and worries are certainly not absent in the lives of these women.

One example comes from a woman who had had an extramarital romance and was beaten by her husband until she was "almost dead." Since then, she "had been afraid to have affairs" (Shostak, 1981, p. 19). Shostak writes about a mother who is worried because her son had become ill (p. 46), about a "general !Kung anxiety about their food supply" (p. 49), about a young child who was "so afraid" because her father had left her alone in the bush (p. 52). However, Barrett is silent about these and other instances of (quite understandable) fearful experiences in the lives of the!Kung.

Core Affect

Unlike emotion, core affect is regulated as a preconceptual primitive process: core affect is a "natural kind." The notion of core affect was introduced by Russell and Barrett (Barrett & Russel, 2009; Russell, 2003) and can be defined as "a neurophysiological state consciously accessible as a simple primitive nonreflective feeling most evident in mood and emotion but always available to consciousness. Although one feeling, core affect can be characterized by two pancultural bipolar dimensions: pleasure-displeasure (valence; feeling good versus bad) and activation (arousal; feeling energetic versus enervated)" (Russell & Barrett, 2009, p. 104). One reason why the term "core" is used for this feeling is that it is constantly present in our lives, although we are not always aware of it. The state is "influenced by a very simple form of meaning analysis—whether stimuli or events are helpful or harmful, rewarding or threatening for a given person at a given point in time and whether an active behavioral response is required" (Barrett, 2006, p. 31).

In some respects, core affect is similar to the concept of a spontaneous good-bad evaluations (SGBE), which are central to the humanistic theory of wellbeing. But in contrast to SGBE, core affect also constitutes the foundation of emotion. Core affect interacts dynamically with the construction of emotional categories to generate an emotional concept as it unfolds in concrete situations. We typically think of a category as a class of things that are treated as equivalent, and to categorize something, Barrett explains, "is to determine what it is, why it is, and what to do with it" (Barrett, 2006, p. 27). As we have seen, Barrett also distinguishes between categories that are "natural" and categories that are conceptual. Core affect is a "natural" category, whereas a concept "can be thought of as a collection of mental representations for a category that people draw on during the process of categorization" (Barrett, 2006, p. 27). Here, Barrett says that the structure and meaning of a conceptual category do not come from something that truly exists in the world but rather from our culture, language, and knowledge structures.

Controversies

Barrett offers a wealth of neuroscientific evidence in support of the claim that no natural categories corresponding to basic emotions exist. Many, however, have no direct bearing on the critical hypotheses she has formulated. For example, Adolphs (2017) agrees with much of what Barrett says about the human brain, such that an emotion is "created by multiple spatiotemporal patterns in varying populations of neurons." But it does not follow that these facts can be used as evidence against basic emotions, which is the conclusion that Barrett draws (Adolphs, 2017, p. 33).

Other inferences made by Barrett are also inconclusive. In the first table presented in Barrett (2016b), the author claims that both Lindquist et al. (2012) and Vytal and Hamann (2010), in two meta-analytic studies mentioned above, show that "Different emotion categories cannot be specifically and consistently localized to distinct populations of neurons within a single region of the human brain" (Barrett, 2016b, p. 4). However, this is only true for Lindquist et al. (2012). As previously reported, Vytal and Hamman argue that "the current meta-analysis results indicate that the key elements of basic emotion views are reflected in neural correlates identified by neuroimaging studies" (Vytal & Hamann, 2010, p. 2864).

Similarly, another meta-study was conducted by a group of constructivist researchers. It concluded that the brain activity patterns they analyzed are consistent with the constructionist approach to emotion (Wager et al., 2015). However, these studies did not analyze models of basic emotions and consequently cannot rule out the possibility that these data are also consistent basic emotion approaches (Kragel & LaBar, 2016). Studies that include such models find not only that is the concept of basic emotion compatible with the available data but also that basic emotion models explain the data better than brain-based models excluding basic emotions. Summarizing their own meta-analysis, Kragel and La Bar therefore concluded that the concept of core affect "is not the primary driver of brain activity that distinguishes discrete emotions. Together, these emerging results suggest that patterns of brain activity indicative of affective dimensions such as arousal and valence may not account for a given brain region's contribution to a specific emotion, such as fear" (Kragel & LaBar, 2016, p. 451). Furthermore, the authors claim that "Results from multiple-category decoding studies are incompatible with theories postulating that specific emotions emerge from the neural coding of valence and arousal" (p. 444).

Other examples of Barrett's idiosyncratic way of interpreting data can be mentioned. In Barrett et al. (2019), for example, studies showing similarities in facial expressions among blind and sighted individuals were called into question. The authors draw heavily on a review by Valente et al. (2018), which thoroughly evaluated 21 studies published between 1932 and 2015 that examined the production of facial expressions of emotion by blind people. This review provides evidence that visual experience is not necessary to spontaneously produce adequate facial expressions for basic emotions such as happiness, anger, and fear. These results are presented along with the authors warning about the limitations of at least some of these studies. Valente et al. also noted that several unanswered questions still exist in this paradigm. Nevertheless, the authors conclude that "studies with blind individuals offer compelling evidence for a non-visually learned and universal source for facial expressions" (p. 494). After all, "Seventeen studies provided evidence that blind and sighted individuals spontaneously produce the same pattern of facial expressions, even if some variations can be found, reflecting facial and body movements specific to blindness or differences in intensity and control of emotions in some specific contexts. This suggests that lack of visual experience does not seem to have a major impact when this behavior is generated spontaneously in real emotional contexts. In contrast, eight studies examining voluntary expressions indicate that blind individuals have difficulty posing emotional expressions" (Valente et al., 2018, p. 483).

The studies reviewed by Valente and colleagues provide a long list of evidence in support of the notion of universal elements in the expressions of emotion. They also raise a series of questions about alternative explanations for the documented evidence that remains to be answered. These studies, like all scientific investigations, have a variety of methodological strengths and weaknesses. However, in their summary of the results from the Valente et al.'s study, Barrett et al. (2019) systematically deflated the evidence in favor of universal emotional mechanisms. Jurist (2019) therefore accuses Barrett of mischaracterizing competing emotion research and for depicting it as "a generic, overgeneralized bogeyman" (p. 195).

It is premature to draw strong conclusions about biological categories of emotion-specific patterns, and neither discrete nor dimensional theories can claim the upper hand. Hence, I take Barrett to mischaracterize the current state of affairs when she announces that "the final nails" have been "driven into the classical view's coffin in this era of neuroscience" (Barrett, 2017a, p. 171).

Feelings and Evaluation

There is a distinction between feelings and emotions, but toward the late twentieth century, the separation gradually disappeared in daily parlor and in some parts of the emotion literature (Alston, 1969). For instance, William James famously suggested that feeling IS the emotion (Damasio & Damasio, 2018; James, 1884). But we should not let the distinction between feelings and emotions go, because the two are truly different (Brown, 1994; Dukes et al., 2021; Ellsworth, 1994; Pribram, 2003; Stein & Hernandez, 2007). In contrast to emotions, feelings are always present when awake; there is always something it feels like to be in a conscious state (Nagel, 1974). In the words of Wundt, we never seem to be in a state "entirely free from feeling" (cited in Barrett & Bliss-Moreau, 2009, p. 169). The ubiquitous presence of feelings is one reason why the humanistic theory of wellbeing considers feelings rather than emotions to be the most relevant core element in affective wellbeing.

At a general level, a feeling state reflects what it is like to have a subjective experience (e.g., Frijda, 2007, p. 210). We feel something when we eat a banana or see a red tomato. We can even feel "being me" (Damasio, 1999; Humphrey, 2006; Lambie & Marcel, 2002; Nagel, 1974). Feelings therefore accomplish something extraordinary because they create a sense of self (Damasio, 2010). Feelings inform us about the conditions of our body parts and signal if they are OK or in need of tending. Feelings provide a moment-to-moment report on the state of life inside an organism; therefore, they are "the feeling of what happens" (Damasio, 1999). In addition, feelings convince us that the things that go on are actually happening to *me*. To see how feelings integrate minds and bodies, consider a patient of the neuropsychologist and psychiatrist Karl Pribram. The patient is called Mrs. C, and due to a sudden damage to her right temporal-parietal cortex, Mrs. C could no longer feel her left arm. She "did not feel anything—nothing at all," according to her own record. The lack of internal physical feelings also created a lack of ownership of the arm. It was as the arm did not belong to her. As a consequence, she started to call her arm Alice (Alice does not live here anymore), and interestingly, she developed a strong dislike for the arm: "It does not look like my arm and does not feel like my arm. I think it is ugly, and I wish it would go away" (Pribram, 2003, p. 127).

In the context of evolution, feelings probably began as a "timid conversation between the chemistry of life and the early version of a nervous system within one particular organism" (Damasio, 2021, p. 71). With the development of a central nervous system, feelings evolved to become a very efficient communicator of goodness and badness, and without a word being spoken, "feelings naturally qualify the life process as conducive or not to well-being and flourishing" (Damasio, 2018, p. 12). In other words, feelings operate as signals that provide organisms with experiences of their own life, and they "collect information about the state of life within the organism, and the 'qualities and intensities' that are manifested by feelings constitute valuations of the process of managing life. (…) The robustness of life is felt as 'plenitude' and 'flourishing'; a balanced life process is translated as 'well-being'" (Damasio, 2021, p. 95).

A feeling is not a unidimensional mental state. As we have seen, Allport (1924) proposed long ago that there are at least two introspective aspects of a feeling state: (1) an affective element of pleasantness or unpleasantness and (2) a distinctive quality of the emotion that differentiates it from other emotions of similar pleasantness level (cited in Ruckmick, 1925, pp. 376–377). This distinction was further elaborated by the biologist Michel Cabanac, who suggested that feelings can be decomposed into at least four dimensions (Cabanac, 1992, 2009, 2010). The first dimension is hedonicity or valence. It runs from pleasure to displeasure and evaluates the usefulness of a situation or a stimulus. To be able to prioritize among competing behaviors, a cue is needed to suggest which is the better. Valence is that cue because it tells us *how good* a stimulus is. The second dimension of a feeling state is quality, which identifies the nature of an object as virtually presented in mental space. It tells us *what* a stimulus is and is sometimes referred to as *qualia*. The distinction between valence and quality can be illustrated by eating chocolate in a state of either hunger or satiety. In a hungry state, the chocolate tastes sweet, and eating it feels pleasant (to most of us). In contrast, eating chocolate after you are full no longer feels pleasant, although the taste is still sweet (Small et al., 2001). The third dimension is intensity, which describes the magnitude of a feeling state. It tells us *how important* a stimulus is. The last dimension is duration, which identifies time. It tells us *how long* a stimulus or situation is present. Cabanac's perspective on the elements of feelings, and particularly his work on the pleasure dimension, will be explained in further detail in Chap. 5.

Evaluations

Feelings provide online reports on the state of our lives, and the valence dimension is a judgment of the quality or wellness of that state. Therefore, the pleasantness of a feeling is an evaluation. But it is not the only evaluation in the toolbox of affects. As elaborated in Chap. 1, evaluations come in many forms, and together, they comprise a set of biologically grounded valuation mechanisms (Tesser & Martin, 1996). Evolutionary speaking, the basic value function came first, and feelings and consciousness came later (Montague, 2007, p. 122). Whether conscious or not, the essence of an evaluation is to ask whether an action or condition enhance or threaten an organism. Is the thing happening "for me or against me?" as Locke formulated it (1969, p. 315).

Most neuroscientific models of the mind include an evaluation component. The French neuroscientist Jean-Pierre Changeux has, for instance, developed what he calls a neuronal workspace model of the mind. The model suggests that five major neuronal circuits or modules have evolved to integrate the stream of information processed by the brain. One of these circuits is referred to as the evaluation circuit, and it represents the brain's simplest representation of valuation. According to Denton (2005, p. 191), the evaluation circuit in Changeux's neuronal workspace model is located in parts of the cingulate cortex, hypothalamus, amygdala, and ventral striatum, and it assesses whether the things happening to us are good or bad.

Others have proposed that the brain's evaluation mechanism is multidimensional. Cacioppo and colleagues offer a theory of evaluation based on a three-dimensional evaluative space, referred to as the "evaluative space model" (Cacioppo & Berntson, 1999; Cacioppo et al., 1993; Norris et al., 2010). The model proposes that positive affect operates in a separate evaluative channel, working relatively independently from negative affect. The positive evaluative channel has evolved in our evolutionary past to make us categorize hospitable environments as attractive. In contrast, the negative affective channel is responsive to aversive information processing and has evolved to make us evaluate hostile environments as unattractive. The two separable channels of evaluations enable quick decisions as to whether one should approach or withdraw from an environment or a situation. However, feelings are a separate dimension in the evaluative space model, and they are supposed to arise as an interaction between the positive affect channel and the negative affect channel. All combinations of positive and negative activation are possible in the model, giving rise to a variety of feelings. However, intense PA tends to suppress NA, and vice versa. If something threatening happens to us, activity in the negative evaluative channel intensifies quickly, and this mechanism is referred to as negativity bias. A quick increase in negative intensity is functional since it is critical to obtain clear warnings about threatening situations. However, as a kind of default feeling, we tend to experience mild positive affect (e.g., Biswas-Diener et al., 2005), a tendency that Cacioppo and colleagues referred to as a positivity offset. The distinction between negativity bias and positivity offset can be illustrated with an analogy to the intercept and slope of regression analyses. The slope of the negativity channel is steeper than that of the positivity channel, which illustrates negativity bias. The intercept of the positivity channel is located above that of the negativity channel, which illustrates the positivity bias (Cacioppo et al., 1997).

An alternative multidimensional model of evaluation was developed by Shizgal (1999), who also employs a channel terminology to account for the creation of values in the human mind. But Shizgal's model is not multidimensional in the sense of having one channel for positive evaluations and another for negative evaluations. Rather, it suggests that valuations are determined by an interplay between one evaluative channel and two nonevaluative channels. The first nonevaluative channel is referred to as perceptual and is constructed to inform us about facts in the world. The perceptual channel indicates what and where something is; for instance, it can update us on the temperature or texture of an object. The second nonevaluative channel keeps score of time. The timing channel helps us predict when or how often an object will be available and thus anticipate when the environmental goodness will next be available. Finally, the third channel in Shizgal's model concerns good-bad evaluations. It is this component that informs a cognitive structure about the attractiveness and unattractiveness of the current physiological state of its owner. It operates without presumption of objective preciseness but provides the perceived facts with intrinsic worth. The good-bad message broadcasted by the evaluative channel might not be conscious, but when it is, we experience it as pleasure or displeasure. Together, the "output of these channels is recorded in multidimensional records that include information of perceptual origin about amount and kind (for example, food, water, or salt), information from the timer about rate and delay, and a subjective assessment of intensity provided by the evaluative channel" (Shizgal, 1999, p. 502).

An important message from Shizgal's model is that a good-bad evaluation is not enough to make a valuation mechanism efficient. Timing is also important. The distribution, or frequency, of "pleasure bursts" (the signals from the evaluation channel) is essential in determining what is important to us. This can be demonstrated in experiments with rats, showing how they change between maximizing "pleasure" and spreading the "pleasure bursts" out in time. These studies show that preferences are based not only on the information distributed by the evaluation channel but also on the rate, delay, and even the kind of stimulus that provides the "pleasure." Multiple coding dimensions are therefore required to capture information about the value of a stimulus. "If only a single dimension were available, then changes in quality would be indistinguishable from changes in intensity" (Shizgal, 1999, p. 513). The finding that the type of stimulus affects the valuation mechanism is essential because it demonstrates that the perceptual channel—signals about what and where something is—affects the valuation process over and above the mere good-bad evaluation. This principle is significant for the humanistic theory of well-being, as will be further detailed in Chap. 7.

A somewhat similar conclusion is drawn by Rangel et al. (2008), who suggest that several valuation systems exist in the brain. For instance, action values are different from outcome valuation, a view that is consistent with the distinction between wanting and liking, which will be discussed in Chap. 5. Briefly, the distinction is that wanting represents the motivational aspect of a "pleasure cycle" and is basically driven by dopaminergic networks in the mesolimbic system in the brain. Liking refers to the hedonic experience of pleasure associated with the consumption of a reward and is anchored in a small set of opioid-regulated "hedonic hotspots" located in the orbitofrontal cortex (OFC), insula, ventral pallidum, and nucleus accumbens (e.g., Kringelbach & Berridge, 2017). This dynamic is beautifully summarized in the title of Barbano and Cador's article "Opioids for hedonic experience and dopamine to get ready for it" (Barbano & Cador, 2007).

Happiness as an Emotion

Chap. 2 showed that the word happiness has many meanings and that one of them is emotional. For example, if people are asked to mention some emotions, happiness is among the first they bring up (Fehr & Russell, 1984; Shaver et al., 1987). When asked which emotion people wish to have for themselves or for their children, most choose happiness (Averill & More, 2000). Children start to use the word happy from about 2 years of age, and at 3, they are able to correctly recognize expressions of happiness almost at the adult level, at least in WEIRD[4] regions of the world (Widen, 2016). Happiness, or a synonym, is also on all the lists of basic emotions. Hence, it seems clear that happiness can refer to a particular emotion.

Describing Emotional Happiness

To better understand what emotional happiness is, it would have been useful to get a good description of what that emotion feels like. After all, the success of science is partly due to the detailed descriptions offered in the process of developing theories (e.g., Craver & Darden, 2013; Haig, 2005; Kagan, 2002; Shapere, 1976). Darwin's theory of evolution, Watson and Crick's theory of the structure of DNA, and Chomsky's theory of syntax are examples of important work that have been based on careful descriptions without any experiments and hypothesis testing

[4]The acronym WEIRD stands for Western, Educated, Industrialized, Rich, and Democratic (Henrich et al., 2010).

involved (Rozin, 2009). Even phenomena as elusive as emotions and feelings require a description of content, i.e., what they feel like, to obtain the pieces in place (e.g., Searle, 2004). However, the task of collecting descriptions of happiness encounters several challenges since both scientific and folk conceptions of happiness vary widely.

For example, Ekman (2003) operates with a dozen or so different kinds of happiness or enjoyment as he also calls it. Taking a yet broader perspective, Lomas (2018) has uncovered 130 unique terms for happiness, and his analysis clearly illustrates that even in the limited sense of being an emotion, happiness cannot escape the curse of the jingle and jangle fallacies. A look at the many ways in which people describe what it feels like to be happy illustrates the problem.

At a general level, it has been argued that happiness[5] roughly corresponds to a positive feeling about a good thing (Ortony et al., 2005). It has, for instance, been observed that happiness typically follows from situations in which something has been achieved or episodes with a desirable outcome. A study by Shaver et al. (1987) reported that 68% of the participants mentioned achievement and desirable outcomes as important sources of happiness. Approximately 40% mentioned that receiving esteem, respect, or praise was a frequent cause of happiness. When asked about their thinking during episodes of happiness, half of the participants reported having a positive outlook and seeing the bright side as a typical mode of thought. Finally, 23% noted that they felt excitement during episodes of happiness, whereas smiling (58%) and hugging (30%) were the most typical expressions of happiness. Another investigation revealed that relations with friends was the most frequent context for which people reported being happy (Scherer, 1986). In that study, almost 40% of all the descriptions of joy and happiness were related to social encounters, which, together with the categories "successful experiences" and "natural experiences," accounted for 62% of all the reported antecedents of joy and happiness.

An examination of the causes and feelings of happiness reported by adolescents (high school students) was provided by Magen (1998). She reports answers such as "The best experience I had in my life was when I stopped smoking marijuana" (p. 74), "One experience that gave me a good feeling was when I did my piano recital" (p. 77), "The best thing that ever happened to me was when I moved from Orlando to Keystone" (p. 80), or "The best experience I ever had was when I was given my first hunting rifle from my parents" (p. 83). Another study asked almost 800 university students from 8 European countries about their experiences of being happy or joyful (Summerfield & Green, 1986). The answers were typically quite short, such as "A guy was present, we were lying on the beach, sunbathing, taking photographs, and saying nice things to each other." Another, even briefer account, was "We talked, laughed, ate, made love, slept" (p. 54). These descriptions are not so different from one that Darwin noticed while observing a 4-year-old girl playing with her peers. The little girl explained to her friends that the secret of happiness is nothing but "laughing, talking, and kissing" (Darwin, 1872, Chap. VIII). Darwin

[5] For simplicity, I'll have the term happiness stand for emotional happiness in this section.

remarked that it would be difficult to give a truer and more practical definition of happiness.

A more careful and introspective investigation of happiness was conducted by Marion Milner, who graduated as a psychologist from the University College in London in 1924. Ten years later, she published *A Life of One's Own*, a remarkable book printed under the pen name of Joanna Field (Field, 1981/1934). Milner's project started when she realized that her "life was not as it ought to be, although from an external viewpoint it was going very well" (p. 173). She therefore decided to map out "the facts of her life" and started in 1926 to keep a diary and to write down "the best thing that had happened during the day." Over the next 7 years, she continued writing down "each day's catch of happiness" (p. 152) and gradually came to realize that happiness came when she was most widely aware of the things that happened around her. Milner noted that "in certain moods the very simplest things, even the glint of electric light on the water in my bath, gave me the most intense delight" (p. 46). Following up on these observations, Milner recognized that happiness was not so much about having success in life. What made her happy "were mostly very small moments of a total change in the way I was perceiving both the outer world and myself" (p. 174). These moments often occurred when she stood aside and looked at her own experience with a wide focus, "wanting nothing and prepared for anything" (Field, 1981/1934, p. 157).

Written in a different key, Davitz (1969) authored a report from a study of 556 US citizens who were asked to describe what happiness felt like for them. The most common response was that happiness consisted of an inner warm glow, a sense of peace and harmony, and warm excitement. Approximately 40% of the sample also recalled that happy feelings involved a sense of accomplishment or fulfillment. A more recent study, Mogilner et al. (2011) reported an age effect in happiness descriptions. Based on 12 million web blogs, Mogilner found that younger people primarily associated happiness with excitement, whereas older people connected happiness with feeling peaceful.

Another narrative about a happy feeling goes like this: "I rolled out of the station with five twenties in my wallet. I was heady with happiness. Since I hadn't yet had my first taste of alcohol, I couldn't compare the feeling to a champagne high, say, but it was the most delightful sensation I'd ever experienced in the front seat of a car. In fact, my cleverness overwhelmed me" (Frank Abagnale, cited in Ruedy et al., 2013, p. 531). What is special with this story is that Abagnale had stolen the money. His pleasure is an example of a so-called cheater's high, i.e., a feeling generated from successfully deceiving others,[6] which reminds us that happy feelings do not necessarily come from morally acceptable conduct.

The above descriptions are from everyday situations (with the report from Abagnale as, hopefully, an exception) and are quite straightforwardly formulated. Other descriptions are less mundane. For instance, the French philosopher Robert

[6] Frank Abagnale is a swindler made famous in the movie *Catch Me If You Can* (Abagnale & Redding, 2000). Wikipedia presents him as an author and conceited felon (https://en.wikipedia.org/wiki/Frank_Abagnale)

Misrahi (1994) has reflected deeply on the feeling of happiness and finds it to be "a radiation of joy over one's existence or over the most vibrant part of one's active past, one's actual present, and one's conceivable future" (cited in Ricard, 2007, p. 18). Matthieu Ricard, a well-known Buddhist and scientist who has been characterized as "the happiest person ever to have existed" (Flanagan, 2007, p. 160), describes happiness as "a deep sense of flourishing that arises from an exceptionally healthy mind. This is not a mere pleasurable feeling, a fleeting emotion, or a mood, but an optimal state of being" (Ricard, 2007, p. 19). Another French writer, Henri Lavedan, described his happiness with the same kind of amazement and sublimity but not as exceptionally healthy as Richard. In my life, Lavedan tells us, "there was nothing missing which is proper to a happy life—even suffering." The quote appears in the work of Wladyslaw Tatarkiewicz, a Polish philosopher and historian well known for his insightful investigations of happiness. Tatarkiewicz noted that Lavedan's life was "not a succession of triumphs nor uninterrupted delight nor excellence; it was the kind of life which brings satisfaction to the man who has lived it" (Tatarkiewicz, 1976, p. 6).

Misrahi and Richard portray happiness as a kind of permanent, almost perfect kind of experience. They are telling us what an ideal life feels like, the sort of happiness that Annas (1993) refers to as a complete life. As such, their descriptions transcend the boundary of emotional happiness. But even if we return to descriptions of happiness as temporary and brief emotional experiences, such as the "laughing, talking, and kissing" kind of happiness that Darwin mentioned, shorter bursts of happiness need not be ordinary. They can be breathtaking and intensely powerful—even decisive. One such example is articulated by Jill Bolte Taylor (2008), whose experiences of being hit by a stroke were briefly introduced in Chap. 1. In more details, Taylor's story began when she woke up in her home in Harvard, USA, on the morning of December 10, 1996, when she was distressed by a sharp pain behind her left eye. Executing her morning routines, she experienced a gradual and strange detachment from her normal cognitive functions. As a neuroscientist, Taylor could notice the details of the changes occurring in her two hemispheres of her brain, as she horrified realized that she was having a massive hemorrhagic stroke. The shocking experience felt "as if the integrity of my mind/body connection had somehow become compromised" (p. 38). Here is a synopsis of her experiences that morning:

> I felt like a genie liberated from its bottle. The energy of my spirit seemed to flow like a great whale gliding through a sea of silent euphoria. Finer than the finest of pleasures we can experience as physical beings, this absence of physical boundary was one of glorious bliss. As my consciousness dwelled in a flow of sweet tranquility, it was obvious to me that I would never be able to squeeze the enormousness of my spirit back inside the tiny cellular matrix. (Taylor, 2008, p. 67)

Notably, Taylor's feeling of extreme pleasure came at the cost of a loss of control of her left hemisphere. As the ultra-intense pleasure took hold of her mind, Taylor lost the sense of being an individual self with goals and plans that otherwise were experienced as so important to her.

> I had spent a lifetime of 37 years being enthusiastically committed to 'do-do-doing' lots of stuff at a very fast pace. On this special day, I learned the meaning of simply 'being'. When I lost my left hemisphere and its language centers, I also lost the clock that would break my moments into consecutive brief instances. Instead of having my moments prematurely stunted, they became open-ended, and I felt no rush to do anything. Like walking along the beach or just hanging out in the beauty of nature, I shifted from the doing-consciousness of my left brain to the being-consciousness of my right brain. I morphed from feeling small and isolated to feeling enormous and expansive. Stopped thinking in language and shifted to taking new pictures of what was going on in the present moment I was not capable of deliberating about past or future-related ideas because those cells were incapacitated. All I could perceive was right here, right now, and it was beautiful. (Taylor 2008, pp. 68–71)

A less dramatic version of a comparable feeling state comes from Erika Leslie, who tells the story of the most profound moments in her life. Leslie is a Norwegian botanist who has spent long periods doing field work in a high mountain area in the southern part of Norway named Finse. During one of her excursions, she had an extraordinarily powerful experience, one that was so strong that she initially decided not to tell anyone about it. However, the feeling continued to return to her, and after 2 years, she disclosed it to her colleague and close friend. The colleague persuades her to publish it as part of an article on the importance of nature and nature experiences. Here is what happened to Erika.

> It had been a fine day. Smells of soil and sun-warmed reindeer lichens surround me. The scenery is beautiful, and there is a sudden tranquility within me and around me. As I sit like this and contemplate the landscape, I register that the internal silence becomes complete. The sense of time disappears. I am just present in the moment, and getting a feeling of eternity I did not realize was possible; a timeless NOW. I feel one with the nature around me—like being a part of a greater wholeness. How long do I sit like this? I don't know—it feels irrelevant. It is one long continuous moment, but at the same time with a strong feeling of being a part of the universe and eternity. (Andersen, 2010, pp. 64, in my translation from Norwegian)

Maslow (1964) would probably refer to the feelings reported by Taylor and Andersen as a peak experience or an oceanic experience. Csikszentmihalyi (1975) would have called them deep flow, while others, such as Keltner (2023), would call them awe. Over the years, the literature has presented many descriptions of how the peak/flow/awe can be experienced, often related to being in nature or as a spiritual epiphany. An early record of such an intense feeling appeared in the twelfth century, when the medieval bishop Isaac of Syria was credited for describing the following peak moment experienced during an episode of reading: "As in a dream, I enter a state when my senses and thoughts are concentrated. Then, when with prolonging of this silence the turmoil of memories is stilled in my heart, ceaseless waves of joy are sent me by inner thoughts, beyond expectation suddenly arising to delight my heart" (cited in Carr, 2010, loc. 1139). Such peak experiences are not as uncommon as one might think, and Richardson (1999) explains that between 28% and 35% of survey participants typically report having had a peak experience at least once in their lives. In one of Richardson's own studies, he quotes the response from a 58-year-old participant to give us an idea of the feeling state in question: "Suddenly I became aware of a blinding light, felt lifted and transported above all problems, conscious of being in contact with the source of all wisdom, aware of the oneness of everything and experiencing a great feeling of relief, joy and a sense of love. The overriding feeling was of having found the truth" (Richardson, 1999, p. 479).

Examples from Fiction

Some writers are better at lining out what emotional states feel like than others, and the refined penmanship of fiction writers can probably teach us a lesson or two about the phenomenological aspects of happiness. Moreover, reading fiction can by itself prompt intense positive feelings (e.g., Nell, 1988). Oatley suggests that fiction can mentally simulate the experiences of the characters in the story, and this simulation activates in our minds the same emotional feeling that we may have in real life (Oatley, 2011, 2012). Fiction further treats themes of psychological importance and can ignite a reflective mode, a way of exploring ideas that stretches beyond the immediate appearance of things. Oatley has advocated that fiction is a model that enables us to see others and ourselves more clearly. Fiction does not claim declarations about the truth; rather, it offers suggestions about how things may fit together (Oatley, 2011). As such, fictional descriptions of happiness may teach us about what a happy feeling could be.

In *Anna Karenina*, Tolstoy provides an intriguing portrayal of a happy moment for Konstantine Levine, one of the main characters in the play. Levine is a farm owner who lives a simple and meaningful life close to the land. This is a lifestyle that Tolstoy, as will be discussed in Chap. 5, found valuable. One morning, when Levine joined the men at harvest to exercise his mowing skills, he entered a state of intense happiness:

> Levine lost all awareness of time and could not have said whether it was late or early now. A change was beginning to come about in his work now that afforded him tremendous pleasure. In the middle of his work moments came over him when he forgot what he was doing and it came easy for him, and during those very minutes his row came out almost as evenly and well as Titus's. However, as soon as he remembered what he was doing and started trying to do better, he immediately felt just how difficult his labor was and the row came out badly. (…) More and more often now came those moments of unconsciousness, when it was possible not to think of what one was doing. The scythe cut by itself. These were happy moments. (Tolstoy, 2014, pp. 231–232)

The feeling of being happy when cut off from the world is a reoccurring issue in fiction. The most famous example is perhaps the celebrated "madeleine moment" in Proust's monumental *Remembrance of Things Past*. Proust writes:

> No sooner had the warm liquid mixed with crumbs touched my palate, than a shudder ran through me, and I stopped, intent upon the extraordinary thing that was happening to me. An exquisite pleasure had invaded my senses, something isolated, detached, with no suggestion of its origin. And at once the vicissitudes of life had become indifferent to me, its disasters innocuous, its brevity illusory – this new sensation having had on me the effect which love has of filling me with a precious essence; or rather this essence was not in me, it was me. (Proust, 1981, p. 48)

The quietness and tranquility narrated in these stories are quite typical of how happiness is described in fiction. Quennell (1988) argues, for instance, that happy moments are typically expressed in novels as resulting either from the quiet enjoyment of some activity or from being together with a loved one. The social element of happiness is well recognized in the scientific literature on wellbeing, whereas in the tranquility part the quiet enjoyment of practicing an activity is less noticeable, although it is not absent (e.g., Haybron, 2008; Lomas, 2021; Vittersø, 2018). However, the extremely intense happiness described as a brief moment by Leslie in Finse, or more permanent in Misrahi's "radiation of joy over one's entire existence," is hardly what the scientific study of wellbeing examines. When Veenhoven defines happiness as a favorable judgment of "the overall quality of one' life-as-a-whole" (Veenhoven, 1984, p. 22) or when Kahneman's fictive character Helen is happy whenever she is "spending time engaged in activities that she would rather have continued than stopped" (Kahneman, 1999, p. 7), the talk is not about Taylor's glide "through a sea of silent euphoria," or Ricard's "deep sense of flourishing that arises from an exceptionally healthy mind."

Happiness as a Basic Emotion

Science aims at explaining the observations we make about the world. To develop a theory of emotions, we thus need to answer questions such as why we have them and how they are assembled. As previously reviewed, one approach to the science of emotion has focused on the notion of basicness. Darwin (e.g., 1872), the intellectual godfather of basic emotions, had happiness on his list of discrete emotions, and all the subsequent basic emotion theories followed Darwin's example here (Keltner, 2009). More precisely, they all listed at least one positive emotion as basic in their respective taxonomies. For example, Tomkins (1962) uses the term enjoyment-joy to name happiness, while others prefer joy[7] (Izard, 1977, 2007) or play (Panksepp, 1998a).

Silvan Tomkins was a basic emotion pioneer who maintained that the smile was an essential element of happiness (or enjoyment-joy in his terminology). Tomkins fathered the facial feedback hypothesis, i.e., the proposal that the activation of certain muscles in the face and the blood flow resulting from these movements can cause or intensify emotions. Facial expressions of emotions were of general importance in his thinking, and when it came to happiness, it was the smile that engaged Tomkins. The "pen-in-the-mouth" research paradigm, in which study participants hold a pen between their teeth to form a smile and presumably then feel happier, grew out of Tomkin's theory. Smiling is also significant in his theory because it facilitates social interaction and social bonding. Another important factor relates to

[7] More recently, Izard (2011) also uses a combination of enjoyment, happiness, and contentment to label the happiness-kind of basic positive emotion in his taxonomy.

the effect smiling has in terms of broadening the spectrum of objects and activities that human beings can enjoy. This effect was subsequently observed empirically by Isen and Daubman (1984).

Happiness as Understood by the "Ekman Group"

Paul Ekman, one of Tomkins' PhD students, has included happiness as one of the "Ekman Six," i.e., the six basic emotions in his theory. Ekman describes happiness as a feeling that is enjoyed and sought by the person experiencing it (Ekman & Cordaro, 2011, p. 365). Like many emotion psychologists, Ekman did not pay much attention to happiness in his early research. But that should change, and Ekman has become more reflective on the issue later in his career.

Ekman uses happiness, or his preferred term enjoyment, in an overarching manner to represent a list of the so-called enjoyable emotions (e.g., Ekman, 2003). One of his lists comprises ten positive, basic emotions: sensory pleasures, amusement, relief, excitement, wonder, ecstasy, rejoicing, and three non-English terms,: fiero, naches, and schadenfreude. The three non-English words are explained as follows: The Italian fiero is a kind of ecstasy that occurs when a challenge has been well overcome. It is more than satisfaction and pride because the accomplishment achieved is very difficult, and the consequent feeling is quite unique. Naches is Yiddish and refers to the "glow of pleasure-plus-pride only a child can give to its parents" (Ekman, 2003, p. 197). German schadenfreude is known to most English speakers as the enjoyment one may feel if someone else has suffered.

Another of Ekman's lists operates with more than a dozen positive emotions. As an extension of the sensory pleasure category, Ekman noted that five different kinds of sensory pleasures should be treated in addition to distinct emotions, one for each sense quality. Thus, visual, tactile, olfactory, auditory, and gustatory pleasures are all examples of basic emotions, and together with the initial 11 happiness emotions on his first list, Ekman ends up with a happiness taxonomy that includes 16 positive emotions. They are all different from each other, and each is triggered by different events, involving different signals and behaviors. Ekman regrets, however, that all these emotions are referred to as happiness. In a recorded conversation with The Dalai Lama, he admits that "if I could have my way, we would get rid of it [the term happiness] from the English language, because it covers so many different things at so many levels."[8]

Others in the so-called Ekman group prefer the term positive emotion over happiness. Keltner and Cowen (2021) identified 11 exemplars of what they name positive basic emotions. The 11 emotions are amusement, awe, compassion, contentment, desire, love, joy, interest, pride, relief, and triumph. A newer version of this view has included 20 positive emotions as basic emotions (Keltner & Oatley, 2022). Shiota et al. (2017) argue that positive emotions "are best described as branches of a

[8] https://www.eiagroup.com/video/types-of-happiness/

"family tree" emerging from a common ancestor mediating adaptive management of fitness-critical resources." The authors maintain that we can no longer assume that all positive emotions have identical response profiles or effects upon motivation and cognition and prefer to define positive emotions "in terms of a common aspect of adaptive function: to facilitate effective management of and response to opportunities, presented by the current environment, to acquire material, social, and/or informational resources that are crucial for promoting fitness" (Shiota et al., 2017, p. 625). More recently, Shiota et al. (2021) have suggested that positive affect and emotion can be organized around three central concepts: "subjectively pleasant affect; approach or appetitive motivation; and emotion states evoked by opportunities and rewards in the environment." The authors label these three groups as positive affect, approach motivation, and positive emotion, respectively.

The Communicative Theory

A previous section established that the communicative theory of emotions is grounded in the idea that "emotions occur at the junctures of plans, when a goal or a plan needs to be reevaluated, perhaps because everything has not fitted together" (Oatley, 1992, p. 348). According to Oatley and Johnson-Laird's theory, most emotions occur when an action tendency is arrested or when a goal unexpectedly becomes urgent and disrupts an ongoing behavior. Happiness seems to be an exception, however, since it occurs when plans run smoothly. Within this framework, happiness is conceptualized as a basic emotion that

> occurs when a goal is achieved and even more frequently when a plan is progressing well, when subgoals are being achieved, and when the probability of a main goal being achieved is increased. Enjoyment occurs where some overall goal is important, as with being in love. It also occurs where there is no pressing overall goal, in states where the mind is listening to music, in creative activities, in play, or when social participation is more important than any end result. Being happy requires that there be no distressing reevaluations, but rather the easy incorporation of new elements into the activity. Enjoyment is therefore less usually the final achievement of a main goal than engagement in what one is doing and the reaching of small subgoals using available resources. (Oatley, 1992, p. 48)

Happiness is also a social emotion, typically fostered by people who are engaged in planning or reaching common goals together. Hence, just as emotions configure an individual's cognitive system, they also structure social relationships. When we are wholeheartedly engaged in what we are doing, by ourselves or with someone else, the characteristic mental tone that identifies happiness occurs. In the capacity to be a basic emotion, the emotional feeling of happiness is, according to Oatley and Johnson-Laird, irreducible and felt separately from pleasure and arousal.

In contrast to some views (e.g., Carver et al., 2014), the communicative theory does not consider happiness a "stopping signal," a notion to be further elaborated below. Rather than ending an activity, happiness is an emotion that stimulates engagement in executing a current plan, to secure the encouragement needed to accomplish work and reach the end of the plan. "According to our formulation, people usually stop not because of a happy emotion but because a goal is reached or an interruption occurs" (Oatley & Johnson-Laird, 1996, p. 366).

Having fun can illustrate how the mechanisms proposed by Oatley and Johnson-Laird's theory work for emotional happiness. Referring to Goffman's essay "Fun in Games" (Goffman, 1961), Oatley points out that it is easier to integrate plans and (sub)goals and have them run smoothly when we play a game with clear rules. Within this framework, we know how to act, what others expect from us, and we understand what is going on. To further enhance engagement in the activity, Goffman introduced the idea that games typically unfold within a "semipermeable membrane." The membrane encloses the game and sets it off from the rest of the world; once inside it, "a distinctive microworld is ordered according to its own rules" (Oatley, 1992, p. 354).

Games are social, and being together is a prototype source of happiness. Social happiness comes in many stripes, but love is particularly intense. Falling in love is usually rated as the strongest source of positive emotions (Argyle, 2001, p. 77). In the early stages of a romantic relation, we not only feel intensely well by just being together with our partner but also engage in making mutual plans, daydreaming about the future, and creating fantasies about a perfect life together. A love relation can grow and expand in ways that fit the template of a plan that is progressing well. More poetically, deep love fills us with "a precious essence" (Proust, 1981, p. 48). Another touching portrayal of a mature love relationship can be read in Tim Russert's bestseller, *Wisdom of Our Fathers* (Russert, 2007). The book is composed of letters from daughters and sons written about their fathers, and one woman writes that shortly after her parents' retirement, her mother became ill and was bedridden for more than a year before she passed away. Her husband spent every day with her until her death. Once she said to him, "I'm so sorry about this, I know we had so many plans for the rest of our life that we won't be able to enjoy now." "What do you mean," he replied. "There's nothing to regret. All I want to do is to be in the same room with you" (cited in Richardson, 2012, p. 27).

Some rejects the idea that romantic love is universal. For instance, it has been proposed that romantic love is a Western and relatively recent invention, dated to 1274 and Dante's autobiographical *La Vita Nuova*, in which Dante falls in love with Beatrice (Johnson-Laird & Oatley, 2000, p. 460). To avoid confusions with the possible nonuniversal nature of romantic love, the communicative theory of emotions refers to the concept of sexual love as a universal and basic emotion, in addition to two other kinds of love, namely, parental love and love for caregivers.

Happiness According to Appraisal Theories

Frijda (2007) is among those who conceptualize happiness within the framework of appraisal theories, articulated as an individual's evaluation of the satisfaction or obstruction of his or her concerns, or "everything we care about," as Frankfurt (1982) calls it. More worldly, Benditt (1974) writes that "to say that happiness-judgments are appraisals amounts to saying that there are certain criteria in accordance with which people are evaluated in respect of their happiness, that these criteria have to do with the conditions and circumstances of a person's life, and that whatever person satisfies these criteria to a high degree is a happy one" (p. 6). Appraisal theorists Stein, Trabasso, and Liwang claim that happiness is the experience of having what one cares to have (Stein et al., 2000, p. 440). In support of this perspective, Lazarus (1991b, 2001) claims that happiness comes from gaining what we desire. More precisely, he maintains that "happiness occurs when we think we are making reasonable progress toward the realization of our goal" (Lazarus, 2001, p. 267). Lazarus assumes that happiness occurs during an activity, while the experiencer has not yet completed a goal but is about to do so.

Other appraisal theorists, such as Smith and Ellsworth (1985), put more emphasis on the rewarding aspect of happiness. To them, happiness is typically experienced after an activity has terminated. As we have seen in the "Emotion" section, Smith and Ellsworth characterize happiness as an emotion that is high in pleasantness and low in effort. Their 1985 study further reported that happiness involves a high level of certainty about the situation and a strong desire to pay attention. It is also frequently observed in social situations, such as being reunited with close friends or relatives after a long absence, being at a party with friends, or going out on a pleasant date (Smith & Ellsworth, 1985, pp. 831–832).

In later work, Smith and colleagues suggested that happiness, together with pride and gratitude, is a so-called benefit-related emotion. This class of positive emotions is beneficial because it is associated with the appraisal of one's circumstances as being relevant and desired. In terms of motivation, happiness prompts an urge to celebrate or savor good moments, which also implies that people in a happy state are not particularly motivated to "persevere in achieving a pending goal. (…) Rather, happiness is evoked by the successful attainment of a goal" (Smith et al., 2014, p. 18). A functional consequence of this celebrating/savoring aspect of happiness is that happiness helps reinforce the efforts that lead to success. The authors argue that if successful behavior is rewarded by strong feelings of happiness, these behaviors are more likely to be repeated in the future.

Happiness as a Constructed Emotion

According to Barrett's constructivist account, people experience an emotion when they conceptualize an instance of affective feeling, which is to say that core affect and conceptualizations of emotion together constitute an emotion (e.g., Barrett, 2006). Hence, it is cultural learning and language that give happiness its specificity. This experience is generated in consistence with Whorf's (1956) strong version of linguistic relativity, which states that language forms the basis of experience (Barrett, 2006, p. 37). Thus, there is no distinct happiness feeling, no specific action readiness, and no particular physiology to characterize happiness. No particular function or evolutionary benefit can be associated with emotional happiness in particular. Even smiles are only associated with happiness through a process of prediction and simulation (e.g., Wager et al., 2015). Ignoring a rich body of historical, cross-cultural, and functional evidence about smiling (e.g., De Waal, 2019; Ekman, 2003), Barrett believes that "smiling was an invention of the Middle Ages, and broad, toothy-mouthed smiles (with crinkling at the eyes, aka the Duchenne smile) became popular only in the eighteenth century as dentistry became more accessible and affordable" (Barrett, 2017a, p. 51).

Barrett argues that happiness is a cultural construction and that it varies too much to constitute something universal:

> You can smile in happiness, sob in happiness, scream in happiness, raise your arms in happiness, clench your fists in happiness, jump up and down doling out high fives in happiness, or even be stunned motionless in happiness. Your eyes might be wide or narrowed; your breathing rapid or slow. You can have the heart-pounding, exciting happiness of winning the lottery or the calm, relaxed happiness of lying on a picnic blanket with your lover. You've also perceived many other people as happy in various ways. Altogether, this motley assortment of experiences and perceptions can involve different actions and inner-body changes, they may feel affectively different, and they can include different sights, sounds, and smells. (Barrett, 2017a, p. 92)

The constructive theory suggests that the concept of happiness is a collection of situated conceptualizations that "guide the emotion categorization process in a flexible and situationally sensitive manner" (Barrett, 2006, p. 33). Barrett presents the following though experiment to give us an idea of how this works: "In the past, you have experienced diverse instances of happiness, may be lying outdoors on a sunny day, finishing a strenuous workout, hugging a close friend, eating a piece of delectable chocolate or winning a competition. Each instance is different from every other, and when the brain creates a concept of happiness to categorize and make sense of the upcoming sensory events, it constructs a population of simulations (as potential actions and perceptions) according to the rules of Bayes' Theorem, whose priors reflect their similarity to the current situation (before the evidence is taken into account). The similarity needs not be perceptual—it can be goal-based. Therefore, the brain constructs an on-line concept of happiness, not in absolute terms but with reference to a particular goal in the situation (to be with friends, to enjoy a meal, to accomplish a task), all in the service of allostasis. This implies that 'happiness' has a specific meaning, but its specific meaning changes from one instance to the next" (Barrett, 2017b, pp. 9–11).

A happy feeling also varies in its amount of pleasure and arousal. It is often high in pleasure but can also be unpleasant. Happiness can also be high or low in arousal. For example, the proud happiness one can experience from the successful performance of a challenging piano concert in front of an audience would be high in both pleasure and arousal. Wishing to share this good experience with a friend, just to find out that she is unavailable produces a low-pleasure kind of happiness (Wilson-Mendenhall et al., 2013). This study provides several examples of how levels of pleasure and arousal can vary in experiences described as happy. However, in all the scenarios, happiness can never be experienced as anything but as valence and arousal. Based on this study, therefore, the possibility that happiness can have a unique feeling quality that unites it over and above core affect was not investigated and therefore cannot be ruled out.

The kind of happiness Barrett does not consider is one that includes a qualia dimension. A phenomenological quality that is distinguishable from valence and arousal. The analogy is that just like sweetness can be experienced as a feeling quality separate from its pleasantness, a happiness quality can also be experienced as distinct from its pleasantness. An equivalent to the chocolate example mentioned in the "Feeling and Evaluation" section, in which sweetness and pleasantness were demonstrated to be separable feeling dimensions, could be the kind of happiness experienced by a mountaineer who finally achieves the goal of the climb. It is conceivable that the mountaineer, after a long and strenuous ascent, reaches the summit completely exhausted and tormented by pain and austere unpleasantness—yet feeling happy about the achievement. The happiness comes from the goal attainment and can be identified as something distinct from the unpleasantness, which results from being exhausted.

The Functions of Emotional Happiness

Emotions are functional. They help us deal with situations in which all the consequences of our actions cannot be fully foreseen (Oatley, 1992, p. 24). They also play important roles as motivators (e.g., Damasio, 2018; Laming, 2000). In this framework, it is commonly assumed that happiness has evolved from a more primitive approach response and that it is associated with an open and expansive orientation (Green et al., 2003; Lang & Bradley, 2013; Plutchik, 1980). Readers who are familiar with the broaden-and-build theory will recognize these aspects in Fredrickson's work. But happiness can also serve other functions. Tomkins (1962) proposed, for instance, that one of the consequences of happiness is that it reduces the effect of negative emotions. Subsequent research has confirmed this assumption (Fredrickson et al., 2000; Moskowitz et al., 2014). Tomkins also forestalled later research with his idea about the rewarding and savoring effects of happiness (Bryant & Veroff, 2006; Ellsworth & Smith, 1988). For example, Lewis (2016, p. 286) reported that when infants as young as 2 months old pulled a string that caused a picture to appear, they showed clear signs of happiness. They associate, in other words, happiness with learning that their action causes something to happen.

At this general level, happiness also enables the formation and negotiation of relationships. Tomasello's theory of human development and morality, briefly presented in Chap. 1, demonstrates how we critically depend on cooperation to do things that we cannot manage alone. In the capacity to be a social emotion, happiness therefore relates to social goals. Being happy is, for instance, likely to elicit cooperation with others (Keltner & Oatley, 2022). Conversely, studies repeatedly show that being social is the kind of context that most frequently elicits emotional happiness (Shaver et al., 1987). In a diary study reported by Duncan and Grazzani-Gavazzi (2004), an average of 42% of the reported episodes of positive emotions occurred in social interactions, whereas 23% of positive emotions occurred when the participants were alone. Self-reported happiness has further been shown to be strongly correlated with time spent with other people (e.g., Cai et al., 2017; Diener et al., 2018; Fredrickson et al., 2008; Hudson et al., 2020; Kahneman et al., 2004).

Distinguishing Kinds of Happiness

Taken broadly, like Ekman does, emotional happiness is an overarching grab-bag concept analogous to that of positive emotions or positive affect. As an alternative, many researchers prefer to use terms such as positive affect or positive emotions, not happiness, as the overarching grab-bag term referring to all the affects considered to be positive. In such a taxonomy, happiness is a kind of positive emotion. But even within this more limited meaning, conceptual disagreements exist about happiness. For example, happiness may be considered a high aroused "go" emotion or, alternatively, as a low aroused "stop" emotion.

Oatley and Johnson-Laird defend the first position, whereas Smith and Ellsworth favor the latter. It was mentioned above that Smith et al. (2014) categorize happiness as a benefit-related emotions. In the same paper, Smith and coauthors group another set of positive emotions into a category named opportunity emotions. Emotions such as interest, challenge/determination, and hope are classified as opportunity emotions because they provide a fundamental basis for learning.

The humanistic theory of wellbeing follows Smith et al. (2014) in this dichotomization of positive emotions and also places happiness in the first, low aroused, category. But the HTW favors the name harmony feelings over benefit-related emotions, partly due to its preference for analyzing feelings rather than emotions in the framework of wellbeing but also because the term benefit applies to a much broader set of emotions. Most emotions are beneficial in some sense. In the HTW, the term harmony feelings is used synonymously with the term hedonic feelings (Chaps. 5 and 7).

The HTW has adopted the term opportunity emotions, although, again, in the slightly altered form of opportunity feelings or interchangeably as eudaimonic feelings (Chaps. 6 and 7). Opportunity feelings comprise feelings such as interest, engagement, immersion, awe, wonder, and some others.

Grouping positive emotions into two broad categories, harmony and opportunity, is an efficient way of separating positive emotions with different functions and phenomenology. But when it comes to happiness, a problem remains because some researchers, such a Smith et al., conceptualize it as a harmony feeling, whereas others, such as Oatley and Johnson-Laird, conceptualize it as an opportunity feeling. Emotional happiness therefore ends up in a jingle-fallacy situation in which the same word is used for an emotion that is either a harmony feeling or an opportunity feeling. The literature on wellbeing exemplifies this dilemma. Myers and Diener (1995) noted, for instance, that "Happiness grows less from the passive experience of desirable circumstances than from involvement in valued activities and progress toward one's goal" (p. 17). Watson (2002, p. 116) is another researcher who places happiness as an opportunity feeling, as he maintains that "it is the process of striving after goals—rather than attaining goals per se—that is crucial for happiness." The evidence provided by Myers and Diener (1995) and Watson (2002) is weak and indirect, however, and a substantial literature rather supports the opposite view, i.e., that a happiness looks more like a harmony feeling than an opportunity feeling.

For example, Fredrickson (2009) reported that when participants were in a positive mood, they created a longer list of what they would like to do, but they did not actually complete the activities on the list. Similar results have been reported by Proffitt (2006), who found that people induced to a happy mood perceived a hill as less steep than people induced to a sad mood, indicating an "easiness bias" in happiness. In an experiment, Gilovich et al. (2005) asked students to predict how long it would take them to complete four academic projects. Half of the participants were randomly allocated to an "agreeable" group, instructed to nodding their heads up and down. The remaining participants formed the control group and were instructed to shake their heads from side to side. While moving their heads, the participants were asked to predict how long it would take them to complete the tasks. The "agreeable" group estimated that they need 5.1 days less than the control group to complete the assignments. Not only did the experimental manipulation influence the estimated completion time, but the agreeable group actually submitted their tasks 6 days after their predicted completion date. In contrast, the control group finished 1 day after their predicted completion date. These results are consistent with the perspective offered by Batson et al. (1992, p. 301), who claim that "positive affect is not likely to motivate action; it is likely simply to be enjoyed." Due to imprecise terminology, however, the above examples are not decisive about the question of whether happiness is a harmony feeling or an opportunity feeling.

Several studies have shown that people in a happy mood are more helpful than people who are less happy. However, the effect is only reported when helping is pleasant and requires little effort (Carlson et al., 1988). These authors reported that happy people were less helpful when altruistic behavior required sustained helpfulness. The correlation between happiness and effortful helping was −0.37. A recent study on helping behavior among job holders also illustrated this tendency. Glomb and coauthors (2011) found that negative mood was the primary elicitor of helping behavior in a work context, while the resulting mood from being helpful was positive.

Categorizing positive affect into harmony feelings and opportunity feelings may still be too broad for proper coverage of the entire spectrum of positive affect. After all, more than 20 positive emotions have been identified as basic (Keltner & Oatley, 2022), and many others exist as nonbasic emotions. But as will be argued in Chap. 7, a taxonomy that operates with the overarching categories of harmony feelings and opportunity feelings may efficiently capture a very important distinction in affective wellbeing. One significant feature captured by this taxonomy is how harmony feelings function as rewards for the fulfillment of stability needs and goal achievement. They also facilitate low-effort activities such as executing plans that are easy to follow or being social in uncomplicated ways. Opportunity feelings, by contrast, motivate effortful activities that can last longer; they can help people to overcome a challenge and, if necessary, motivate a postponement of immediate need gratification.

An innovative study by Thagard (2002) illustrates these mechanisms. Thagard analyzed the variety of emotions associated with the distinct phases of scientific activities. Reading James Watson's famous story of the discovery of the chemical structure of DNA (Watson, 1999), Thagard observed that when Watson and Crick struggled to understand the puzzle in front of them, feelings such as interest, curiosity, and wonder arose. Feelings such as pleasure, happiness, and beauty, on the other hand, typically occurred when Watson described how new facts were discovered or when important hypotheses were justified.

Interest as an Emotion

Interest is less of a prototypical emotion than happiness; some classification systems do not even include it as an emotion. An important reason is that interest often has been treated as motivational or cognitive rather than as affective (Hidi, 2006; Silvia, 2006). For example, Ekman considers interest to be a cognitive state of focused attention rather than an emotion (e.g., Ekman & Cordaro, 2011).[9] However, the practice of excluding interest from the domain of emotions is not only due to the (somewhat anachronistic) distinctions between affect and cognition (e.g., Ellsworth, 2003); it can also be explained by a jingle-fallacy concerning interest as referring to an emotion or interest as referring to a topic. People can be interested in particular topic, such as old cars, French vines, and country music (Bathgate et al., 2014; Silvia & Kashdan, 2009). Being interested in a topic is different than feeling interested when learning something new or when trying to overcome a challenge. Thus, emotional interest is not the same as topic interest (Renninger & Hidi, 2016).[10] In the capacity of being a something we feel, interest can be considered a knowledge emotion (Silvia, 2014), an opportunity-related emotion (Smith et al., 2014), an emotion of attraction (Oatley, 1992), or even a self-transcendent emotion (Pizarro et al., 2021).

[9] Phoebe Ellsworth, who was Ekman's research assistant when the basic structure of the "Ekman's six" was carved out, has later regretted the decision to not include interest as a basic emotion. "If I had only six to choose, I would have dropped surprise and kept interest," she now admits (Ellsworth, 2003, p. 84).

[10] State and trait are the common vocabulary in emotion research. In the literature on interest, however, it is not uncommon to use the terms individual and situational interest to refer to dispositional (trait) and situational (state) version of interest (e.g., Renninger & Hidi, 2016).

The History

Etymologically, *inter esse* comes from Latin and is laid out as "to be between" or "to take part in," and that is a rather precise description of what it feels like to be in a state of emotional interest. Interestingness seems to generate the experience of being between something, for example, something familiar and something new (Teigen, 1987), or between things that are too simple and things that are too difficult (Eckblad, 1963; Rathunde, 1993). Moreover, according to the English and English's dictionary (English & English, 1958), interest refers to "a tendency to engage in an activity for the gratification of engaging therein" (cited in Teigen, 1985, p. 224) or the "feeling of wanting to investigate," as Izard (1977, p. 216) puts it.

As a popular topic in the early days of psychology, emotional interest was studied by pioneers such as Ebbinghaus, James, Dewey, and Bartlett. In an early review, Arnold (1906) proposed that interest has evolved as a signal of a possible pleasure that lies ahead. Arnold's insight was almost a prophetic prediction of the knowledge to be established in neuroscience a century later. However, his observation about the differences between feelings of interest and feelings of pleasure has mainly been overlooked in the literature on wellbeing. But this distinction was debated extensively in the early psychological literature. For example, Ebbinghaus (1885/1964) acknowledged the functional role interest held in attention and remembering. James (1890) and Bartlett (1932) recognized the important part of interest in learning and human development. John Dewey even developed a comprehensive theory of emotional interest in the beginning of the twentieth century (Dewey, 1913). Dewey considered interest to be experienced during undisturbed and absorbing action, a "unified action," as he termed it (Dewey, 1895, p. 31). An important message from this analysis was that if we try to understand something new, the feeling of interest makes the learning process appears effortless. This idea was later soaked up in the concept of flow (Csikszentmihalyi, 1975), and the descriptions of deeply felt interest and flow overlap in important respects.

With the dominance of behaviorism, studies of emotions were basically replaced with studies of motivation. Feelings of interest came to be studied under the heading of intrinsic motivation. For example, when Dashiell (1925) observed explorative behavior in non-hungry rats, a phenomenon that could not be explained by the concept of drive reduction, he speculated that the rats must be motivated by a different mechanism, which Dashiell referred to as an "instinct of curiosity." Deci and Ryan (1985) provided a comprehensive review of the studies conducted by Dashiell and others classified as the forerunners for their own research into intrinsic motivation, known as self-determination theory (SDT). Whereas the SDT grew out of the research on motivation in the 1960s (see Chap. 6), another paradigm born in the same period looked as interest as an affect. A dominant scholar in this camp was Silvan Tomkins.

Tomkins

Tomkins categorized interest as a primary affect or a basic emotion in today's vocabulary (e.g., Frijda, 1986) and considered it as "the affect which has been most seriously neglected" (Tomkins, 1962, p. 337). Recall that Tomkins held emotional experiences to be generated by muscular feedback and that happiness is evoked by a reduction in muscular firings. In contrast, interest is activated by an increase in the rate of neural firing. Moreover, Tomkins saw interest as an emotion related to exploration, attention, and learning. To acquire knowledge of a new object, for instance, it is necessary to attack the problem over time. Almost any object is too large a bite to be swallowed whole, and this creates some problems in the perception of unfamiliar stimuli; they need to be perceived interchangeably in some detail and as a whole unity. Attention must therefore be upheld long enough to achieve both the details and the unity of an unfamiliar object. The function of interest is thus to maintain the attention needed to comprehend a complex object and to committing the experiencer to long-term psychological goals. The absence of interest would therefore "jeopardize intellectual development no less than the destruction of brain tissue" (Tomkins, 1962, p. 343).

Tomkins argued clearly in favor of separating happiness (or pleasure) and interest because he considered interest to be the emotion dealing with engagement of new and complex aspects of the world, whereas happiness deals with rewarding goal achievement and building attachment to familiar environments.

Berlyne

Tomkins' thinking was highly theoretical, but the idea that interest is associated with learning and complex information processing has gradually been supported by empirical evidence. Early contributions came from Berlyne, sometimes considered the father of the modern study of emotional interest (Silvia et al., 2009). In his formative years, Berlyne (1949) thought that interest must reflect both feelings and attention, and 25 years of research convinced him that things are experienced as "interesting to the extent that they contain information that cannot be absorbed immediately but seems likely to be absorbed relatively speedily through perceptual and intellectual effort" (Berlyne, 1974a, p. 179).

Berlyne's account of emotional interest sprang out of his general theory of affective responses. At least two different versions of the theory were developed, both using arousal as the pivotal explanatory factor. Arousal was generated by three factors Berlyne argued: the first is the psychophysical characteristics of the stimulus (e.g., intensity, pitch, brightness, and saturation); the second is the ecological characteristics such as the meaningfulness or signal value of the stimulus; and the third is the collative characteristics of a stimulus. The term collative refers to a comparison (collation) between two or more elements and reflects the degree of discrepancy between them. The four most common collative variables in Berlyne's theory are novelty, uncertainty, conflict, and complexity (e.g., Berlyne, 1963, p. 287).

In his early years, Berlyne considered the relation between arousal and preferences to be linear and negative. The more arousal a situation generates, the less we prefer it. This assumption was consistent with the drive reduction theories that dominated psychology before the cognitive revolution, and a preference was alternately operationalized as pleasure and interest. However, Berlyne was gradually forced to reformulate his original thoughts, and the revised theory included three neural systems. The first was the primary reward system, which generates positive affect whenever the arousal potential increases. The second, referred to as the primary aversion system, engenders negative affect when the arousal potential increases. Finally, the threshold for the reward system was supposed to be lower than the threshold for activating the aversion system. In sum, the reward system drove preferences up at low levels of arousal, and the aversion system pulled them downward at higher levels of arousal, creating an inverted U-shaped function between arousal and preference.

The U-shaped principle was easily demonstrated for pleasant feelings. Berlyne collected much data to show that when one of the collative properties of a situation increased from low to moderate, self-reports of pleasure increased (e.g., Berlyne, 1960, 1971). As arousal continued to increase, however, pleasantness decreased, presumably because the aversive system became activated. But the pattern for interest was different. Berlyne therefore considered interest to be the feeling we experience when we examine a particular thing, a specific exploration, as he called it. The function of specific exploration is to reduce the arousal generated by the collative variables, which occurs when novel and complex patterns are inspected. By examining the unknown, uncertainty is reduced, as is the conflict potential. Thus, the unpleasantness of the arousal generated by collative variables will be reduced by exploring novel or complex stimuli.

Berlyne is often taken to defend the idea that the relation between complexity and interest forms an inverted U. That is not correct. In fact, Berlyne argued that the relationship between collative variables and interest is linear. Pleasure, by contrast, was curvilinearly related to complexity in Berlyne's theory: "Pleasingness and equivalent attributes usually vary nonmonotonically with complexity, producing an inverted U-shaped curve or else a curve with several peaks, while interestingness tends to ride monotonically as complexity rises, at least to very high levels are reached" (Berlyne, 1974a, p. 176).

The relations Berlyne proposed between arousal and feelings are currently considered to be an oversimplification and are no longer supported. As noted by Martindale (1984), the theory requires that any two stimuli with the same arousal potential must be equally preferred. To illuminate the shortcomings of that idea, Martindale presents the following thought experiment. Suppose that the amount of arousal produced when a mother sees her baby can be determined. Furthermore, suppose that the intensity of a pure tone could be adjusted to produce the same amount of arousal. Berlyne's theory predicts that the mother will prefer her baby and the tone equally (Martindale, 1984, p. 55).

Neuroscientific Approaches

Panksepp

Jaak Panksepp (e.g., Panksepp, 1998a; Panksepp & Biven, 2012) was the first neuroscientist to identify the physiological basis of emotional interest (Renninger & Hidi, 2016). As briefly explained in the section "Basic Emotions," Panksepp refers to interest as a SEEKING system, and he argues that it explains the urge all mammals have to explore their environments. Importantly, the feeling experienced during such explorative activities is not pleasure but interest. "When fully aroused, SEEKING fills the mind with interest and motivates organisms to move their bodies seemingly effortlessly in search of the things they need, crave, and desire" (Panksepp, 2012, p. 35). Panksepp therefore describes the feeling produced in a SEEKING state as "intense interest," "engaged curiosity," and "eager anticipation" (Panksepp, 1998b, p. 149). Interest further generates and sustains a search for higher meaning, curiosity, and intellectual pursuits. It even helps in connecting and creating abstract thinking (Panksepp & Biven, 2012, p. 143).

In more details, Panksepp suggested that the most important neurochemical ingredient in the SEEKING system is dopamine, and drugs that typically stimulate the system are psychostimulants such as amphetamines and cocaine. SEEKING is anchored in the mesolimbic/cortical circuits, stretching "through the ventrolateral regions of the diencephalon—areas of the brain called the medial forebrain bundle (MFB) of the lateral hypothalamus (LH) which contains many neurochemically specific tracts." (Panksepp, 1998a, p. 146). Rather than inducing pleasure, activity in these structures produces a highly energized state of physical power and engagement with the world. Being in a state of SEEKING means being eager to pursue a variety of goal-directed activities (Panksepp, 1998a, pp. 150–151).

As we will see in Chap. 5, the pleasure system plays a quite different role in the government of behavior. It sustains the regulation of bodily processes, including feeding, drinking, and temperature regulation. Stimuli that promote a return to the homeostatic set point are routinely experienced as pleasurable, while those that impair homeostasis are unpleasant. Therefore, rather than feeling excited and curious, as was the case in the SEEKING system, the pleasure state is dominated by satisfaction.

Panksepp further noted that the results from the so-called intracranial self-stimulation (ICSS) studies speak in favor of SEEKING as a basic emotion. The ICSS became known with the studies by James Olds and his graduate student Peter Milner (Olds & Milner, 1954). Untrained in laboratory routines and borrowing a primitive laboratory from Donald Hebb at McGill University in Canada, the two psychologists started a search for learning structures in the central nervous system. In the early phase of their study, the two erroneously administered electrical shock to the wrong part of a rat's brain and thus stumbled upon one of the most fascinating phenomena ever discovered in biopsychology. What they quite serendipitously found was that if rats, wired to a self-administered device that provided electrical stimulation to particular areas of their brains, were given the choice to stimulate themselves, they would become almost unstoppable. Rather than eating, drinking, or having sex, the rats preferred to press the lever that provided electrical signals thousands of times in a row. Olds (1956) reported that some self-stimulating rats could press a lever at a rate of up to 2000 times per hour, forsaking food, water, sleep, and sex until they collapsed from exhaustion. This procedure rapidly became popular and has been used by various researchers on monkeys, dolphins, rabbits, goldfish, dogs, chickens, and even humans. On one occasion, a dolphin was reported to have pushed the lever "too rapidly, [which] caused a seizure, [and then the dolphin] became unconscious, respiration failed, and he died" (Dror, 2016, p. 236).

Although Olds and Milner initially named these brain regions "reinforcing structures" (1954, p. 425), these structures were quickly referred to as "pleasure centers" (Dror, 2016; Olds, 1956). These centers were so named because the animals actively sought to be stimulated by activating them (Berridge, 1999, p. 537). The idea that ICSS produces pleasure has since been stuck in much of the psychological literature. For instance, Kahneman (2011) talks about how classic studies on ICSS demonstrated that self-stimulation produced "sensations of intense pleasure" (p. 384). However, the idea that such craving behavior is driven by pleasant feelings is misleading. What seems to have escaped the attention of most observers of ICSS is that the behavior displayed by the rats in these states does not look very similar to what we think of as pleasant behavior. Rather than the rewarding, consuming, and fairly laidback activities associated with pleasure, self-stimulating animals typically look excessively exited, even crazed, when they work for this kind of stimulation. As explained in Chap. 5, the term wanting seems more appropriate than pleasure for these kinds of activities (e.g., Berridge, 1999).

In a dramatic and shockingly unethical research program, the psychiatrist Robert Heath of Tulane University in New Orleans applied the ICSS paradigm to humans. Without much concern for the legal rights of psychiatric patients, he hooked dozens of schizophrenics and other patients in his psychiatry ward up to an ICSS apparatus (Frank, 2018). With this procedure, he hoped to cure their pathologies, which, at that time, included homosexuality. But even if a variety of feeling states were reported by Heath's patients, they were rarely described as pleasant (Heath, 1963, 1964). Thus, Panksepp (1998a) suggested that terms such as intense interest and engaged curiosity better reflect the feeling systems involved in ICSS behavior, a conclusion that is consistent with the observations Oliver Sacks presented in his bestselling book *Awakenings* (Sacks, 1990).

Pribram

Another neuroscientific model of interest as a feeling has been advanced by Pribram (2003). The theory claims that brief, episodic, and mild changes in expectations are experienced as interesting and novel, whereas more severe disruptions are disturbing. Pribram further speaks of a comfort-effort dimension and claims that "when a conflict between maintenance and change needs to be mediated, the mediation can become stressful and demand effort; when little mediation is needed, behavior is regulated by pre-established context, becomes more or less automatic, and when experienced feels comfortable" (Pribram, 2003, p. 128). Pribram also suggested that chemicals such as endorphins (a morphine-like substance) are involved in feelings of temperature and pain and that dopamine is involved in the feeling of effectiveness, while enkephalins are involved in feelings of interest. It is also interesting to note that the hedonic mechanisms in Pribram's model are sensitive only to quantities and that they are not involved in the identification of the so-called qualitative aspects of the outer worlds, such as shapes, colors, or location in time and space. Pribram claims that comfort is the inverse of coordinated effort and that the feeling of state interest is the result of the dopaminergic system. Feelings of familiarity imply stabilization, that is, a feeling of a reasonable amount of stability and a smooth transition from one state to another (Pribram, 2003, p. 125).

Appraisal Theories of Interest

Some attention has been devoted to analyzing emotional interest within the framework of appraisal theories. For example, Ellsworth and Smith (1988) observed that interest contrasts with happiness in regard to effort. Interest is typically associated with moderate levels of effort, whereas happiness is associated with low levels. Ellsworth and Smith also proposed that interest was characterized by high levels of pleasure, although, as we have seen, much evidence has already been reported against this idea. Based on these updated observations, Paul Silvia developed a more comprehensive appraisal theory of interest (Silvia, 2006). The theory proposes that interest involves two major appraisals—novelty checks and coping potential. Novelty-complexity appraisals refer to a class of disruptive variables that appear if an event is new, uncertain, complex, or contradictory. Coping potential appraisals refer to the ability to understand new, complex things and thus indicate resources, power, abilities, and control in relation to an event. The feeling that follows from high levels of coping potential is described by Silvia as interest. In studies of art, for instance, "feeling able to understand art is associated with finding art interesting" (Silvia, 2005, p. 90).

Since the association between novelty-complexity and interest often shows up as curvilinear, Silvia suggests that a two-factor model is necessary to account for emotional interest. The first factor is linearly and positively associated with interest. Silvia proposes that this factor is represented by variables such as complexity, novelty, uncertainty, and conflict, i.e., Berlyne's collative variables. The second factor needed to create an inverted-U is a moderator that changes the linear trend from positive to negative, which Silvia refers to as "the hinge between interest and disinterest" (Silvia, 2006, p. 53). In Silvia's approach, this second factor is represented by coping potential appraisals, a concept that broadly refers to "estimates of resources, power, abilities, and control in relation to an event" (Silvia, 2005, p. 90). The combination of novelty-complex appraisals and coping potential appraisals unfolds as follows: When facing an unfamiliar or ambiguous event, people with high coping potential believe that they will be able to understand the complexity. Therefore, interesting events may be described as events that people do not quite understand but nevertheless judge to be understandable. It thus seems that interest kicks in for people with coping potential but only after an initial moment of uncertainty.

Theories Inspired by Piaget

Piaget, in his extensive work on the generalizable structures of human action, integrated both cognitive and motivational elements into his concept of a schema (e.g., Eckblad, 1981). Less acknowledged are the affective elements involved in Piaget's conceptualization of schemas, partly because they were never taken to be the target of his analyses. However, thanks to scholars such as Ginsburg and Opper (1969), Eckblad (1981), and Mandler (1984), summaries of Piaget's thinking about the role of emotions in intellectual activity are available.

Feelings of interest were particularly important to Piaget since he considered them to facilitate learning (Ginsburg & Opper, 1969, p. 223). Piaget argued that interest operates differently than other positive affects, which primarily serve the regulation of physiological needs (e.g., Piaget, 1952). By separating interest from other positive feelings, Piaget offered a theory that opposed the two dominating theories of his time, i.e., Freud's psychodynamic theory of personality and Hull's drive reduction theory. Rather than considering the principal human motivation to be an escape from unconscious conflicts or arousal, Piaget emphasized that infants do not always try to avoid increased stimulation. To the contrary, they often seek it. When capable of performing a particular activity, infants tend to intrinsically perform it by practicing the steps involved in the procedure (Ginsburg & Opper, 1969, p. 33). The explanation Piaget offered to account for these observations was functional. To be effective, the action sequences inherent in a schema must be exercised, which means that a mechanism that makes the rehearsal of the sequences intrinsically motivating gives organisms an evolutionary advantage. According to Piaget's theory then, biology ensures that the execution of immature schemes can be driven at least partly by emotional interest. The activity thus became rewarding in and by itself. From where comes this reward, Piaget asked, before answering, "from functioning as such" (Piaget, 1952, p. 42). In other words, it feels good to function well. But the feeling of exercising complex or immature schemes is not pleasure, but interest.

Piaget suggested that we become interested in things that are moderately novel to us. Objects that are too familiar do not capture our attention, and objects that are too unfamiliar do not resonate with our schemas. He thus stated a moderate novelty principle asserting that interest stems from engagement with environments that are somewhat novel and therefore provide incongruities and conflicts with existing cognitive structures. These new observations do not assimilate easily, as they are met with "a resistance which is imposed by the reality of the objects themselves" (Ginsburg & Opper, 1969, p. 59).

Building on Piaget's insights, George Mandler (e.g., Mandler, 1982, 1984) differentiates between feelings of pleasure and feelings of interest by suggesting that congruence is related to the former, whereas incongruity produces interest. To Mandler, schema congruity is an inherently positive affective experience, whereas incongruity is attention-grabbing and thus interesting. Together with William Gaver, he elaborated on these ideas in a paper entitled *Play it Again, Sam* (Gaver & Mandler, 1987). Here, the authors point out that, in principle, plain assimilation of information into a schema requires virtually no mental effort, while massive accommodation may demand extensive processing. Listening to music serves as a good example. Simple music, Gaver and Mandler argue, fits our existing schema well and therefore often becomes popular. Listening to it typically elicits pleasant feelings. Great works of music, by contrast, are more complex, and it is the right amount of complexity that makes it both great and interesting. The point is that complexity cannot be easily assimilated, and that is precisely why it becomes interesting.

Similarly, Karl Halvor Teigen (e.g., Teigen, 1986, 1987) has developed a model of emotional interest grounded in the idea that information cannot be interesting unless it contains something new and informative. By hypothesizing that interestingness depends on perceived informativeness, Teigen proposed that the combination of novelty and familiarity engenders interest. The prospect of absorbing a new element of something that is already familiar is interesting. Information is not interesting when one is told something one already knows (familiarity without novelty) or something completely new (novelty without familiarity). However, something appears interesting if some part of the information corresponds to an existing knowledge structure (is familiar) and another part of it does not correspond to the existing knowledge (is novel). In several nicely designed experiments, Teigen (1985) illustrated these principles by showing, for instance, that the preferences of first-term psychology students were linearly related to psychologists according to their familiarity (as judged by an independent sample of students). For second-year students, on the other hand, the preference function is curved, indicating that with increasing prior knowledge, some psychologists are just too well known to be maximally attractive to read about.

Eckblad

Gudrun Eckblad's work on emotional interest is articulated in her scheme theory, a work inspired by Piaget and that draws heavily on the concepts of schema, assimilation, and accommodation (Eckblad, 1981). A schema refers to the structure of an action and is defined as an organized sequence of operations (p. 18). A schema operates by incorporating input from the environment, what we call assimilation. All schemas comprise certain standards or expectations, and when the input is consistent with the expectations, the schema is in equilibrium. In contrast, if the input does not match these expectations, the schema enters a state of disequilibrium, and a structural change is needed. This is the process of accommodation (p. 22).

The degree of misfit between inputs and expectations is referred to as assimilation resistance (AR). The unique feature of Eckblad's theory is that AR can not only motivate behavior but also cause certain feelings. This happens when a schema becomes "spontaneously active." A full account of the notion of a spontaneously active schema is a bit technical but has, somewhat simplified to do with what Piaget-labeled circular reactions. A major feature of these reactions is that the goal of the activity is embedded within the activated schema. According to scheme theory, this is the essence of intrinsic motivation. The motivating mechanism is embedded in the activity itself; it comes from exercising a schematic routine or "from functioning as such," as Piaget formulated it.

Eckblad describes the features of a spontaneous active schema in Chap. 2 of *Scheme Theory* (Eckblad, 1981). One of her examples comes from a young baby who moves her hands around, thus exercising schema A. By chance, the hand hits a rattle that makes a sound. A vague expectation that certain hand movements cause the rattle to make a sound becomes a new schema, which will run spontaneously until the sequence, including the predicted sound, becomes well-rehearsed and familiar. The level of AR, both in terms of muscle movements, standards, and expectations, decreases and will at some point no longer keep the scheme active. Another scheme/activity takes over.

The sequence entails two phases, one familiar and one new. Thus, some elements in Eckblad's model resemble the two elements in Teigen's theory of interest. In the first stage, the schema directs one's attention to something familiar. In the second stage, novel or incongruous features of the situation stand out as important. Thus, spontaneously active schemas operate in the range between something familiar and something novel, i.e., while incorporating input that creates varying degrees of assimilation resistance. In these situations, the spontaneously active scheme gains nearly exclusive control over the resources of the organism, which means that the organism is concentrated on the task at hand and has a high distractibility threshold (Eckblad, 1981, pp. 40–41).

As AR increases, qualitatively different feelings are created. Pleasure is the typical feeling of low levels of AR, whereas interest gradually increases as the level of AR increases. Very high levels of AR produce a feeling of being challenged, while too high levels become overwhelming and result in feelings such as frustration, anger, or fear. The assumption made in Eckblad's theory is that *Pleasure* < *Interest* < *Challenge* < *Complex* in terms of assimilation resistance. The relationship between AR and feelings is curvilinear in the sense that a feeling will intensify with increasing AR up to an optimal level for that feeling quality before its intensity starts decreasing. Thus, each feeling state has "a single-peaked preference function for any given complexity dimension" (Eckblad, 1981, p. 97).

Differences Between Interest and Happiness/Pleasure

In Act II of *A Midsummer Night's Dream,* Shakespeare lets Oberon, the king of the fairies, squeeze the juice from a small flower into the eye of his sleeping wife Titania. The juice will make her fall in love with the first creature she sees upon waking. In analyzing this act, Oatley (2011) suggests that strangeness makes the scene interesting. Shakespeare could have made it more familiar, by, for instance, letting Titania be hit by Cupid's arrow rather than a drop of juice. But Cupid's arrow was already a cliché when the play was written; thus, introducing an unknown juice rather than the familiar arrow to initiate the upcoming love story makes the scene more interesting (Oatley, 2011, p. 14).

As the previous pages have testified, there is much to support Oatley's interpretation of Shakespeare's love story. People do seem to find simple or familiar things pleasant and moderately complex or new things interesting. For example, studies of the affective response to problem-solving have shown that people tend to rank complex polygons as interesting and simple polygons as enjoyable. An early study was conducted by Day (1967), who had participants rank polygons of varying complexities. He found that pleasure decreased as complexity increased, whereas interest increased. Similar results were reported by Aitken (1974), Walker (1980), and Reeve (1989).

More recently, Silvia has replicated and extended these findings (e.g., Silvia, 2006). In one study, participants were presented with polygons of varying complexities and were either asked to select the images they found most pleasant or the images they found most interesting. The interesting images were significantly more complex than the pleasant images (Silvia, 2005). Turner and Silvia (2006) analyzed people's responses to a set of classical paintings. Basically, they observed that disturbing pictures were highly interesting but unpleasant, whereas calming pictures were highly pleasant but uninteresting. Using multilevel modeling, they also found that interest and pleasantness were unrelated and that the appraisal of novelty-complexity had opposite relationships with interest and pleasantness. In another set of studies, Reeve (1993) found that films rated as equally joyful could vary in their degree of interest. Relatedly, a study by Iran-Nejad (1987) revealed that some stories are pleasant but not interesting, while others are interesting but not pleasant. However, a third category was found to be both interesting and pleasant. Straume and Vittersø (2012) reported that complex work situations predicted an increase in inspiration but a decrease in happiness. Relatedly, Delle Fave et al. (2011) noted that some activities, such as work, can be meaningful but not pleasant. As discussed in Chap. 6, similar results have been presented by Baumeister (2018) and Bauer (2016).

A sophisticated study by Eckblad (1981) elegantly illustrates the difference between interest and pleasure. Eckblad had 32 students predict black and white patterns within a quadratic display of 8 × 8 cells, varying in complexity. An example of such a pattern is shown in Fig. 3.1, panel A. As shown in the figure, each quadrat comprises a combination of 64 white and black cells. The participants predicted the color of each of the 64 cells, starting in the upper left corner and moving row-wise

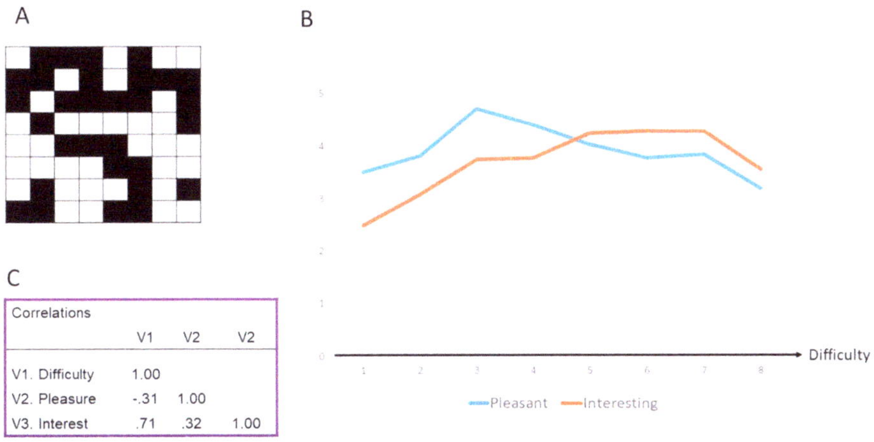

Fig. 3.1 Pleasure and interest as functions of difficulty in Eckblad's experiment

to the right. The quadrat depicted in Fig. 3.1 is generated at random and is the most difficult of all tasks. In fact, it is unpredictable and only solvable by chance. In the simplest task, the first four cells in each row are white, and the remaining four are black.

After guessing black or white for all eight cells in a row, participants rated how much pleasantness, interestingness, and complexity they felt while executing this part of the task. Eckblad also kept scores of the number of errors made by each participant and on when the last erroneous guess was made. This procedure was repeated for a total of 24 quadrats of varying complexities. Using this procedure, Eckblad confirmed that pleasure and interest were curvilinearly related to task complexity but at increasingly higher levels of difficulty (Fig. 3.1, panel B). The correlations between experienced pleasant, interest, and difficult was also as expected (panel C), with a moderate and negative correlation between difficulty and pleasure ($r = -0.31$) and a strong and positive correlation between difficulty and interest ($r = 0.71$).

On average, pleasure peaked at perceived complexity level 4, while interest peaked at complexity level 5. Both the easiest task and the most difficult task were rated as the most boring and the most unpleasant. Unsurprisingly, complexity was correlated with errors. Less obviously, however, was the finding that participants preferred some difficulty—even at the cost of performing more errors. This result may indicate that people do not always prefer easy and perfect things in life; some difficulties and error-making are also valued in our lives.

Much of my own research has been devoted to examining the distinction between interest and other opportunity feelings, on the one hand, and happiness and other harmony feelings, on the other (see Vittersø, 2016, for an overview). Indicators of harmony feelings, (pleasure, tranquility, contentment, and happiness), and indicators of opportunity feelings, (interest, engagement, immersion, and wonder/awe) typically load on two distinct factors. In terms of functionality, Vittersø et al. (2009)

hypothesized and found that systematically thinking about a happy moment generates interest, whereas mental replaying generates pleasantness. Participants who were randomly assigned to a group that systematically analyzed a happy moment increased feelings of interest, while the level of pleasantness remained unchanged. A panel study by Vittersø and Søholt (2011) showed that life satisfaction predicted harmony feelings but not opportunity feelings. Conversely, personal growth predicted opportunity feelings but not harmony feelings. A third example comes from Vittersø et al. (2010), who measured happiness and interest before and during a problem-solving task. The participants reported higher levels of happiness before they engaged in the task as compared with happiness during the task. The opposite was found for interest, which was more intensely experienced during the task than before the task.

Another distinction between interest and happiness/pleasure can be observed in facial expressions. In the Reeve (1993) study mentioned above, the author also identified a set of facial expressions that were uniquely associated with emotional interest. Later studies have verified the distinctiveness of the facial expressions of interest, as in a study by Cordaro et al. (2018), demonstrating that interest does not share the smile component with other positive emotions. In contrast with the expressions of most other positive affect, interest and awe are "characterized by distinctive patterns of eyebrow lifts, mouth movements, and forward movement of the head and/or torso" (Shiota et al., 2017, p. 620).

In summary, interest is different from happiness in several ways. The essence of the distinction is well captured by Izard and Ackerman (2000), who remarked that interest seems to sustain active engagement in an activity, whereas "happiness follows from achievement of a goal, mastery, or some incongruous event" (p. 258). Interest and other opportunity feelings often operate independently, and sometimes even antagonistically, with happiness and other harmony feelings. Unfortunately, this distinction has not received much attention in the wellbeing literature, although Oishi's recent studies on the distinction between happiness and psychological richness excellently replicate and extend the arguments made in the long-standing tradition of research on emotional interest that have been reviewed in the present section (e.g., Oishi & Westgate, 2022).

References

Abagnale, F. W., & Redding, S. (2000). *Catch me if you can: The true story of a real fake*. Broadway Books.

Adolphs, R. (2017). Reply to Barrett: Affective neuroscience needs objective criteria for emotions. *Social Cognitive and Affective Neuroscience, 12*(1), 32–33. https://doi.org/10.1093/scan/nsw155

Adolphs, R., & Anderson, D. J. (2018). *The neuroscience of emotion: A new synthesis [Kindle]*. Princeton University Press.

Aitken, P. P. (1974). Judgments of pleasingness and interestingness as functions of visual complexity. *Journal of Experimental Psychology, 103*(2), 240–244. https://doi.org/10.1037/h0036787

Allport, F. H. (1924). *Social psychology*. Houghton.
Alston, W. P. (1969). Feelings. *The Philosophical Review, 78*(1), 3–34.
Andersen, H. (2010). Den dype naturfølelsen. *Fjell og Vidde, 3*, 62–67.
Anglim, J., Horwood, S., Smillie, L. D., Marrero, R. J., & Wood, J. K. (2020). Predicting psychological and subjective well-being from personality: A meta-analysis. *Psychological Bulletin, 146*, 279–323. https://doi.org/10.1037/bul0000226
Annas, J. (1993). *The morality of happiness [Kindle]*. Oxford University Press.
Argyle, M. (2001). *The psychology of happiness* (2nd ed.). Routledge.
Arnold, F. (1906). The psychology of interest (I). *Psychological Review, 13*(4), 221–238. https://doi.org/10.1037/h0075836
Arnold, M. (1960). *Emotion and personality*. Columbia University Press.
Arnold, M., & Gasson, J. A. (1954). Feelings and emotions as dynamic factors in personality integration. In M. Arnold & J. A. Gasson (Eds.), *The human person* (pp. 294–313). Ronald.
Averill, J. R., & More, T. A. (2000). Happiness. In M. Lewis & J. Haviland-Jones (Eds.), *Handbook of emotions* (2nd ed., pp. 663–676). Guilford.
Barbano, M. F., & Cador, M. (2007). Opioids for hedonic experience and dopamine to get ready for it. *Psychopharmacology, 191*, 497–506.
Barrett, L. F. (2006). Solving the emotion paradox: Categorization and the experience of emotion. *Personality and Social Psychology Review, 10*(1), 20–46.
Barrett, L. F. (2013). Psychological construction: The Darwinian approach to the science of emotion. *Emotion Review, 5*(4), 379–389. https://doi.org/10.1177/1754073913489753
Barrett, L. F. (2016a). Navigating the science of emotion. In H. L. Meiselman (Ed.), *Emotion measurement* (pp. 31–63). Woodhead Publishing. https://doi.org/10.1016/B978-0-08-100508-8.00002-3
Barrett, L. F. (2016b). The theory of constructed emotion: An active inference account of interoception and categorization. *Social Cognitive and Affective Neuroscience, 12*(1), 1–23. https://doi.org/10.1093/scan/nsw154
Barrett, L. F. (2017a). *How emotions are made: The secret life of the brain [Kindle]*. Houghton Mifflin Harcourt.
Barrett, L. F. (2017b). The theory of constructed emotion: An active inference account of interoception and categorization. *Social Cognitive and Affective Neuroscience, 12*(1), 1–23. https://doi.org/10.1093/scan/nsw154
Barrett, L. F. (2018). Emotions are constructed with interoception and concepts within a predicting brain. In A. S. Fox, R. C. Lapate, A. J. Shackman, & R. J. Davidson (Eds.), *The nature of emotion. Fundamental questions [Kindle]* (pp. 34–38). Oxford University Press.
Barrett, L. F., Adolphs, R., Marsella, S., Martinez, A. M., & Pollak, S. D. (2019). Emotional expressions reconsidered: Challenges to inferring emotion from human facial movements. *Psychological Science in the Public Interest, 20*(1), 1–68. https://doi.org/10.1177/1529100619832930
Barrett, L. F., & Bliss-Moreau, E. (2009). Affect as a psychological primitive. In M. P. Zanna (Ed.), *Advances in experimental social psychology* (Vol. 41, pp. 167–218). Academic Press. https://doi.org/10.1016/S0065-2601(08)00404-8
Barrett, L. F., Lindquist, K. A., & Gendron, M. (2007). Language as context for the perception of emotion. *Trends in Cognitive Sciences, 11*(8), 327–332. https://doi.org/10.1016/j.tics.2007.06.003
Barrett, L. F., & Russel, J. A. (2009). Circumplex models. In D. Sander & K. R. Scherer (Eds.), *The Oxford companion to emotive and the affective sciences* (pp. 85–88). Oxford University Press.
Barrett, L. F., & Russell, J. A. (2014). *The psychological construction of emotion*. Guilford.
Bartlett, F. C. (1932). *Remembering*. Cambridge University Press.
Bates, J. E. (2000). Temperament as an emotion construct: Theoretical and practical issues. In M. Lewis & J. M. Haviland-Jones (Eds.), *Handbook of emotions* (2nd ed., pp. 382–396). The Guilford Press.
Bathgate, M. E., Schunn, C. D., & Correnti, R. (2014). Children's motivation toward science across contexts, manner of interaction, and topic. *Science Education, 98*(2), 189–215. https://doi.org/10.1002/sce.21095

Batson, C. D., Shaw, L. L., & Oleson, K. C. (1992). Differentiating affect, mood and emotion: Toward functionally based conceptual distinctions. In M. S. Clark (Ed.), *Review of personality and social psychology* (Vol. 13, pp. 294–326).

Bauer, J. J. (2016). Eudaimonic growth: The development of the goods in personhood (or: Cultivating a good life story). In J. Vittersø (Ed.), *Handbook of eudaimonic well-being* (pp. 147–174). Springer. https://doi.org/10.1007/978-3-319-42445-3_10

Baumeister, R. F. (2018). Happiness and meaningfulness as two different and not entirely compatible versions of the good life. In J. P. Forgas & R. E. Baumeister (Eds.), *The social psychology of living well* (pp. 21–33). Routledge.

Benditt, T. (1974). Happiness. *Philosophical Studies: An International Journal for Philosophy in the Analytic Tradition, 25*(1), 1–20. https://doi.org/10.2307/4318819

Berlyne, D. E. (1949). 'Interest' as a psychological concept. *British Journal of Psychology General Section, 39*(4), 184–195. https://doi.org/10.1111/j.2044-8295.1949.tb00219.x

Berlyne, D. E. (1960). *Conflict, arousal, and curiosity*. McGraw-Hill.

Berlyne, D. E. (1963). Complexity and incongruity variables as determinants of exploratory choice and evaluative ratings. *Canadian Journal of Psychology, 17*, 274–290.

Berlyne, D. E. (1971). *Aesthetics and psychobiology*. Appleton.

Berlyne, D. E. (1974a). Novelty, complexity, and interestingness. In D. E. Berlyne (Ed.), *Studies in the new experimental aesthetics: Steps toward and objective psychology of aesthetic appreciation* (pp. 175–180). Wiley.

Berlyne, D. E. (Ed.). (1974b). *Studies in the new experimental aesthetics: Steps toward an objective psychology of aesthetic appreciation*. Wiley.

Berridge, K. C. (1999). Pleasure, pain, desire and dread: Hidden core processes of emotion. In D. Kahneman, E. Diener, & N. Schwarz (Eds.), *Well-being: The foundations of hedonic psychology* (pp. 527–559). Russell Sage Foundation.

Berscheid, E. (1990). Contemporary vocabularies. In B. S. Moore & A. M. Isen (Eds.), *Affect and social behavior* (pp. 22–38). Cambridge University Press.

Biswas-Diener, R., Vittersø, J., & Diener, E. (2005). Most people are pretty happy, but there is cultural variation: The Inughuit, the Amish, and the Maasai. *Journal of Happiness Studies, 6*, 205–226.

Bojanowska, A., & Piotrowski, K. (2021). Two levels of personality: Temperament and values and their effects on hedonic and eudaimonic well-being. *Current Psychology, 40*(3), 1185–1193. https://doi.org/10.1007/s12144-018-0043-0

Brown, T. (1994). Affective dimensions of meaning. In W. F. Overton & D. S. Palermo (Eds.), *The Nature and ontogenesis of meaning* (pp. 177–190). Lawrence Erlbaum.

Bryant, F. B., & Veroff, J. (2006). *Savoring; A new model of positive experience*. Lawrence Erlbaum.

Buss, A. H., & Plomin, R. (1975). *A temperament theory of personality development*. Wiley-Interscience.

Cabanac, M. (1992). Pleasure: The common currency. *Journal of Theoretical Biology, 155*(2), 173–200. https://doi.org/10.1016/S0022-5193(05)80594-6

Cabanac, M. (2009). *The fifth influence. The dialectics of pleasure*. iUniverse.

Cabanac, M. (2010). The dialectics of pleasure. In M. L. Kringelbach & K. C. Berridge (Eds.), *Pleasures of the brain* (pp. 113–124). Oxford University Press.

Cacioppo, J. T., & Berntson, G. G. (1999). The affect system: Architecture and operating characteristics. *Current Directions in Psychological Science, 8*, 133–137.

Cacioppo, J. T., Crites, A. L., Berntson, G. G., & Cole, M. G. H. (1993). If attitudes affect how much stimuli are processed, should they not affect the event-related brain potential? *Psychological Science, 4*(2), 108–111.

Cacioppo, J. T., Gardner, W. L., & Berntson, G. G. (1997). Beyond bipolar conceptualization and measure: The case of attitudes and evaluative space. *Personality and Social Psychology Review, 1*(1), 3–25.

Cai, D., Zhu, M., Lin, M., Zhang, X. C., & Margraf, J. (2017). The bidirectional relationship between positive mental health and social rhythm in college students: A three-year longitudinal study [original research]. *Frontiers in Psychology, 8*. https://doi.org/10.3389/fpsyg.2017.01119

Carlson, M., Charlin, V., & Miller, N. (1988). Positive mood and helping behavior: A test of six hypotheses. *Journal of Personality and Social Psychology, 55*(2), 211–229.

Carr, N. (2010). *The shallows: What the Internet is doing to our brains [Kindle]*. Norton.

Carver, C. S., Scheier, M. F., & Johnson, S. L. (2014). Origins and functions of positive affect. A goal regulation perspective. In J. Gruber & J. T. Moskowitz (Eds.), *Positive emotion: Integrating the light sides and dark sides* (pp. 34–51). Oxford University Press.

Celeghin, A., Diano, M., Bagnis, A., Viola, M., & Tamietto, M. (2017). Basic emotions in human neuroscience: Neuroimaging and beyond [review]. *Frontiers in Psychology, 8*(1432). https://doi.org/10.3389/fpsyg.2017.01432

Cloninger, C. R. (1987). A systematic method for clinical description and classification of personality variants. *Archives of General Psychiatry, 44*, 573–588.

Clore, G. L., & Schiller, A. J. (2016). New light on the affect–cognition connection. In L. F. Barrett, M. Lewis, & J. M. Haviland-Jones (Eds.), *Handbook of emotions* (pp. 532–546). Guilford.

Clore, G. L., & Schnall, S. (2005). The influence of affect on attitude. In D. Albarracín, B. T. Johnson, & M. P. Zanna (Eds.), *The handbook of attitudes* (pp. 437–489). Routledge.

Cordaro, D. T., Sun, R., Keltner, D., Kamble, S., Huddar, N., & McNeil, G. (2018). Universals and cultural variations in 22 emotional expressions across five cultures. *Emotion, 18*(1), 75–93. https://doi.org/10.1037/emo0000302

Cowen, A. S., & Keltner, D. (2020). What the face displays: Mapping 28 emotions conveyed by naturalistic expression. *American Psychologist, 75*, 349–364. https://doi.org/10.1037/amp0000488

Cowen, A. S., Keltner, D., Schroff, F., Jou, B., Adam, H., & Prasad, G. (2021). Sixteen facial expressions occur in similar contexts worldwide. *Nature, 589*(7841), 251–257. https://doi.org/10.1038/s41586-020-3037-7

Cowen, A., Sauter, D., Tracy, J. L., & Keltner, D. (2019). Mapping the passions: Toward a high-dimensional taxonomy of emotional experience and expression. *Psychological Science in the Public Interest, 20*(1), 69–90. https://doi.org/10.1177/1529100619850176

Craver, C. F., & Darden, L. (2013). *In search of mechanisms: Discoveries across the life sciences [Kindle]*. University of Chicago Press.

Csikszentmihalyi, M. (1975). *Beyond boredom and anxiety*. Jossey-Bass.

Damasio, A. (1994). *Descartes' error. Emotion, reason, and the human brain*. Avon Books.

Damasio, A. (1999). *The feeling of what happens: Body and emotion in the making of consciousness*. Avon Books.

Damasio, A. (2010). *Self comes to mind: Constructing the conscious brain [Kindle]*. Pantheon Books.

Damasio, A. (2018). *The strange order of things: Life, feeling, and the making of culture [Kindle]*. Pantheon Books.

Damasio, A. (2021). *Feeling & knowing: Making minds conscious [Kindle]*. Pantheon.

Damasio, A., & Damasio, H. (2018). Emotions and feelings. William James then and now. In A. S. Fox, R. C. Lapate, A. J. Shackman, & R. J. Davidson (Eds.), *The nature of emotion. Fundamental questions [Kindle]* (pp. 1–6). Oxford University Press.

Darwin, C. (1859). *The origin of species by means of natural selection*. http://www.gutenberg.org/files/2009/2009-h/2009-h.htm.

Darwin, C. (1872). *The expression of the emotions in man and animals*. University of Chicago Press. http://www.gutenberg.org/files/1227/1227-h/1227-h.htm

Dashiell, J. F. (1925). A quantitative demonstration of animal drive. *Journal of Comparative Psychology, 5*, 205–208.

Davidson, R. J. (1998). Affective style and affective disorders: Perspectives from affective neuroscience. *Cognition and Emotion, 12*(3), 307–330.

Davidson, R. J. (2018). Reactivity, recovery, regulation the three R's of emotional responding. In A. S. Fox, R. C. Lapate, A. J. Shackman, & R. J. Davidson (Eds.), *The nature of emotion. Fundamental questions [Kindle]* (pp. 1–6). Oxford University Press.

Davidson, R. J., & Begley, S. (2012). *The emotional life of your brain [Kindle]*. Hodder & Stoughton.

Davitz, J. R. (1969). *The language of emotion*. Academic Press.

Day, H. (1967). Evaluations of subjective complexity, pleasingness and interestingness for a series of random polygons varying in complexity. *Perception & Psychophysics, 2*, 281–286.

De Pauw, S. S. W., Mervielde, I., & Van Leeuwen, K. G. (2009). How are traits related to problem behavior in preschoolers? Similarities and contrasts between temperament and personality. *Journal of Abnormal Child Psychology, 37*(3), 309–325. https://doi.org/10.1007/s10802-008-9290-0

De Waal, F. (2019). *Mama's last hug: Animal emotions and what they tell us about ourselves [Kindle]*. WW Norton & Company.

Deci, E. L., & Ryan, R. M. (1985). *Intrinsic motivation and self-determination in human behavior*. Plenum Press.

Delle Fave, A., Brdar, I., Freire, T., Vella-Brodrick, D., & Wissing, M. (2011). The eudaimonic and hedonic components of happiness: Qualitative and quantitative findings. *Social Indicators Research, 100*(2), 185–207. https://doi.org/10.1007/s11205-010-9632-5

Denton, D. (2005). *The primordial emotions: The dawning of consciousness*. Oxford University Press.

Dewey, J. (1895). The theory of emotions II: The significance of emotions. *Psychological Review, 2*, 13–32.

Dewey, J. (1913). *Interest and effort in education*. Riverside.

DeYoung, C. G. (2015). Openness/intellect: A dimension of personality reflecting cognitive exploration. In *APA handbook of personality and social psychology, Volume 4: Personality processes and individual differences* (pp. 369–399). American Psychological Association. https://doi.org/10.1037/14343-017

Diener, E. (1998). Subjective well-being and personality. In D. F. Barone & M. Hersen (Eds.), *Advanced personality* (pp. 311–334). Plenum.

Diener, E., & Lucas, R. E. (1999). Personality and subjective well-being. In D. Kahneman, E. Diener, & N. Schwarz (Eds.), *Well-being: The foundations of hedonic psychology* (pp. 211–229). Russell Sage Foundation.

Diener, E., & Lucas, R. E. (2000). Subjective emotional well-being. In M. Lewis & J. M. Haviland-Jones (Eds.), *Handbook of emotions* (2nd ed., pp. 325–337). The Guilford Press.

Diener, E., & Lucas, R. E. (2018). Personality traits: Required reading. In R. Biswas-Diener & E. Diener (Eds.), *Handbook of subjective well-being* (pp. 279–296). DEF Publishers.

Diener, E., Scollon, C. N., & Lucas, R. E. (2009). The evolving concept of subjective well-being. The multifaceted nature of happiness. In E. Diener (Ed.), *Assessing well-being. The collected works of Ed Diener* (pp. 67–100). Springer.

Diener, E., Seligman, M. E. P., Choi, H., & Oishi, S. (2018). Happiest people revisited. *Perspectives on Psychological Science, 13*(2), 176–184. https://doi.org/10.1177/1745691617697077

Diener, E., Suh, E. M., Lucas, R. E., & Smith, H. L. (1999). Subjective well-being: Three decades of progress. *Psychological Bulletin, 125*(2), 276–302. https://doi.org/10.1037/0033-2909.125.2.276

Dror, O. E. (2016). Cold war "super-pleasure": Insatiability, self-stimulation, and the postwar brain. *Osiris, 31*(1), 227–249. https://doi.org/10.1086/688162

Dukes, D., Abrams, K., Adolphs, R., Ahmed, M. E., Beatty, A., Berridge, K. C., Broomhall, S., Brosch, T., Campos, J. J., Clay, Z., Clément, F., Cunningham, W. A., Damasio, A., Damasio, H., D'Arms, J., Davidson, J. W., de Gelder, B., Deonna, J., de Sousa, R., et al. (2021). The rise of affectivism. *Nature Human Behaviour, 5*(7), 816–820. https://doi.org/10.1038/s41562-021-01130-8

Duncan, E., & Grazzani-Gavazzi, I. (2004). Positive emotional experiences in Scottish and Italian young adults: A diary study. *Journal of Happiness Studies, 5*(4), 359–384. https://doi.org/10.1007/s10902-004-0666-8

Ebbinghaus, H. (1885/1964). *Memory: A contribution to experimental psychology* (T. H. A. Ruger & C. E. Bussenius, Trans.). Dover (Original work published in 1885).

Eckblad, G. (1963). The attractiveness of uncertainty. *Scandinavian Journal of Psychology, 4*, 1–13.

Eckblad, G. (1981). *Scheme theory*. Academic Press.
Ekkekakis, P. (2013). *The measurement of affect, mood, and emotion. A guide for health behavioral research*. Cambridge University Press.
Ekman, P. (1980). Universal facial expressions of emotion. *Journal of Personality and Social Psychology, 39*, 1125–1134.
Ekman, P. (1992). An argument for basic emotions. *Cognition and Emotion, 6*(3–4), 169–200. https://doi.org/10.1080/02699939208411068
Ekman, P. (1994). All emotions are basic. In P. Ekman & R. J. Davidson (Eds.), *The nature of emotion. Fundamental questions* (pp. 15–19). Oxford University Press.
Ekman, P. (2003). *Emotions revealed: Recognizing faces and feelings to improve communication and emotional life*. Henry Holt.
Ekman, P., & Cordaro, D. (2011). What is meant by calling emotions basic. *Emotion Review, 3*(4), 364–370. https://doi.org/10.1177/1754073911410740
Ekman, P., & Davidson, R. J. (Eds.). (1994). *The nature of emotion. Fundamental questions*. Oxford University Press.
Elfenbein, H. A., & Ambady, N. (2002). On the universality and cultural specificity of emotion recognition: A meta-analysis. *Psychological Bulletin, 128*(2), 203–235. https://doi.org/10.1037/0033-2909.128.2.203
Eliot, G. (1985). *Middlemarch*. Bantham Books. (Original work published 1871–1872).
Ellsworth, P. C. (1994). William James and emotion: Is a century of fame worth a century of misunderstanding? *Psychological Review, 101*(2), 222–229.
Ellsworth, P. C. (2003). Confusion, concentration, and other emotions of interest: Commentary on Rozin and Cohen (2003). *Emotion, 3*(1), 81–85. https://doi.org/10.1037/1528-3542.3.1.81
Ellsworth, P. C., & Smith, C. A. (1988). Shades of joy: Patterns of appraisal differentiating pleasant emotions. *Cognition and Emotion, 2*(4), 301–331.
English, H. B., & English, A. C. (1958). *A comprehensive dictionary of psychological and psychoanalytical terms*. Longmans, Green.
Fehr, B., & Russell, J. A. (1984). Concept of emotion viewed from a prototype perspective. *Journal of Experimental Psychology: General, 113*(3), 464–486. https://doi.org/10.1037/0096-3445.113.3.464
Field, J. (1981/1934). *A life of one's own*. J. P. Tarcher. (Original work published in 1934).
Flanagan, O. (2007). *The really hard problem. Meaning in a material world*. The MIT Press.
Fox, A. S., Lapate, R. C., Shackman, A. J., & Davidson, R. J. (Eds.). (2018). *The nature of emotion: Fundamental questions [Kindle]*. Oxford University Press.
Frank, L. (2018). *The pleasure shock: The rise of deep brain stimulation and its forgotten inventor [Kndle]*. Penguin.
Frankfurt, H. (1982). The importance of what we care about. *Synthese, 53*, 257–272.
Fredrickson, B. L. (2009). *Positivity: Groundbreaking research to release your inner optimism and thrive [Kindle]*. Crown Publishers.
Fredrickson, B. L., Cohn, M. A., Coffey, K., Pek, J., & Finkel, S. M. (2008). Open hearts build lives: Positive emotions, induced through meditation, build consequential personal resources. *Journal of Personality and Social Psychology, 95*(5), 1045–1062.
Fredrickson, B. L., Manusco, R. A., Braningan, C., & Tugade, M. M. (2000). The undoing effect of positive emotions. *Motivation and Emotion, 24*(4), 237–258.
Freud, S., & Breuer, J. (1895). *Studies on hysteria. The Pelican Freud Library*. Penguin (current edition 1974).
Frevert, U. (2016). The history of emotion. In L. F. Barrett, M. Lewis, & J. M. Haviland-Jones (Eds.), *Handbook of emotions* (pp. 49–65). Guilford Publications.
Frijda, N. H. (1986). *The emotions*. Cambridge University Press.
Frijda, N. H. (1999). Emotions and hedonic experience. In D. Kahneman, E. Diener, & N. Schwarz (Eds.), *Well-being: the foundations of hedonic psychology* (pp. 190–210). Russell Sage Foundation.
Frijda, N. H. (2007). *The laws of emotions*. Lawrende Erlbaum Associates.

Gaver, W. W., & Mandler, G. (1987). Play it again Sam: On liking music. *Cognition and Emotion, 1*(3), 259–282.
Gendron, M., & Feldman Barrett, L. (2009). Reconstructing the past: A century of ideas about emotion in psychology. *Emotion Review, 1*(4), 316–339. https://doi.org/10.1177/1754073909338877
Gilovich, T. D., Epley, N., & Hanko, K. (2005). Shallow thoughts about the self: The automatic components of self-assessment. In M. D. Alicke, D. Dunning, & J. Krueger (Eds.), *The self in social judgment* (5th ed., pp. 67–84). Psychology Press.
Ginsburg, H., & Opper, S. (1969). *Piaget's theory of intellectual development. An introduction*. Prentice-Hall.
Glomb, T. M., Bhave, D. P., Miner, A. G., & Wall, M. (2011). Doing good, feeling good: Examining the role of organizational citizenship behaviors in changing mood. *Personnel Psychology, 64*(1), 191–223. https://doi.org/10.1111/j.1744-6570.2010.01206.x
Goffman, E. (1961). Fun in games. In *Encounters: Two studies in the sociology of interaction* (pp. 15–81). Bobbs-Merrill.
Green, J. D., Sedikides, C., Saltzberg, J. A., Wood, J. V., & Forzano, L.-A. B. (2003). Happy mood decreases self-focused attention. *British Journal of Social Psychology, 42*(1), 147–157. https://doi.org/10.1348/014466603763276171
Haidt, J. (2012). *The righteous mind: Why good people are divided by politics and religion [Kindle]*. Penguin Books.
Haig, B. D. (2005). An abductive theory of scientific method. *Psychological Methods, 10*, 371–388.
Haybron, D. M. (2008). *The pursuit of unhappiness. The elusive psychology of well-being*. Oxford University Press.
Heath, R. G. (1963). Electrical self-stimulation of the brain. *American Journal of Psychiatry, 120*(6), 571–577.
Heath, R. G. (Ed.). (1964). *The role of pleasure in behavior. A symposium by 22 authors*. Harper & Row Publishers.
Henrich, J., Heine, S. J., & Norenzayan, A. (2010). The weirdest people in the world? *Behavioral and Brain Sciences, 33*, 61–83.
Hidi, S. (2006). Interest: A unique motivational variable. *Educational Research Review, 1*(2), 69–82. https://doi.org/10.1016/j.edurev.2006.09.001
Hilgard, E. R. (1980). The trilogy of mind: Cognition, affection, and conation. *Journal of the History of the Behavioral Sciences, 16*(2), 107–117. https://doi.org/10.1002/1520-6696(198004)16:2<107::AID-JHBS2300160202>3.0.CO;2-Y
Hudson, N. W., Lucas, R. E., & Donnellan, M. B. (2020). Are we happier with others? An investigation of the links between spending time with others and subjective well-being. *Journal of Personality and Social Psychology, 119*(3), 672–694. https://doi.org/10.1037/pspp0000290
Humphrey, N. (2006). *Seeing red. A study in consciousness*. The Belknap Press of Harvard University Press.
Huntsinger, J. R., Isbell, L. M., & Clore, G. L. (2014). The affective control of thought: Malleable, not fixed. *Psychological Review, 121*(4), 600–618. https://doi.org/10.1037/a0037669
Inzlicht, M., Bartholow, B. D., & Hirsh, J. B. (2015). Emotional foundations of cognitive control. *Trends in Cognitive Sciences, 19*(3), 126–132. https://doi.org/10.1016/j.tics.2015.01.004
Iran-Nejad, A. (1987). Cognitive and affective causes of interest and liking. *Journal of Educational Psychology, 79*(2), 120–130.
Isen, A. M., & Daubman, K. A. (1984). The influence of affect on categorization. *Journal of Personality and Social Psychology, 47*(6), 1206–1217.
Izard, C. E. (1977). *Human emotions*. Plenum Press.
Izard, C. E. (2007). Basic emotions, natural kinds, emotion schemas, and a new paradigm. *Perspectives on Psychological Science, 2*(3), 260–280. https://doi.org/10.1111/j.1745-6916.2007.00044.x
Izard, C. E. (2011). Forms and functions of emotions: Matters of emotion–cognition interactions. *Emotion Review, 3*(4), 371–378. https://doi.org/10.1177/1754073911410737
Izard, C. E., & Ackerman, B. P. (2000). Motivational, organizational, and regulatory functions of discrete emotions. In M. Lewis & J. M. Haviland-Jones (Eds.), *Handbook of emotions* (pp. 253–264). The Guilford Press.

James, W. (1884). What is an emotion? *Mind, 9*, 188–205.
James, W. (1890). *Principles of psychology*. Henry.
Johnson-Laird, P. N., & Oatley, K. (2000). Cognitive and social construction in emotions. In M. Lewis & J. M. Haviland-Jones (Eds.), *Handbook of emotions* (pp. 458–475). The Guilford Press.
Jurist, E. (2019). Review of How emotions are made: The secret life of the brain. *Journal of Theoretical and Philosophical Psychology, 39*(3), 193–198. https://doi.org/10.1037/teo0000098
Kagan, J. (1994). Distinctions among emotions, moods, and temperamental qualities. In P. Ekman & R. J. Davidson (Eds.), *The Nature of emotion. Fundamental questions* (pp. 74–78). Oxford University Press.
Kagan, J. (1998). *Galen's prophecy. Temperament in human nature*. Westview Press.
Kagan, J. (2002). *Surprise, uncertainty, and mental structures*. Harvard University Press.
Kagan, J. (2018). The bases for preservation of emotional biases. In A. S. Fox, R. C. Lapate, A. J. Shackman, & R. J. Davidson (Eds.), *The nature of emotion. Fundamental questions [Kindle]* (pp. 66–71). Oxford University Press.
Kahneman, D. (1999). Objective happiness. In D. Kahneman, E. Diener, & N. Schwarz (Eds.), *Well-being: The foundations of hedonic psychology* (pp. 3–25). Russell Sage Foundation.
Kahneman, D. (2011). *Thinking, fast and slow*. Penguin Books.
Kahneman, D., Krueger, A. B., Schkade, D., Schwarz, N., & Stone, A. (2004). A survey method for characterizing daily life experience: The Day Reconstruction Method. *Science, 305*(5702), 1776–1780. https://doi.org/10.1126/science.1103572
Keltner, D. (2009). *Born to be good: The science of meaningful life [Kindle]*. Norton.
Keltner, D. (2023). *Awe: the new science of everyday wonder and how it can transform your life*. Penguin Press.
Keltner, D., & Cowen, A. (2021). A taxonomy of positive emotions. *Current Opinion in Behavioral Sciences, 39*, 216–221. https://doi.org/10.1016/j.cobeha.2021.04.013
Keltner, D., & Oatley, K. (2022). Social functions of emotions in life and imaginative culture. *Evolutionary Studies in Imaginative Culture, 6*(1), 1–20. https://doi.org/10.26613/esic.6.1.263
Keltner, D., Oatley, K., & Jenkins, J. M. (2014). *Understanding emotions* (3rd ed.). Wiley.
Keltner, D., Oatley, K., & Jenkins, J. M. (2019). *Understanding emotions* (4th ed.). Wiley.
Kesebir, P., & Diener, E. (2008). In pursuit of happiness: Empirical answers to philosophical questions. *Perspectives on Psychological Science, 3*(2), 117–125. https://doi.org/10.1111/j.1745-6916.2008.00069.x
Kirby, L. A. J., & Robinson, J. L. (2017). Affective mapping: An activation likelihood estimation (ALE) meta-analysis. *Brain and Cognition, 118*, 137–148. https://doi.org/10.1016/j.bandc.2015.04.006
Kleinginna, P. R., & Kleinginna, A. M. (1981). A categorized list of emotion definition, with suggestions for a consensual definition. *Motivation and Emotion, 5*, 345–379.
Kragel, P. A., & LaBar, K. S. (2016). Decoding the nature of emotion in the brain. *Trends in Cognitive Sciences, 20*(6), 444–455. https://doi.org/10.1016/j.tics.2016.03.011
Kranzbühler, A.-M., Zerres, A., Kleijnen, M. H. P., & Verlegh, P. W. J. (2020). Beyond valence: A meta-analysis of discrete emotions in firm-customer encounters. *Journal of the Academy of Marketing Science, 48*(3), 478–498. https://doi.org/10.1007/s11747-019-00707-0
Kringelbach, M. L., & Berridge, K. C. (2017). The affective core of emotion: Linking pleasure, subjective well-being, and optimal metastability in the brain. *Emotion Review, 9*(3), 191–199. https://doi.org/10.1177/1754073916684558
Lambie, J. A., & Marcel, A. J. (2002). Consciousness and the variety of emotion experience: A theoretical framework. *Psychological Review, 109*(2), 219–259.
Laming, D. R. J. (2000). On the behavioural interpretation of neurophysiological observation. *Behavioral and Brain Sciences, 23*(2), 209–209. https://doi.org/10.1017/S0140525X00392421
Lang, P. J., & Bradley, M. M. (2013). Appetitive and defensive motivation: Goal-directed or goal-determined? *Emotion Review, 5*(3), 230–234. https://doi.org/10.1177/1754073913477511
Lazarus, R. S. (1966). *Psychological stress and the coping process*. McGraw-Hill.
Lazarus, R. S. (1991a). Cognition and motivation in emotion. *American Psychologist, 46*(4), 352–367.

Lazarus, R. S. (1991b). *Emotion and adaptation*. Oxford University Press.
Lazarus, R. (1994). The stable and unstable in emotions. In P. Ekman & R. J. Davidson (Eds.), *The nature of emotion. Fundamental questions* (pp. 79–85). Oxford University Press.
Lazarus, R. S. (2001). Relational meaning and discrete emotions. In K. R. Scherer, A. Schorr, & T. Johnstone (Eds.), *Appraisal processes in emotion. Theory, methods, research* (pp. 37–67). Oxford University Press.
Lench, H. C., Flores, S. A., & Bench, S. W. (2011). Discrete emotions predict changes in cognition, judgment, experience, behavior, and physiology: A meta-analysis of experimental emotion elicitations. *Psychological Bulletin, 137*(5), 834–855. https://doi.org/10.1037/a0024244
Lewis, M. (2016). The emergence of human emotion. In L. F. Barrett, M. Lewis, & J. M. Haviland-Jones (Eds.), *Handbook of emotions* (pp. 272–292). Guilford Publications.
Lindquist, K. A., Wager, T. D., Kober, H., Bliss-Moreau, E., & Barrett, L. F. (2012). The brain basis of emotion: A meta-analytic review. *Behavioral and Brain Sciences, 35*(3), 121–143. https://doi.org/10.1017/S0140525X11000446
Locke, E. A. (1969). What is job satisfaction? *Organizational Behavior and Human Performance, 4*(4), 309–336. https://doi.org/10.1016/0030-5073(69)90013-0
Lomas, T. (2018). *Translating happiness: A cross-cultural lexicon of well-being [Kindle]*. MIT Press.
Lomas, T. (2021). Life balance and harmony. *International Journal of Wellbeing, 11*(1). https://doi.org/10.5502/ijw.v11i1.1477.
Lucas, R. E., & Diener, E. (2015). Personality and subjective well-being: Current issues and controversies. In *APA handbook of personality and social psychology, Volume 4: Personality processes and individual differences* (pp. 577–599). American Psychological Association. https://doi.org/10.1037/14343-026
Magen, Z. (1998). *Exploring adolescent happiness. Commitment, purpose, and fulfillment*. Sage.
Mandler, G. (1982). The structure of values: Accounting for taste. In M. S. Clark & S. T. Fiske (Eds.), *Affect and cognition. The seventeenth annual carnigie symposium on cognition* (pp. 3–36). Lawrence Erlbaum.
Mandler, G. (1984). *Mind and body. Psychology of emotion and stress*. W.W. Norton & Company.
Mandler, G. (1993). Approaches to a psychology of value. In M. Hechter, L. Nadel, & R. E. Michod (Eds.), *The origin of values* (pp. 229–258). Aldine de Gruyter.
Martindale, C. (1984). The pleasure of though: A theory of cognitive hedonism. *The Journal of Mind and Behavior, 5*(1), 40–80.
Maslow, A. (1964). *Religions, values and peak-experiences*. Ohio State University Press.
Matsumoti, D., & Ekman, P. (2009). Basic emotions. In D. Sander & K. R. Scherer (Eds.), *The Oxford companion to emotive and the affective sciences* (p. 104). Oxford University Press.
Miron, M. S. (1969). What is it that is being differentiated by the semantic differential? *Journal of Personality and Social Psychology, 12*(3), 189–193.
Misrahi, R. (1994). *Le bonheur, essai la joie*. Optiques, Hatier.
Mogilner, C., Kamvar, S. D., & Aaker, J. (2011). The shifting meaning of happiness. *Social Psychological and Personality Science, 2*(4), 395–402. https://doi.org/10.1177/1948550610393987
Montague, R. (2007). *Your brain is (almost) perfect: How we make decisions [Kindle]*. Dutton.
Moors, A. (2009). Theories of emotion causation: A review. *Cognition and Emotion, 23*(4), 625–662. https://doi.org/10.1080/02699930802645739
Moors, A. (2012). Comparison of affect program theories, appraisal theories, and psychological construction theories. In P. Zachar & R. D. Ellis (Eds.), *Categorical versus dimensional models of affect: A seminar on the theories of Panksepp and Russell* (pp. 257–278). John Benjamins.
Moors, A., Ellsworth, P. C., Scherer, K. R., & Frijda, N. H. (2013). Appraisal theories of emotion: State of the art and future development. *Emotion Review, 5*(2), 119–124. https://doi.org/10.1177/1754073912468165
Morris, W. N. (1999). The mood system. In D. Kahneman, E. Diener, & N. Schwarz (Eds.), *Well-being: The foundations of hedonic psychology* (pp. 169–189). Russell Sage Foundation.

Moskowitz, J. T., Clark, M. S., Ong, A. D., & Gruber, J. (2014). The role of positive affect on thinking and decision-making. A tribute to Alice Isen. In J. Gruber & J. T. Moskowitz (Eds.), *Positive emotion: Integrating the light sides and dark sides* (pp. 72–77). Oxford University Press.
Myers, D. G., & Diener, E. (1995). Who is happy? *Psychological Science, 6*(1), 10–19.
Nagel, T. (1974). What is it like to be a bat? *Philosophical Review, 83*, 435–450.
Nell, V. (1988). *Lost in a book*. Yale University Press.
Norris, C. J., Gollan, J., Berntson, G. G., & Cacioppo, J. T. (2010). The current status of research on the structure of evaluative space. *Biological Psychology, 84*(3), 422–436. https://doi.org/10.1016/j.biopsycho.2010.03.011
Nussbaum, M. C. (2001). *Upheavals of thought*. Cambridge University Press.
Oatley, K. (1992). *Best laid schemes. The psychology of emotions*. Cambridge University Press.
Oatley, K. (2004). Emotional intelligence and the intelligence of emotions. *Psychological Inquiry, 15*(3), 216–236.
Oatley, K. (2011). *Such stuff as dreams. The psychology of fiction*. Wiley-Blackwell.
Oatley, K. (2012). *The passionate muse. Exploring emotion in stories*. Oxford University Press.
Oatley, K. (2018). *Our minds, our selves: A brief history of psychology [Kindle]*. Princeton University Press.
Oatley, K., & Jenkins, J. M. (1996). *Understanding emotions*. Blackwell.
Oatley, K., & Johnson-Laird, P. N. (1987). Towards a cognitive theory of emotions. *Cognition and Emotion, 1*(1), 29–50.
Oatley, K., & Johnson-Laird, P. N. (1996). The communicative theory of emotions: Empirical tests, mental models, and implications for social interaction. In L. L. Martin & A. Tesser (Eds.), *Striving and feeling. Interactions among goals, affect, and self-regulation* (pp. 363–394). Lawrence Erlbaum.
Oatley, K., & Johnson-Laird, P. (2011). Basic emotions in social relationships, reasoning, and psychological illnesses. *Emotion Review, 3*(4), 424–433. https://doi.org/10.1177/1754073911410738
Oishi, S., & Westgate, E. C. (2022). A psychologically rich life: Beyond happiness and meaning. *Psychological Review, 129*(4), 790–811. https://doi.org/10.1037/rev0000317
Olds, J. (1956). Pleasure centers in the brain. *Scientific American, 195*(4), 105–117. http://www.jstor.org/stable/24941787
Olds, J., & Milner, P. (1954). Positive reinforcement produced by electrical stimulation of septal area and other regions of rat brain. *The Journal of Comparative Physiological Psychology, 47*, 419–427.
Ortony, A., Clore, G. L., & Collins, A. (1988). *The cognitive structure of emotions*. Cambridge University Press.
Ortony, A., Clore, G. L., & Collins, A. (2022). *The cognitive structure of emotions [Kindle]*. Cambridge University Press.
Ortony, A., Norman, D. A., & Revelle, W. (2005). Affect and proto-affect in effective functioning. In J. M. Fellous & M. A. Arbib (Eds.), *Who needs emotions* (pp. 173–202). Oxford University Press.
Panksepp, J. (1994). The basics of basic emotions. In P. Ekman & R. J. Davidson (Eds.), *The nature of emotion. Fundamental questions* (pp. 20–24). Oxford University Press.
Panksepp, J. (1998a). *Affective neuroscience. The foundations of human and animal emotions*. Oxford University Press.
Panksepp, J. (1998b). The quest for long term happiness: to play or not to play, that is the question. *Psychological Inquiry, 9*(1), 56–66.
Panksepp, J. (2000). Emotions as natural kinds within the mammalian brain. In M. Lewis & J. M. Haviland-Jones (Eds.), *Handbook of emotions* (pp. 137–156). The Guilford Press.
Panksepp, J. (2012). In defence of multiple core affects. In P. Zachar & R. D. Ellis (Eds.), *Categorical versus dimensional models of affect: A seminar on the theories of Panksepp and Russell* (pp. 31–78). John Benjamins.
Panksepp, J., & Biven, L. (2012). *The archaeology of mind. Neuroevolutionary origins of human emotions*. Norton.
Piaget, J. (1952). *The origins of intelligence in children*. International Universities Press.

Pizarro, J. J., Basabe, N., Fernández, I., Carrera, P., Apodaca, P., Man Ging, C. I., Cusi, O., & Páez, D. (2021). Self-transcendent emotions and their social effects: Awe, elevation and Kama Muta promote a human identification and motivations to help others. *Frontiers in Psychology, 12*, 709859.

Plamper, J. (2015). *The history of emotions: An introduction [Kindle]*. Oxford University Press.

Plutchik, R. (1980). *Emotion. A psychoevolutionary synthesis*. Harper & Row.

Plutchik, R., & Kellerman, H. (Eds.). (1980). *Theories of emotion, vol. 1 of Emotion: Theory, research, and experience*. Academic Press.

Power, M., & Dalgleish, T. (2015). *Cognition and emotion. From order to disorder* (3rd ed.). Psychology Press.

Pribram, K. H. (2003). Forebrain psychophysiology of feelings: Interest and involvement. *International Journal of Psychophysiology, 48*(2), 115–131. https://doi.org/10.1016/S0167-8760(03)00049-7

Proffitt, D. R. (2006). Embodied perception and the economy of action. *Perspectives on Psychological Science, 1*(2), 110–122.

Proust, M. (1981). *Remembrance of things past* [À la recherche du temps perdu] (C. K. Scott Moncrief & T. Kilmartin, Trans.). Vintage Books.

Quennell, P. (1988). *The pursuit of happiness*. Oxford University Press.

Rangel, A., Camerer, C., & Montague, P. R. (2008). A framework for studying the neurobiology of value-based decision making. *Nature Reviews Neuroscience, 9*(7), 545–556. https://doi.org/10.1038/nrn2357

Rathunde, K. (1993). The experience of interest: A theoretical and empirical look at its role in adolescent talent development. *Advances in Motivation and Achievement, 8*, 59–98.

Reeve, J. (1989). The interest-enjoyment distinction in intrinsic motivation. *Motivation and Emotion, 13*(2), 83–103.

Reeve, J. (1993). The face of interest. *Motivation and Emotion, 17*(4), 353–375.

Reisenzein, R. (1992). A structuralist reconstruction of Wundt's three-dimensional theory of emotion. In H. Westmeyer (Ed.), *The structuralist program in psychology. Foundations and applications* (pp. 141–189). Hogrefe & Huber.

Renninger, K. A., & Hidi, S. (2016). *The power of interest for motivation and engagement [Kindle]*. Routledge.

Ricard, M. (2007). *The art of happiness. A guide to developing life's most important skill*. Atlantic Books.

Richardson, A. (1999). Subjective experience: Its conceptual status, method of investigation, and psychological significance. *The Journal of Psychology, 133*(5), 469–485. http://search.proquest.com/docview/213827001?accountid=17260

Richardson, F. C. (2012). On psychology and virtue ethics. *Journal of Theoretical and Philosophical Psychology, 32*(1), 24–34. https://doi.org/10.1037/a0026058

Roseman, I. J. (1984). Cognitive determinants of emotions: A structural theory. In *Review of personality and social psychology; Vol 5. Emotions, relationships, and health*. Sage.

Roseman, I. J., & Smith, C. A. (2001). Appraisal theory: Overview, assumptions, varieties, controversies. In K. R. Scherer, A. Schorr, & T. Johnstone (Eds.), *Appraisal processes in emotion. Theory, methods, research* (pp. 3–34). Oxford University Press.

Rozin, P. (2009). What kind of empirical research should we publish, fund, and reward?: A different perspective. *Perspectives on Psychological Science, 4*(4), 435–439. https://doi.org/10.1111/j.1745-6924.2009.01151.x

Ruckmick, C. A. (1925). The psychology of pleasantness. *Psychological Review, 32*(5), 362–383.

Ruedy, N. E., Moore, C., Gino, F., & Schweitzer, M. E. (2013). The cheater's high: The unexpected affective benefits of unethical behavior. *Journal of Personality and Social Psychology, 105*(4), 531–548. https://doi.org/10.1037/a0034231

Russell, J. A. (2003). Core affect and the psychological construction of emotion. *Psychological Review, 110*(1), 145–172.

Russell, B. (2011). Introduction to a special section on basic emotion theory. *Emotion Review, 3*(4), 363. https://doi.org/10.1177/1754073911411606

Russell, J. A., & Barrett, L. F. (1999). Core affect, prototypical emotional episodes, and other things called emotion: dissecting the elephant. *Journal of Personality and Social Psychology, 76*(5), 805–819.

Russell, J. A., & Barrett, L. F. (2009). Core affect. In D. Sander & K. R. Scherer (Eds.), *The Oxford companion to emotive and the affective sciences* (p. 104). Oxford University Press.

Russert, T. (2007). *Wisdom of our fathers: Lessons and letters from daughters and sons.* Random House.

Sacks, O. (1990). *Awakenings*. Macmillan: Picador.

Salovey, P., & Mayer, J. (1990). Emotional intelligence. *Imagination, Cognition and Personality, 9*, 185–211.

Scarantino, A. (2016). The philosophy of emotions and its impact on affective science. In L. F. Barrett, M. Lewis, & J. M. Haviland-Jones (Eds.), *Handbook of emotions* (pp. 3–48). Guilford Publications.

Schachter, S., & Singer, J. E. (1962). Cognitive, social and physiological determinants of emotional state. *Psychological Review, 69*(5), 379–399.

Scherer, K. R. (1984). Emotion as a multi-component process: A model and some cross-cultural data. In P. Shaver (Ed.), *Review of personality and social psychology 5. Emotions, relationships, and health.* Sage.

Scherer, K. R. (1986). Studying emotions empirically: Issues and a paradigm for research. In K. R. Scherer, H. G. Wallbott, & A. B. Summerfield (Eds.), *Experiencing emotions: A cross-cultural study* (pp. 3–27). Cambridge University Press.

Scherer, K. R. (1988). Criteria for emotion antecedent appraisal: A review. In J. Kuhl, M. Kazen-Saad, V. Hamilton, G. Bower, & N. Frijda (Eds.), *Cognitive perspectives on emotion and motivation* (pp. 89–126). Kluwer. https://link.springer.com/chapter/10.1007%2F978-94-009-2792-6_4

Scherer, K. R. (1994). Towards a concept of "modal emotions". In P. Ekman & R. J. Davidson (Eds.), *The nature of emotion. Fundamental questions* (pp. 25–31). Oxford University Press.

Scherer, K. R. (2009). The dynamic architecture of emotion: Evidence for the component process model. *Cognition and Emotion, 23*(7), 1307–1351. https://doi.org/10.1080/02699930902928969

Scherer, K. R., Schorr, A., & Johnstone, T. (Eds.). (2001). *Appraisal processes in emotion. Theory, methods, research.* Oxford University Press.

Schimmack, U., & Crites, S. L. (2005). The structure of affect. In D. Albarracín, B. T. Johnson, & M. P. Zanna (Eds.), *The handbook of attitudes* (pp. 397–435). Lawrence Erlbaum.

Schweder, R. A. (1994). "You're not sick, you're just in love": Emotion as an interpretive system. In P. Ekman & R. J. Davidson (Eds.), *The nature of emotion. Fundamental questions* (pp. 32–44). Oxford University Press.

Searle, J. R. (2004). *Mind. A brief introduction.* Oxford University Press.

Shapere, D. (1976). The influence of knowledge on the description of facts. *Philosophy of Science Association, 2*, 281–298.

Shaver, P., Schwartz, J., Kirson, D., & O'Connor, C. (1987). Emotion knowledge: Further exploration of a prototype approach. *Journal of Personality and Social Psychology, 52*(6), 1061–1086. https://doi.org/10.1037/0022-3514.52.6.1061

Shiner, R. L. (2018). Personality as lasting individual differences in emotions. In A. S. Fox, R. C. Lapate, A. J. Shackman, & R. J. Davidson (Eds.), *The nature of emotion. Fundamental questions [Kindle]* (pp. 61–64). Oxford University Press.

Shiner, R. L., & DeYoung, C. G. (2013). The structure of temperament and personality traits: A developmental perspective. In P. D. Zelazo (Ed.), *The Oxford handbook of developmental psychology, Vol. 2: Self and other* (pp. 113–141). Oxford University Press. https://doi.org/10.1093/oxfordhb/9780199958474.013.0006

Shiota, M. N., Campos, B., Oveis, C., Hertenstein, M. J., Simon-Thomas, E., & Keltner, D. (2017). Beyond happiness: Building a science of discrete positive emotions. *American Psychologist, 72*(7), 617–643. https://doi.org/10.1037/a0040456

Shiota, M. N., Sauter, D. A., & Desmet, P. M. A. (2021). What are 'positive' affect and emotion? *Current Opinion in Behavioral Sciences, 39*, 142–146. https://doi.org/10.1016/j.cobeha.2021.03.007

Shizgal, P. (1999). On the neural computation of utility: Implications from studies of brain stimulation reward. In D. Kahneman, E. Diener, & N. Schwarz (Eds.), *Well-being: the foundations of hedonic psychology* (pp. 502–526). Russell Sage Foundation. http://cogprints.org/740/1/Well-Being_v4_15.html

Shostak, M. (1981). *Nisa. The life and words of an !Kung woman*. Vintage Books.

Siegel, E. H., Sands, M. K., Van den Noortgate, W., Condon, P., Chang, Y., Dy, J., Quigley, K. S., & Barrett, L. F. (2018). Emotion fingerprints or emotion populations? A meta-analytic investigation of autonomic features of emotion categories. *Psychological Bulletin, 144*(4), 343–393. https://doi.org/10.1037/bul0000128

Silvia, P. J. (2005). What is interesting? Exploring the appraisal structure of interest. *Emotion, 5*(1), 89–102.

Silvia, P. J. (2006). *Exploring the psychology of interest*. Oxford University Press.

Silvia, P. J. (2014). Knowledge emotions: Feelings that foster learning, exploring, and reflecting. In R. Biswas-Diener & E. Diener (Eds.), *Noba textbook series: Psychology*. DEF Publishers. https://doi.org/nobaproject.com

Silvia, P. J., Henson, R. A., & Templin, J. L. (2009). Are the sources of interest the same for everyone? Using multilevel mixture models to explore individual differences in appraisal structures. *Cognition and Emotion, 23*(7), 1389–1406. https://doi.org/10.1080/02699930902850528

Silvia, P. J., & Kashdan, T. B. (2009). Interesting things and curious people: Exploration and engagement as transient states and enduring strengths. *Social and Personality Compass, 3*(5), 785–797.

Simon, H. A. (1967). Motivational and emotional controls of cognition. *Psychological Review, 74*(1), 29–39.

Small, D. M., Zatorre, R. J., Dagher, A., Evans, A. C., & Jones-Gotman, M. (2001). Changes in brain activity related to eating chocolate. From pleasure to aversion. *Brain, 124*, 1720–1733.

Smith, C. A., & Ellsworth, P. C. (1985). Patterns of cognitive appraisal in emotion. *Journal of Personality and Social Psychology, 48*(4), 813–838. https://doi.org/10.1037/0022-3514.48.4.813

Smith, C. A., & Lazarus, R. S. (1990). Emotion and adaptation. In L. Pervin (Ed.), *Handbook of personality: Theory and research*. Guildford.

Smith, C. A., & Lazarus, R. S. (1993). Appraisal components, core relational themes, and the emotions. *Cognition and Emotion, 7*(3–4), 233–269. https://doi.org/10.1080/02699939308409189

Smith, C. A., Tong, E. M. W., & Ellsworth, P. C. (2014). The differentiation of positive emotional experience as viewed through the lens of appraisal theory. In M. M. Tugade, M. N. Shiota, & K. N. Kirby (Eds.), *Handbook of positive emotions* (pp. 11–27). Guilford.

Steel, P., Schmidt, J., & Shultz, J. (2008). Refining the relationship between personality and subjective well-being. *Psychological Bulletin, 134*(1), 138–161.

Stein, N. L., & Hernandez, M. W. (2007). Assessing understanding and appraisals during emotional experience. The development and use of Narcoder. In J. A. Coan & J. J. B. Allen (Eds.), *Handbook of emotion elicitation and assessment* (pp. 298–317). Oxford University Press.

Stein, N. L., Trabasso, T., & Liwang, M. D. (2000). A goal appraisal theory of emotional understanding: Implications for development and learning. In M. Lewis & J. M. Haviland-Jones (Eds.), *Handbook of emotions* (pp. 436–457). The Guilford Press.

Straume, L. V., & Vittersø, J. (2012). Happiness, inspiration and the fully functioning person: Separating hedonic and eudaimonic well-being in the work place. *Journal of Positive Psychology, 7*(5), 387–398. https://doi.org/10.1080/17439760.2012.711348

Su, R., Tay, L., & Diener, E. (2014). The development and validation of the Comprehensive Inventory of Thriving (CIT) and the Brief Inventory of Thriving (BIT). *Applied Psychology: Health and Well-Being, 6*(3), 251–279. https://doi.org/10.1111/aphw.12027

Summerfield, A. B., & Green, E. J. (1986). Categories of emotion-eliciting events: A qualitative overview. In K. R. Scherer, H. G. Wallbott, & A. B. Summerfield (Eds.), *Experiencing emotions: A cross-cultural study* (pp. 50–65). Cambridge University Press.

Tatarkiewicz, W. (1976). *Analysis of happiness*. Nijhoff.

Taylor, J. B. (2008). *My stroke of insight [Kindle]*. Hodder & Stoughton.

Teigen, K. H. (1985). The novel and the familiar: Sources of interest in verbal information. *Current Psychology, 4*(3), 224–238. https://doi.org/10.1007/bf02686573

Teigen, K. H. (1986). Old truths or fresh insights? A study of students' evaluations of proverbs. *British Journal of Social Psychology, 25*(1), 43–49. https://doi.org/10.1111/j.2044-8309.1986.tb00700.x

Teigen, K. H. (1987). Intrinsic interest and the novelty–familiarity interaction. *Scandinavian Journal of Psychology, 28*(3), 199–210.

Tesser, A., & Martin, L. (1996). The psychology of evaluation. In E. T. Higgins & A. W. Kruglanski (Eds.), *Social psychology. Handbook of basic principles* (pp. 400–431). The Guildford Press.

Thagard, P. (2002). The passionate scientist: Emotion in scientific cognition. In P. Carruthers, S. Stich, & M. Siegal (Eds.), *The cognitive basis of science* (pp. 235–250). Cambridge University Press.

Tolstoy, L. (2014). *Anna Karenina* (M. Schwartz, Trans.). Yale University Press. (Original work published 1878).

Tomkins, S. S. (1962). *Affect, imagery, consciousness. Vol. 1. The positive affects*. Springer.

Tomkins, S. S. (1963). *Affect, imagery, consciousness. Vol. 2. The negative affects*. Springer.

Turner, S. A., Jr., & Silvia, P. J. (2006). Must interesting things be pleasant? A test of competing appraisal structures. *Emotion, 6*(4), 670–674.

Valente, D., Theurel, A., & Gentaz, E. (2018). The role of visual experience in the production of emotional facial expressions by blind people: A review. *Psychonomic Bulletin & Review, 25*(2), 483–497. https://doi.org/10.3758/s13423-017-1338-0

Veenhoven, R. (1984). *Conditions of happiness*. Kluwer Academic.

Viñas, F., González, M., Malo, S., García, Y., & Casas, F. (2014). Temperament and personal well-being in a sample of 12 to 16 year-old adolescents. *Applied Research in Quality of Life, 9*(2), 355–366. https://doi.org/10.1007/s11482-013-9242-x

Vittersø, J. (2016). The feeling of excellent functioning: Hedonic and eudaimonic emotions. In J. Vittersø (Ed.), *Handbook of eudaimonic well-being* (pp. 253–276). Springer. https://doi.org/10.1007/978-3-319-42445-3_17

Vittersø, J. (2018). Do it! Activity theories and the good life. In E. Diener, S. Oishi, & L. Tay (Eds.), *Handbook of well-being*. DEF Publishers. https://doi.org/nobascholar.com

Vittersø, J., & Nilsen, F. (2002). The conceptual and relational structure of subjective well-being, neuroticism, and extraversion: Neuroticism is again found to be the important predictor of happiness. *Social Indicators Research, 57*(1), 89–118.

Vittersø, J., Overwien, P., & Martinsen, E. (2009). Pleasure and interest are differentially affected by replaying versus analyzing a happy life moment. *The Journal of Positive Psychology, 4*(1), 14–20. https://doi.org/10.1080/17439760802060602

Vittersø, J., & Søholt, Y. (2011). Life satisfaction goes with pleasure and personal growth goes with interest: Further arguments for separating hedonic and eudaimonic well-being. *Journal of Positive Psychology, 6*(4), 326–335. https://doi.org/10.1080/17439760.2011.584548

Vittersø, J., Søholt, Y., Hetland, A., Thorsen, I. A., & Røysamb, E. (2010). Was Hercules happy? Some answers from a functional model of human well-being. *Social Indicators Research, 95*(1), 1–18. https://doi.org/10.1007/s11205-009-9447-4

Vytal, K., & Hamann, S. (2010). Neuroimaging support for discrete neural correlates of basic emotions: A voxel-based meta-analysis. *Journal of Cognitive Neuroscience, 22*(12), 2864–2885. https://doi.org/10.1162/jocn.2009.21366

Wager, T. D., Kang, J., Johnson, T. D., Nichols, T. E., Satpute, A. B., & Barrett, L. F. (2015). A Bayesian model of category-specific emotional brain responses. *PLoS Computational Biology, 11*(4), e1004066. https://doi.org/10.1371/journal.pcbi.1004066

Walker, E. L. (1980). *Psychological complexity and preference. A hedhodge theory of behavior.* Brooks-Cole.
Watson, J. (1999). *The double helix. A personal account of the structure of DNA*. Penguin Books.
Watson, D. (2000). *Mood and temperament*. The Guilford Press.
Watson, D. (2002). Positive affectivity: The disposition to experience pleasurable emotional states. In *Handbook of positive psychology* (pp. 106–119). Oxford University Press.
Watson, D., Clark, L. A., & Tellegen, A. (1988). Development and validation of brief measures of positive and negative affect: The PANAS scales. *Journal of Personality and Social Psychology, 54*(6), 1063–1070. https://doi.org/10.1037/0022-3514.54.6.1063
Watson, D., Wiese, D., Vaidya, J., & Tellegen, A. (1999). The two general activation systems of affect: Structural findings, evolutionary considerations, and psychobiological evidence. *Journal of Personality and Social Psychology, 76*(5), 820–838.
Whorf, B. L. (1956). *Language, thought, and reality*. Technology Press of MIT.
Widen, S. C. (2016). The development of children's concepts of emotion. In L. F. Barrett, M. Lewis, & J. M. Haviland-Jones (Eds.), *Handbook of emotions* (pp. 307–318). Guilford Publications.
Wilson-Mendenhall, C. D., Barrett, L. F., & Barsalou, L. W. (2013). Neural evidence that human emotions share core affective properties. *Psychological Science, 24*(6), 947–956. https://doi.org/10.1177/0956797612464242
Zachar, P. (2012). Introduction. In P. Zachar & R. D. Ellis (Eds.), *Categorical versus dimensional models of affect: A seminar on the theories of Panksepp and Russell* (pp. 1–30). John Benjamins.
Zajonc, R. B. (1980). Feelings and thinking: Preferences need no inferences. *American Psychologist, 35*(2), 151–175. https://doi.org/10.1037/0003-066X.35.2.151

Chapter 4
Life Satisfaction

Introduction

When animals are satisfied, they tend to fall asleep. (Panksepp & Biven, 2012, p. 85)

The word satisfaction comes from the Latin *satis* (enough) and *facere* (to do or make) and was once used to express an opportunity to defend one's honor. In the European upper classes of the seventeenth and eighteenth centuries, it was not uncommon to hear the phrase "I demand the satisfaction of a gentleman," illustrating that duels were not always fought to kill the opponent but to satisfy or restore one's honor (Millingen, 2022). When the concept of satisfaction was introduced as an object of scientific studies in the early twentieth century, however, it had little to do with restoring the honors of gentlemen. For example, Kurt Lewin initiated a paradigm that looked at satisfaction in the context of aspiration research. In this new context, satisfaction came to mean things such as the fulfillment of needs and desires or the ability to live up to one's expectations (Carlquist et al., 2016).

The current wellbeing literature is more specifically concerned with the concept of satisfaction with life, although satisfaction with life domains, such as job satisfaction or leisure satisfaction, is also relevant. A small sample of definitions of life satisfaction is provided in Table 4.1.

The first four definitions are cognitive or computational in the sense that life satisfaction is supposed to comprise a comparison between one's life as currently lived or perceived and some ideal or standard for one's life. The next definitions are less concrete with respect to the cognitive element assumed to be involved; rather, life satisfaction is taken to be an evaluation or appraisal. As we have seen in Chap. 3, evaluations can be conscious or unconscious, and they can be affective or cognitive. Within this evaluative framework, life satisfaction is typically considered to be reflective and broad and to concern one's life as a whole (definitions 5 and 6). The evaluation can regard the *quality* of one's life (definition 8) or how *happy* one's life is (definition 9). Satisfaction can even be a cognitive experience (definition 1) or a transcendent experience (definition 10). However, the latter definition does not refer

J. Vittersø, *Humanistic Wellbeing*, https://doi.org/10.1007/978-3-031-69292-5_4

Table 4.1 Some definitions of life satisfaction

Definition	Source
1. A cognitive experience in which the individual compares his perception of his present situation to a situation which he aspired to, expected, or felt he deserved	Campbell et al. (1976, p. 119)
2. A function of perceived discrepancies between what one has and wants, relevant others have, the best one has had in the past, expected to have 3 years ago, expects to have after 5 years, deserves, and needs	Michalos (1985, p. 348)
3. A personal assessment of one's condition compared to an external reference standard or to one's aspirations	McDowell (2006, p. 521)
4. A comparison of one's circumstances with what is thought to be an appropriate standard	Diener et al. (1985, p. 71)
5. A report of how a respondent evaluates or appraises his or her life taken as a whole. It is intended to represent a broad, reflective appraisal that a person makes of his or her life	Diener (2006, p. 401)
6. A life satisfaction judgment is the assessment a person makes of how well his or her life is going overall	Tiberius (2014, p. 3591)
7. A reflective assessment on a person's life or some specific aspect of it	OECD (2013, p. 9)
8. Happiness or life satisfaction denotes the degree to which people judge the overall quality of their life as a whole favorably	Veenhoven (1988, p. 334)
9. A component of subjective wellbeing that reflects the cognitive evaluation of whether one is happy with one's life	Cheung and Lucas (2014, p. 2809)
10. A state of blessed contentment, nirvana, mystical enlightenment, peace, tranquility, a sense of something beyond your existence	Berns (2010, loc. 3108)

to life satisfaction but rather to satisfaction as a feeling and was included in the table to illustrate that the term satisfaction sometimes refers explicitly to an affective concept.

Life satisfaction is often used interchangeably with happiness. Veenhoven's formulation (definition 8) is one example, and a similar approach is taken by Tsurumi et al. (2021). These authors define life satisfaction as "a cognitive conceptualization of happiness" (p. 2501). A combination of happiness and satisfaction also appeared in Andrews and Withey's classic texts from 1976: *Social Indicators of Well-Being*. The book introduced the Delighted–Terrible scale, which asks: "How do you feel about your life as a whole…?" and offers the following response options: (1) terrible, (2) unhappy, (3) mostly dissatisfied, (4) mixed, (5) mostly satisfied, (6) pleased, and (7) delighted.

Relatedly, in *The Quality of American Life*—another classic from 1976—Campbell, Converse, and Rodgers aspired to bridge the gap between satisfaction as affect and satisfaction as cognition. The authors argued that life satisfaction comprises a phenomenological component, a kind of judgmental feeling or cognitive experience (p. 8). Campbell and colleagues even talked about satisfaction as an "experience of pleasure" that "hinge upon the relationship of current experience to past experience" (p. 184). However, the process that generated the experience was cognitive and could be "precisely defined as the perceived discrepancy between aspiration and achievement, ranging from the perception of fulfillment to that of deprivation" (Campbell et al., 1976, p. 8).

These examples illustrate that life satisfaction can be seen as an affective indicator of wellbeing, as well as a cognitive indicator. Both approaches will be examined next.

Life Satisfaction as Affective Wellbeing

The term satisfaction can be affective in the sense of being a feeling. For example, the English Dictionary (Dictionary & Lexico) explains that one meaning of satisfaction is the pleasure derived from the fulfillment of one's wishes, expectations, or needs. The MacMillan dictionary defines satisfaction as "the feeling of pleasure that you get when you achieve or obtain something that you want." The Oxford Dictionary of English offers several definitions, and one considers satisfaction to be "the sense of achievement and the fulfillment of a need."

Similarly, and in contrast to mainstream SWB research, the general psychology literature frequently categorizes satisfaction as an affective concept. For example, to explain the mechanism behind his law of effect, Thorndike (1927) referred to the term "satisfyingness," which is characterized as a hedonic concept in the sense of describing a state of pleasure (Beebe-Center, 1932). In motivational psychology, satisfaction is also considered to be affective and rewarding. Trope (1986, p. 352) suggested that "success produces positive esteem-related affect (e.g., pride, satisfaction)." Here, satisfaction is considered to be something we experience after a need or desire has been fulfilled or after a goal has been achieved. The self-determination theory (SDT; Ryan & Deci, 2017) provides a comprehensive account of these mechanisms. The theory will be discussed in detail in Chap. 6, but briefly, it considers satisfaction to be a hedonic reward mechanism that kicks in when a psychological need has been fulfilled. According to the SDT, satisfaction is a feeling that follows from need fulfillment and goal achievement, i.e., something that occurs after an act of behavior has been completed: "The reward (and hence, satisfaction) is the feeling of competence and self-determination which results from having done that" (Deci, 1975, p. 104). Ekman (2003) similarly considers satisfaction to be affective and describes it as a feeling that typically occurs "when everything seems right in the world, when there is nothing we feel we need to do" (p. 193). As a final example, Casebeer (2003) categorizes satisfaction as a "higher-order emotion."

These descriptions are about satisfaction more generally, and not about satisfaction with life as a whole, which is the concept of interest in the mainstream wellbeing literature. But even for life satisfaction, we can find affective definitions. Some of these were mentioned in the above review of the happiness as life satisfaction discussion in the 1970s and 1980s. More recently, Crisp (2017) has noted that within positive psychology, life satisfaction is sometimes given "some kind of hedonistic account" (p. 3). An example in case is a paper by Kaiser and Oswald (2022), in which self-reported life satisfaction is referred to as a measure of a feeling state.

With more analytical detail, a qualitative study by Ralph et al. (2012) asked Britons about their interpretations of a commonly used self-report question in life satisfaction research: "Overall, how satisfied are you with your life nowadays?" Most participants took the item to be a positive statement, although a few identified it as neutral or even negative. The researchers categorized the positive responses into three clusters. Interestingly, all of them defined life satisfaction as affective. The three meanings applied to life satisfaction were (a) feeling one's needs have been completely met, (b) peace and contentment felt in life, or (c) happiness felt in life. The number of respondents in the study was small ($N \approx 40$), so the results cannot be easily generalized to a broader population. Nevertheless, the answers reflect the views of at least some people, and they match the results from other and more powerful examinations like those reported by Ross et al. (1986) who used a "think aloud" procedure to allow participants to report on their life satisfaction, happiness, and domain satisfaction. The researchers specifically asked how the participants decided whether they were satisfied with their lives. Between 41% and 53% of the responses were categorized as affective. Examples of affective responses included statements such as "I am feeling very smug, very satisfied right now, I enjoy being with my family, I enjoy cooking"; "You get mad if you are dissatisfied"; "I get panicky and shaky sometimes"; and "Well, I feel good."

A conceptual analysis of the term life satisfaction was also provided by Carlquist et al. (2018). Based on qualitative responses from 276 Norwegians, the authors found that the term life satisfaction ("livstilfredshet" in Norwegian) has a multitude of meanings, which were categorized into financial aspects, health, nourishment, material aspects, and psychological conditions. The latter category reflects both cognitive and affective meanings, with responses such as harmony, calmness, contentment, joy, enjoyment, and absence of worries.

The affective element of life satisfaction has also been identified in quantitative examinations. In a creative study by Røysamb et al. (2018), the facets of the five factor model of personality were used as predictors of self-reported life satisfaction. Among the 30 personality facets, only depression, anxiety, positive emotions, and activity were significantly related to life satisfaction. As the authors commented, the highly emotional nature of these facets is noteworthy. Similarly, Kainulainen et al. (2018) found that the affective component (pleasure) predicts more life satisfaction variance than does the cognitive component (getting things you want from life). The robust finding that neuroticism is the strongest predictor of life satisfaction (Anglim et al., 2020; Steel et al., 2008; Vittersø & Nilsen, 2002) also speaks to the affective argument in conceptual debates about life satisfaction.

The perspective of satisfaction as a feeling is also dominant in studies on work satisfaction (Weiss, 2002). For example, an authority such as Locke (1969) defines job satisfaction as "the pleasurable emotional state resulting from the appraisal of one's job as achieving or facilitating the achievement of one's job value" (p. 316).

In the philosophical literature on wellbeing, Sumner (1996) argues that happiness can be articulated in terms of life satisfaction and that life satisfaction is a concept that comprises both cognitive and affective components. The affective component is defined as the presence of positive emotions, whereas the cognitive component is defined as a judgment about a life that is going well, according to the standards for the person whose life it is.

The psychologist Robert Cummins stands out as a vibrant defender of the position that life satisfaction is affective. He argues that a survey item such as "How satisfied are you with your life as a whole?" is predominantly affective (e.g., Capic et al., 2020). A series of studies provide empirical support for this claim, such as Davern et al. (2007), who reported that 66% of the variance in life satisfaction measures is emotional. To account for these observations, Cummins proposed that the variance of life satisfaction measures can be divided into two components. One is a stable mood affect called Homeostatically Protected Mood (HPMood), and the other is emotion. HPMood is a biologically determined positive mood that comprises the most basic experienced feelings (Cummins, 2010). It represents the unchanging, affective-mood setpoint for each person, which is at a constant level within that range. These two mechanisms led Cummins to conclude that satisfaction with life is "dominated by its affective content" (Cummins & Weinberg, 2015, p. 239).

Schwarz and Strack have also written extensively on the role of mood in judgments about life satisfaction (e.g., Schwarz & Strack, 1991, 1999; Strack et al., 1991). The authors argue that mood may affect self-reported life satisfaction, but they maintain that the informational value of mood becomes important only for self-reported life satisfaction when affect appears salient in the reporter's awareness. This makes life satisfaction an unstable indicator of wellbeing because affect can easily be manipulated into a survey participant's awareness through experimental manipulation. This was illustrated in the "weather study" (Schwarz & Clore, 1983), a telephone survey in which participants were interviewed on either warm and sunny days or on rainy spring days. Participants called on sunny days reported higher levels of both "momentary happiness" (a proxy for mood) and life satisfaction than did those called on rainy days. However, no difference in life satisfaction was found in comparison with a group for whom the weather was explicitly mentioned before the interviewer started questioning the participants. Mood was unaffected by the experimental manipulation and remained high for sunny days and low for rainy days. Schwarz and Strack suggest that participants in bad moods eliminate the "default assumption" of taking good moods as an indicator of high life satisfaction. Rather, the participants attributed their low mood to bad weather and turned to other sources of information when judging their life satisfaction.

Finally, Veenhoven also finds good reasons to assume that overall life satisfaction is mostly inferred from affective experience. One of the reasons is that "life-as-a-whole is not a suitable object for calculative evaluation. Life has many aspects, and there is usually not one clear-cut ideal model to compare with" (Veenhoven, 2013, p. 208).

Life Satisfaction as Cognitive Wellbeing

In his 1984 *Psychological Bulletin* article on subjective wellbeing, Diener downplayed the affective part of life satisfaction and proposed to define the concept as "a cognitive judgmental evaluation of one's life" (Diener, 1984, p. 550). He has also referred to life satisfaction as "a cognitive sense of satisfaction with life" (Diener & Suh, 1997, p. 200). Two other definitions proposed by Diener are presented in Table 4.1.

During his long career as a wellbeing researcher, Sirgy (2012) has also argued that life satisfaction should be considered a cognitive component of wellbeing, whereas happiness is an affective component (p. 35). Steptoe et al. (2015, p. 641) have suggested that survey questions about life satisfaction are "likely to demand *substantial thinking* (italics added), including aggregation over time and comparison with self-selected standards." The number of researchers who reason along similar lines is large and includes Krasko et al. (2022), Lomas et al. (2021), Lucas et al. (1996), Luhmann et al. (2012), OECD (2013), and Stiglitz et al. (2009).

Many philosophers also distinguish between affective wellbeing (i.e., happiness) and cognitive wellbeing (i.e., life satisfaction). Haybron considers life satisfaction to be a rational affirmation of the question of whether things are generally going well for a person: "The rational part of life satisfaction *competes* (italics added) with the emotional part involved in happiness, defined in this context to be an emotional response to a life when things are generally experienced as going well. We might say that life satisfaction chiefly concerns the endorsement of the intellect, whereas happiness concerns the endorsement of the emotional aspects of the self" (Haybron, 2008, p. 111). Similarly, Feldman (2010) concludes that happiness and satisfaction are quite different concepts and that a person therefore can be happy without being satisfied, and vice versa. To support this view, Feldman presents an imagined person who has no reason to be discontented with her life and consequently reports high levels of life satisfaction. Nevertheless, this person is not necessarily happy because she is never in a cheerful mood and never enjoys anything.

Computations

What do SWB researchers mean by declaring that life satisfaction is cognitive? Generally, cognition is associated with non-affective mental activities such as problem solving, remembering, and analyzing. But none of these processes are evaluative. So how can these cognitive processes determine whether a life is good or bad? One answer suggests that a cognitive evaluation can be made by means of computations as a step-by-step sequence of logical comparisons of predefined standards for a good life against the actual life a person is leading. This approach is exemplified in the first definitions of Table 4.1. Historically, Fritz Heider argued that the meaning of satisfaction gives itself according to the formula "desire and obtaining x are sufficient conditions of pleasure"[1] (Heider, 1958, p. 130). To Heider, this connection is a priori, what in semantics is referred to as an "analytic proposition." Analytic propositions are true by virtue of their meaning, as in defining a bachelor as an unmarried adult. As discussed in Chap. 1, analytic propositions cannot be justified or falsified by empirical observations (e.g., Putnam, 2004).

Katzell (1964) offers a technical formulation of the analytic approach and suggests that a given amount of object–value discrepancy will produce different degrees of satisfaction, depending on the importance of the value they represent for the individual. Katzell's formula is:

$$S = \frac{1-(X-V)}{V}$$

where S = satisfaction, X = the amount of stimulus, and V = the amount most desired. This is "analogous to a Weber function for evaluation, e.g., the more of something one wants, the less 'noticeable' will be a given amount of deficit" (cited in Locke, 1969, p. 323). Katzell's equation visualizes the principal problem for the computational approach, which is that it overestimates the capacity individuals have for making complex, cognitive comparisons.

When these tedious and time-consuming computational mechanisms are fleshed out in more detail, the trustworthiness of the perspective must be questioned. This becomes even more evident in Davis' (1981) proposal to compute the level of happiness in a person's life. Davis uses the term happiness rather than life satisfaction, but the analytical reasoning he details for estimating the gap between one's current conditions in life and one's preferred conditions applies to both concepts.

Davis considers happiness to be a combination of three things: beliefs (b), desires (d), and thinking or "a thought predicate" (P). Happiness is the linear combination of these ingredients, calculated as

$$h_A^t = \sum_{i=1}^{n} b(P_i)\,d(P_i), \text{where } P_1 \ldots P_n \text{ is an enumeration of all thoughts A is thinking.}$$

Here, h_A^t represents person A's happiness at time t. To the extent that A is aware of his or her happiness, A must continuously think through every proposition he or she is contemplating at the moment, multiply the degree (quantified as a number) to which the thought is believed by the degree (again quantified as a number) to which it is desired, and add up all the products. The sum, according to Davis, is person A's degree of happiness at time t.

To put the effort needed to calculate the information requested in the above proposals in perspective, consider an illustration provided by Johnson-Laird et al. (2004). The authors explain that if one wants to compare 100 dual propositions, the time needed for the calculation is much longer than the universe has existed. The analysis would take approximately 4 quadrillion years, or 4^{16} years—given that each

[1] In this context, Heider is using pleasure as a synonym for satisfaction.

possibility was checked in a millionth of a second. Although comparing dual propositions is not directly comparable to weighting and multiplying beliefs, desires, and "utiles," the analogy is not totally irrelevant. After all, the fundamental issue of about wellbeing is for the most part a dual decision: good or bad. As it has been suggested that a conscious moment lasts 2–3 s (Tononi, 2004) and given that a billion seconds is almost 32 years, a human coming to age must calculate the satisfaction of more than a billion conscious moments to cover their "life as a whole."

The models and procedures proposed by Katzell and Davis are extreme versions of the idea that judgments of life satisfaction are generated as cognitive computations. To my knowledge, mainstream SWB researchers do not think of life satisfaction along these lines. Yet, the examples illustrate the fundamental problem in the computational approach to life satisfaction, which is the enormous amount of cognitive processing it requires. Even more modest versions of the comparison hypothesis about life satisfaction encounter these issues. For example, Michalos' multiple discrepancies theory suggests that "Reported net satisfaction is a function of perceived discrepancies between what one has and wants, relevant others have, the best one has had in the past, expected to have 3 years ago, expects to have after 5 years, deserves and needs" (Michalos, 1985, p. 347).

Relatedly, Andrews and Withey (1976) proposed that a cognitive evaluation of life satisfaction could proceed as a mental add-up of a series of judgments of life domains. The authors proposed that a cognitive evaluation could be made along three levels of specificity so that a series of distinct evaluative "criteria" could be combined with any applicable life domain. The model can then be represented as a matrix, with the criteria located along the columns and the life conditions, or domains, along the rows. Each cell mean in the matrix reflects a particular decision (for example, satisfaction with achieved success, safety, joy, or any other relevant evaluation a person may make) related to a particular domain (such as house, job, family life, or any other relevant domain in a person's life). Each row mean reflects the sum of all possible evaluative decisions that can be made for a particular domain, and each column mean reflects the sum of a particular decision across all the possible decisions. Resembling statistical analyses of variance (where the rightmost bottom cell of the matrix summarizes the "grand mean"), the concept of life satisfaction is also represented as the "grand mean" in the Andrews and Withey matrix. Unlike the mathematical preciseness of an ANOVA table, however, both common sense and empirical evidence suggest that the cell means of a cognitive evaluation described by Andrews and Withey hardly add up to the row means and column means. Neither will the row means nor the column means amount to an overall "grand mean." Empirical estimates suggest that approximately half of the variance in global life satisfaction can be accounted for by domain satisfactions (McLean et al., 2020; Tomyn & Cummins, 2011).

Diener and his colleagues have also suggested that life satisfaction reflects a process in which individuals "examine the conditions in their lives, weigh the importance of these conditions, and then evaluate their lives on a scale ranging from dissatisfied to satisfied" (Diener et al., 2009, p. 196). Similarly, Pavot and Diener write that life satisfaction is "a judgmental process, in which individuals assess the quality of their lives on the basis of their own unique set of criteria. A comparison of one's perceived life circumstances with a self-imposed standard or set of standards is presumably made, and to the degree that conditions match these standards, the person reports high life satisfaction" (Pavot & Diener, 1993, p. 164). Moreover, when the Satisfaction With Life Scale was introduced (Diener et al., 1985), the aim was to measure "a comparison of one's circumstances with what is thought to be an appropriate standard" (p. 71). However, the details of these comparisons are not accounted for.

But Diener has also endorsed a different perspective on life satisfaction, one that defines the concept as a global or overall evaluation. Definition 5 in Table 4.1 ("life satisfaction as a report of how a respondent evaluates or appraises his or her life taken as a whole, intended to represent a broad, reflective appraisal that a person makes of his or her life") is an example. A reminiscent idea is advocated in Diener and Seligman (2004), who write that "well-being includes pleasure, engagement, and meaning, and the concept of life satisfaction may reflect all of these" (p. 4).[2] In the next section, I refer to this approach as the "all things considered myth" of life satisfaction research.

The "All Things Considered" Myth

As far as I know, the "all things considered" verdict in empirical wellbeing research started with Gurin et al. (1960), known as the developers of an early and influential happiness scale. The introduction to the survey item has become a classic way of measuring overall happiness and life satisfaction, and it is spelled out like this: "Taking all things together, how would you say things are these days?" The response options in the Gurin et al. scale are (1) very happy, (2) pretty happy, and (3) not too happy. Ever since this formula was introduced, wellbeing researchers have been surprisingly loyal to the idea that humans can express the realization of everything they value in a single number. Large study programs and numerous researchers are now committed to this paradigm (e.g., Clark et al., 2018; Helliwell et al., 2021). The World Values Survey and the European Social Survey use a version of this phrase in their questionnaires, which in both surveys runs: "All things considered, how satisfied are you with your life as a whole these days?" The Office for National Statistics in Britain (ONS) asks "Overall, how satisfied are you with your life nowadays?" as part of their National Well-being Programme (Ralph et al., 2012). Both the "all ting considered" and the "overall" phrases are also recommended by the OECD (2013) as a default setup for wellbeing surveys.

Helliwell and colleagues argue that the response people give to questions about life satisfaction "is based on their focus on life as a whole, thereby permitting

[2] This quote is a bit confusing, considering that Diener also has suggested that "A person's subjective well-being cannot be fully assessed by a single measure such as life satisfaction" (Diener et al., 2012, p. 140).

economics, health, trust, freedom and social relations to be *consistently* (italics added) taken into account, using survey-based life evaluations as the research base to establish *what matters most* (italics added)" (Helliwell et al., 2014, p. 3). A similar way of thinking is adopted in the prestigious report from the Sarkozy Commission, which shares the notion of satisfaction as an evaluation of all things that matter. The authors conclude that life satisfaction is "a convenient shortcut and potentially provides a natural way to aggregate various experiences in a way that reflects *people's own preferences* (italics added). Furthermore, this approach makes it possible to reflect *the diversity* (italics added) of people's views about what is important in their lives" (Stiglitz et al., 2009, p. 245). Another example of this reasoning is provided by Diener and Tov (2012). Because life satisfaction is a state in which a person believes that life is going well, "it reflects *the many different values* (italics added) that are strived for by the individual" (p. 137). Oishi is more specific in suggesting how reflective values are included in self-reports of life satisfaction: "even if different individuals and cultures hold different views of happiness, the subjective judgments, as long as they are well informed, provide a good clue into how well or poorly their lives are going. Hedonists might judge their lives based on how much pleasure they feel each day, while moralists might judge their lives based on how virtuous their lives have been" (Oishi, 2012, p. 12). Similarly, Diener et al. (2012) hypothesized that life satisfaction "can be influenced both by hedonic and what are called eudaimonic aspects of life" (p. 334).

However, what kind of arguments can defend the omnipresent "all things considered" doctrine? More precisely, how can the doctrine be accommodated to current knowledge about the limits of human cognitive processing capacities? It can certainly not be defended on the basis of response time. Survey participants spend only a few seconds answering a question about life satisfaction, hardly more than they need to answer questions about their current mood (Robinson & Clore, 2002; Vittersø et al., 2009).

Several possible answers to the "all things considered" puzzle were proposed by Diener and his colleagues about 20 years ago. In response to the fact that human cognition is inept at processing the information needed to compare "all things" in a person's lives, Diener and Lucas (2000) introduced the evaluative theory of wellbeing. The theory suggests that only some evaluative comparisons enter the mental computation that produces the responses to life satisfaction measures. Diener and Lucas referred to this more limited proportion of information evaluated in survey responses as "chronically accessible information."

The empirical support for the idea of chronically accessible information was reviewed in Diener (2013). The authors argue that 74% of the variance in life satisfaction is due to chronically accessible information. But this number basically refers to how much stable mood contributes to life satisfaction (see Eid & Diener, 2004) and if mood is the dominating mechanism in life satisfaction, the cognitive nature of life satisfaction is in trouble. Other studies from the Diener camp point more directly to cognitive content in their account for the chronically accessible information. For example, Schimmack et al. (2002) reported that college students frequently and consistently use information about their family, relationships with friends, romantic life, and academic success to assess their satisfaction with life. Thus, Schimmack et al. proposed that self-reports on life satisfaction draw on three types of information: (1) a temporarily accessible source that is salient in one assessment situation but not in other situations, (2) chronically accessible sources that provide variable information, and (3) chronically accessible sources that provide stable information (Schimmack et al., 2002, p. 348). The model was able to account for a series of empirical observations, such as temporal fluctuations in satisfaction measures (Schwarz & Clore, 1988); how satisfaction may vary as a function of changeable internal and external circumstances, such as changes in mood (Schwarz & Clore, 1983), health, or income (Pagán-Rodrıguez, 2012); and the relatively high stability of life satisfaction measured over time (Diener, 2012; Pavot & Diener, 1993). In support of their model, Schimmack and colleagues also reported several studies in which domain satisfaction correlated with life satisfaction but only when the domain was judged as important by the participant. In other words, domains reported as important were more strongly correlated with life satisfaction than domains rated as less important. This can be taken as evidence that people do keep prestored evaluations about important aspects of their lives readily accessible and that these evaluations are prompted in survey responses about satisfaction. However, the valuation questions in the Schimmack et al. (2002) studies were asked *after* the life satisfaction questions, so the researchers did not really test whether the values were prestored and thus activate before the life satisfaction responses were given.

Oishi (2012) has presented some arguments in favor of the accommodated "all things considered" doctrine inherent in Diener and Lucas' evaluation theory. Oishi reasoned that responses to life satisfaction items can be both quick and reliable, given that the evaluation required to produce them is well practiced. If people frequently reflect upon the quality of their lives, they will also have easy access to the relevant information used to guide their snap judgments about life satisfaction. If we think more often about important than unimportant circumstances in our lives, the former comes to mind more easily when we respond to survey questions about life satisfaction. This is not an unreasonable suggestion since studies show that most people think about happiness quite often. In an early investigation, Freedman (1978, p. 4) noted that "people are very interested in happiness and seem to enjoy talking about it." A study reported by Andrews and Withey more systematically asked a US sample if they believed that the adult population maintained some form of running evaluation about their lives, and the results revealed that "the majority of respondents agreed that some evaluation is kept by most people" (Andrews & Withey, 1976, p. 65). This result accords with one of Andrews and Withey's own investigations. After having asked thousands of survey participants to evaluate the quality of their life-as-a-whole, this study concluded that people are able and willing to give such answers "promptly and with apparent ease" (Andrews & Withey, 1976, p. 64). Diener (2000) collected cross-cultural data to show that these results seem to be generalizable to most countries. Asking participants how often they think about happiness on a scale from 1 (never) to 7 (very much) revealed a county average between 5 and 6 in most nations. Diener asked the same question about life satisfaction and obtained comparable results. The average across the 17 nations was 5.3 for happiness and 5.1 for life satisfaction.

Some critiques against this conclusion have been voiced. For example, Freedman observed that people tended to "avoid thinking about happiness too seriously" (Freedman, 1978, p. 5). Few people, he claims, "spend much time considering the elements that may go into happiness" (p. 10). Hence, the fact that people regularly think briefly about happiness does not support the assumption that they reflect upon it deeply or in the sense of "all things considered." Freedman's observation is also corroborated in more recent research. Tetlock (1992) found that in a survey context, people typically behave as cognitive misers, i.e., they are reluctant to make deeper analyses of the items they are answering. The same conclusion was drawn by Gilovich et al. (2005), who found that the answers given in surveys are produced relatively spontaneously and automatized and do not result from carefully thinking about each question. This tendency seems to increase as the topic under evaluation becomes more complex (Buchanan, 2007; Mercier & Sperber, 2017).

Heuristics

Studies of the information processing strategies utilized by survey participants reveal systematic use of heuristics. In the context of a questionnaire, heuristic judgments mean that a question is substituted for another, and in the case of life satisfaction studies, it means that the extremely complex "all things considered" part is replaced with something simpler. For example, Kahneman (2011) argues that people who respond to wellbeing questions do not engage in careful examination when they evaluate their life. Rather, they use heuristics such as mood and thus substitute the question "How satisfied are you with your life as a whole?" with the question "What is my mood right now?"

Early findings about heuristics and how they are applied by survey participants were reported by Sherman and Corty (1984, p. 218). They found that participants typically develop their answers at the time the question is asked, rather than thoroughly running through their existing knowledge about the topic. Similarly, Schwarz and Strack (1991, p. 28) argue that many survey responses can "be considered constructions to a particular question posed at a particular time." It is also known that participants who are asked to make holistic judgments about multidimensional stimuli use fewer cues than they claim to use (Slovic & Lichtenstein, 1971). Other studies have shown that cognitive processes are simplified as a consequence of increased information complexity (e.g., Payne, 1982).

A response heuristic with relevance for life satisfaction studies is the focusing illusion. It describes how our evaluation of something is affected by first being primed to focus on that something. It is a cognitive trap in the sense that when you do focus on something, its importance increases as *a consequence* of the mere thinking about it. "Nothing in life is as important as you think it is when you are thinking about it" (Kahneman, 2011, p. 402). The essence of the focusing illusion is

WYSIATI (What You See Is All There Is). Basically, the slogan illustrates that people who evaluate their wellbeing normally put too much emphasis on what they are currently attending to and too little emphasis on all the other determinants of life satisfaction. This illusion explains several peculiar and unexpected findings in the wellbeing literature. A well-known example is that people seem to believe that the weather in California increases the life satisfaction of those living there, whereas the weather in midwestern states such as Ohio and Michigan causes as decrease in the life satisfaction of Midwesterners (Schkade and Kahneman, 1998). However, their study revealed no difference in self-reported life satisfaction between the two regions. Directing one's attention to the weather makes these conditions salient, but on a day-to-day basis, "living in California is like having ten toes: nice but not something one thinks much about" (Kahneman, 2011, p. 404).

Another heuristic in wellbeing research is the so-called Lake Wobegon effect, the tendency to overestimate one's capabilities. The name comes from the fictional town created by Garrison Keillor and known from the US radio program *A Prairie Home Companion* and the novel *Lake Wobegon Days*. In the Wobegon community, all children are known to be "above average" (Kruger, 1999), and this better-than-average effect plays out in surveys about life satisfaction—and in many other areas in life. For example, in his study of more than 100,000 Americans, Freedman (1978, p. 38) found that only 13% described themselves as less happy or satisfied than the average US American. Similarly, Michalos (1980) found that survey participants who first compared their lives with that of an average citizen scored higher on a subsequent wellbeing item than when this item came after a comparison of their current life with "their own all-time high." Michalos suggested that this might be taken as evidence for a "better-than-average effect." Another early "Lake Wobegon effect" was demonstrated by Andrews and Withey when they asked participants to estimate their nearest neighbor's global wellbeing and found a scale point difference of −0.30 compared to the participants' own global wellbeing (the mean scores were 5.12 for their neighbor versus 5.42 for themselves). Andrews and Withey referred to this effect as "an interesting bias in perception," but today, most of us would probably refer to it as a better-than-average effect. Similar effects were reported in other life domains, such as participants typically considered themselves to have a better family life, to have more fun, and to be more accepted than others—operationalized than their neighbors. However, there were a few exceptions to this pattern. Ironically, most Americans believed that their nearest neighbor perceived the neighborhood as better than the participants did. The greatest difference was for politics. Here, people very clearly estimated that their neighbors were more satisfied with the national government than they were themselves (Andrews & Withey, 1976, p. 241).

In their classic book *The American Soldier*, Stouffer et al. (1949) found that combatants' satisfaction was more related to their reference group than to the actual degree of hardship they experienced. Stouffer and coworkers further observed that members of the Air Corps expressed less satisfaction with the possibilities for promotions than did members of the Military Police, despite the higher rate of promotions in the Air Corps. The authors suggested that soldiers in different branches adopt different frames of reference when evaluating their promotion opportunities (cited in Ross et al., 1986, p. 83).

Other biases that might influence self-reported life satisfaction include the tendency of optimists to update their beliefs more in response to information that is good rather than bad. In a study by Sharot et al. (2011), highly optimistic individuals "exhibited reduced tracking of estimation errors that called for negative update in right inferior prefrontal gyrus. These findings indicate that optimism is tied to a selective update failure and diminished neural coding of undesirable information regarding the future" (p. 1475). Given that optimism correlates with life satisfaction (e.g., Diener et al., 2018), it is not surprising that satisfied people seem to overreport their life wellbeing (Prati & Senik, 2022). This mechanism has been further described by Lyubomirsky and Ross (1999). These authors followed students' transition from high school to college and compared the likeability of colleges between participants high and low in life satisfaction, or "chronically happy" and "chronically unhappy" individuals, as Lyubomirsky and Ross called them. In a two-wave follow-up study, ratings of likeability measured immediately after the students had sent in their college applications were compared with likeability ratings measured after the students had been informed if the colleges had accepted or rejected them. The chronically happy students changed their likeability in a flexible way. Colleges that accepted them were more attractive at Time 2 than at Time 1. In contrast, the colleges that rejected them were less attractive at Time 2 than at Time 1. These changes were not observed for the chronically unhappy students. These results are interesting in themselves, but for the present purpose, it is important that current mood was unrelated to the observed changes in likeability. The flexible use of evaluative standards was not generated by the affective dimension of wellbeing.

Affective and Cognitive Overlaps and Distinctions

Thus far, I have presented two overarching approaches to the study of life satisfaction. One considers life satisfaction to be an affective concept, and the other considers it a cognitive concept. This distinction is an old heritage, returning to classic Greek thinkers. For example, Plato considered the mind to comprise three independent dimensions, translated to English as cognitive, affective, and motivational. This tripartite structure was adopted by psychologists and have remained popular until recently (e.g., Okon-Singer et al., 2015; Scott et al., 1979). Consequently, much psychology was inspired by a model of the mind that strictly separated cognitive and affective processes, and a review by LeDoux (1998) shows how scientists working in the wake of the cognitive revolution typically excluded emotions from the concept of cognition, as exemplified in the work by central theoreticians such as Fodor (1975) and Neisser (1967). In the 1960s and 1970s, almost everything had a "cognitive" and an "emotional" dimension, and models of wellbeing were no exception (e.g., Andrews & Withey, 1976; Campbell et al., 1976; Diener, 1984; Veenhoven, 1984).

There are differences between cognition and affect (e.g., Mischel & Shoda, 1995; Rolls, 2018), but they are not self-governing or independent, as suggested by Plato and the first generation of cognitive scientists. To the contrary, it has been argued that "it is by no means clear that the distinction between emotion and cognition is one that can or ever should be made" (Gray, 1990, p. 269). Today's scholars typically argue that there is no such thing as a "non-affective thought," and modern psychology has abandoned a strict separation between cognition and affect. For example, Phelps (2006) explained that "it has become increasingly apparent that the neural circuitry of emotion and cognition interact from early perception to decision making and reasoning." Affect plays a role in perception and cognition, even when people cannot feel its influence (e.g., Duncan & Barret, 2007). Barrett (2015, p. 500) explains that "cognition and emotion are still considered separate processes in the mind and brain, but there's growing evidence that the brain does not respect this division—every psychological theory in which emotions and cognitions battle each other, or in which cognitions regulate emotions, is wrong." Hence, Plato's idea of a strict independence between cognition and emotions is considered a relic of the past. The critical question today is how cognition and emotion interact rather than how strict domains of cognitive and emotional components can be mapped (e.g., Okon-Singer et al., 2018; Shackman & Lapate, 2018).

Consider the Capgras syndrome, a very rare condition involving the inability to integrate information about persons into a stable person representation. This inability causes in the bearer of the syndrome a delusion of misperceiving a familiar person as an unknown imposter (Ramachandran, 2011; Sacks, 1998). Some Capgras patients are not able to recognize a close relative such as their mother or spouse, and when the familiar person appears, they are accused of being an intruder. Ramachandran and Hirstein (1999) suggested that the cause may be an affective defect localized in the connections between the cortex and the amygdala. Under normal circumstances, this connection evokes a "warm fuzzy emotional response" when seeing someone dear. "We suggested that in the absence of limbic activation—the 'glow' of recognition—there is no incentive for the brain to link successive views of a face, so that the patient treats a single person as several people" (pp. 31–32). Hence, the concept of a mother is neither "purely cognitive," nor "purely affective."

Something similar can apply for life satisfaction as well: it is not a feeling or a mood but is affected by a valuation mechanism that is not cognitive in the classical sense. Hence, I believe that Cummins' theory of Homeostatically Protected Mood got it wrong and that life satisfaction cannot be reduced to mood and emotions. I also think that Seligman is mistaken in dismissing life satisfaction from his wellbeing theory because, as he argues, it is basically an affective concept determined by positive mood (Seligman, 2011).

Seligman refers to studies by Norbert Schwarz and colleagues to justify his removal of life satisfaction as an essential element in wellbeing. Schwartz research was briefly reviewed in the "Life Satisfaction as Affective Wellbeing" section, and one of his early demonstrations of the influence of mood on life satisfaction was presented in his doctoral thesis. Here, Schwartz observed that participants who randomly found a dime on a copy machine before answering a wellbeing questionnaire reported a marked increase in their life satisfaction compared with those who did not find a dime (e.g., Schwarz et al., 1987). The model suggests that finding a dime increases mood, which in turn increases life satisfaction.

Numerous studies offering empirical support for this "mood as information" argument have since been published by Schwarz and others, yet the impact of current mood on life satisfaction is not as strong as these authors seem to assume. It has, to the contrary, been difficult to replicate the "mood of the day" effect on life satisfaction (Lucas, 2018; Yap et al., 2016). One important study by Eid and Diener (2004) showed that the correlation between current mood and life satisfaction was relatively inconsistent and so small that less than 2% of the occasion-specific variance in life satisfaction could be explained by current mood effects. Moreover, the variability in life satisfaction was much smaller than the variability in mood. Eid and Diener reported that between 74% and 83% of the variance in life satisfaction responses was due to stable life satisfaction rather than situation-specific factors, such as current mood. However, the study did show that the correlation between stable mood and life satisfaction was quite strong ($r = 0.74$). This result indicates that affective traits, but not affective states, influence people's life satisfaction. Other studies using happiness as a proxy for mood have reported comparable results. Sirgy (2012) found that life satisfaction and happiness have between 50% and 60% of their variance in common, an estimate that corresponds roughly to other studies finding a correlation between life satisfaction and happiness to be between 0.70 and 0.80 (e.g., Glatz & Eder, 2020; Glatzer, 1984; Schimmack & Oishi, 2005). These results are basically from WEIRD cultures (Henrich et al., 2010); however, thus, when data from a broader sample of countries are analyzed, the relation between affect and life satisfaction fluctuates more. For example, one study found that the correlation between life satisfaction and affect varied from 0.22 in Nigeria to 0.57 in Germany, with an average cross-national correlation of 0.41 (Suh et al., 1998).

But even if two variables are highly correlated, one cannot assume that they reflect the same underlying concept. As noted by Borsboom et al. (2004), the correlation between lightning and thunder is almost perfect, yet the two phenomena are not identical. Studies by Schimmack and collaborators illustrate how this may apply to the relationship between satisfaction and affect. In one set of analyses, Schimmack et al. (2008) revealed not only that indicators of affective wellbeing and life satisfaction loaded on separate factors but also that the two forms of wellbeing were influenced differently by a set of predictors. The effect of personality was stronger on affective wellbeing than on cognitive wellbeing, whereas the effect of unemployment and religion showed the opposite pattern. Similarly, Luhmann et al. (2012) found that people tend to attribute their life satisfaction to general life circumstances, whereas they attribute affect to specific everyday activities and events. These studies are but some very few examples of the many empirical studies suggesting that life satisfaction and affect are separate, although not uncorrelated, dimensions of wellbeing.

Diener also commented on the separation of life satisfaction and affect in his autobiography: "My own assessment is that I am extremely high in life satisfaction, but I am only average in levels of positive moods" (Diener, 2008, p. 6). Another founding figure in wellbeing research, Alex Michalos, has also pointed out that people can vary somewhat independently in their levels of happiness and satisfaction. He designed a two-by-two table with high versus low life satisfaction along the horizontal line and low versus high happiness along the vertical line. He named people in one cell *frustrated* (low happiness and low satisfaction) and those in another cell *aspirers* (high happiness and low satisfaction). Individuals in the third cell were called *resigned* (low happiness and high satisfaction), and the final group was named *achievers* (high happiness and high satisfaction). In an empirical test of the setup, Michalos (1980) found that aspirers were practically non-existing, comprising only 2 persons out of 353 (i.e., 0.6%). There were some frustrated persons (13%) and some resigned (almost 15%), but most people ended up as achievers (71%).

A more indirect argument about the distinction between affective wellbeing and life satisfaction comes from the extensive study of Henry Molaison, an amnestic patient known in the literature as HM. Due to severe epileptic seizures, an experimental brain surgery was offered for HM in 1953, when he was 27 years old. The operation damaged the central areas of his brain, and HM consequently lost the ability to form new memories. However, he remained highly intelligent, so even if he could forget a conversation that took place minutes before, he was still able to solve challenging crossword puzzles (Corkin, 2014, p. xviii). The psychiatrist George Murray performed a careful examination of HM and formed the impression of a fairly harmonious person who was "always smiling and had a relatively warm interaction with me" (cited in Corkin, 2014, p. 111). HM was also perceived by those who knew him as "easygoing, generous and altruistic" (p. xvii). Nevertheless, there were some troubling elements in his life. For example, when Murray asked HM whether he liked himself, he answered with a cautious smile: "Yes and no." When asked if he felt hopeless, HM, again smilingly, replied, "Yes, and mostly no" (p. 112). HM's wellbeing showed signs of being bothered by his brain damage—troubled by what we perhaps can call a shallow existential living. HM could, for instance, not articulate a life goal for himself, which was a source of frustration. Thus, something seemed to be lacking in HM's mental wellbeing, despite his momentary cheerful mood and smiling appearance. As recalled from Chap. 3, Shizgal (1999) has pointed out that we need to remember things to form and evaluate important goals in our lives. We must be able to mimic scenarios and uphold a cognitive account of how we are doing with regard to our goals, and we need episodic memory to create and execute plans. In other words, we need cognition to plan for a route that leads from the current state to a higher-valued state and to appreciate the achievement, and we need cognition to make relevant evaluations of these achievements. "Essential to such tasks is a readily accessible ('working') memory store in which critical information is held on-line. Working memory also plays an essential role in models that find efficient routes to goals" (Shizgal, 1999, p. 508). In other words, it is unlikely that we can fully process a plan and appreciate successful goal achievement without support from some of the cognitive elements in our minds.

My final example for why life satisfaction is more than affect is from Jill Bolte Taylor. As described in Chapters 1 and 3, Taylor gave a detailed account of her experiences as a stroke patient, culminating in an intense feeling that was "finer than the finest of pleasures" (Taylor, 2008, p. 67). After her recovery, Taylor also reflected on the absence of achievement motivation during her intense moment of ecstatic pleasantness. During the stroke, she was trapped in an ecstatic feeling of pleasure while at the same time being physically powerless and unable to follow a string of logical thought. Her experience made it clear that not only is there a distinction between the pleasure of here-and-now and the satisfaction of getting things done but also that we sometimes have to choose between the two. Contemplating the distinction between peaks of intense pleasure and the satisfaction of goal achievement, Taylor asked herself, "Could I rejoin the rat race without becoming a rat again?" (p. 82).

It is interesting to note that when Seligman went from his "authentic happiness" theory to his newer "flourishing" theory (Seligman, 2011), he also abandoned the view that life satisfaction is the essence of wellbeing (e.g., Diener & Seligman, 2004; Seligman, 2002). In contrast, Kahneman did the opposite move when he turned from his "objective happiness" theory to his "two-dimensional self" theory (Kahneman, 2011; Kahneman & Riis, 2005). According to Kahneman's revised terminology, two kinds of selves are relevant for wellbeing. One is the experiencing self, which is sensitive to feelings. The other is the remembering self, which is sensitive to thinking and judgments. The difference can be explained as a distinction between affective wellbeing (being happy *in* your life) and judgmental wellbeing (being happy *with* your life). In a chapter in Brockman's readable book *What Have You Changed Your Mind About?*, Kahneman (2009) explains how he came to think differently about the affective and cognitive elements of wellbeing. After much pondering the problem of the hedonic treadmill, i.e., the tendency to adopt one's experienced pleasures to the circumstances, Kahneman realized that the situational adjustment of pleasure is different from the situational adjustment of life satisfaction. In other words, there is not one treadmill but two (see also Kahneman, 1999). The things your feelings adopt to are not the same as those your satisfaction adopts to. On the hedonic treadmill, a person's pleasure adapts to the situation that generates it, resulting in a reduced feeling of pleasure. In the satisfaction treadmill, the experienced pleasantness remains steady, but the standards applied to evaluate one's life satisfaction change. The bottom line of the shift in Kahneman's perspective is that pleasure is different from satisfaction and both are important in a good life.

> In part because of these findings I have changed my mind about the definition of well-being. The goals that people set for themselves are so important to what they do and how they feel about it that an exclusive focus on experienced well-being is not tenable. We cannot hold a concept of well-being that ignores what people want. On the other hand, it is also true that a concept of well-being that ignores how people feel as they live and focuses only on how they feel when they think about their life is also untenable. We must accept the complexities of a hybrid view, in which the well-being of both selves is considered. (Kahneman, 2011, p. 401)

Life Satisfaction, Stability, and Cognitive Ease

The humanistic theory of wellbeing assumes that both pleasure and life satisfaction[3] originate from spontaneous good–bad evaluations (SGBE). As will be recalled from Chap. 1, SGBE are quick assessments that humans continuously make about themselves and their environments. Thus, even if pleasure and satisfaction are different, they may have functional similarities. For instance, both are associated with easy information processing, which is typical for System 1 thinking (e.g., Kahneman, 2011; Montague, 2007). Cognitive ease is in turn related to feelings of familiarity, goodness, and effortlessness. This argument suggests that high life satisfaction is associated with things that are easy.

Two schools of thoughts are involved in this debate, and they resemble the two perspectives on emotional happiness presented in Chap. 3. Just as emotional happiness can occur from need fulfillment and goal achievement, life satisfaction can also result when something valuable has been accomplished. In accordance with the idea that happiness is a "stop" signal, life satisfaction can be perceived as a state of "having" (e.g., Allport, 1955; Vittersø, 2018). Opposing this position, arguments have been raised in favor of happiness as a "go" signal and, similarly, that life satisfaction reflects a mental state that tends to initiate activity. Thus, life satisfaction is better conceptualized as a state of "doing," rather than a state of "having."

The HTW is basically teamed up with the "stop/having" perspective and argues that high life satisfaction reflects successful management of stability needs. Satisfaction motivates us to keep things as they are; dissatisfaction motivates us to change the current situation. This, however, is not to say that satisfied people are inactive, since they clearly are not (e.g., Kushlev et al., 2020). But the stability hypothesis does suggest that life satisfaction is more commonly associated with easy rather than complex mental and physical activities.

Against the stability assumption in the HTW, some arguments favor the idea that high life satisfaction is associated with the "doing" perspective. In this view, high life satisfaction reflects approach motivation and stimulates effortful striving. For example, Kesebir and Diener (2008) argue that life satisfaction does not emanate from ease, "but from striving for and making progress toward goals derived from one's most-prized values. Feelings of meaning, purpose, and fulfillment thus typically trump pleasure as predictors of happiness" (p. 121). As reviewed in Chap. 3, wellbeing researchers such as Watson (2002) and Myers and Diener (1995) have also suggested that life satisfaction, or overall happiness, motivates individuals to become involved and activated to make progress toward their goals. In the early days of empirical wellbeing studies, researchers such as Klinger (1975), Palys and Little (1983), Emmons (1986), and Cantor (1990) similarly contributed conceptual and empirical support for the "go/doing" perspective on life satisfaction.

---

[3] In this and the next section, the term happiness is frequently used as a synonym for life satisfaction. The reason is that much of the literature I cite uses the term happiness in the same sense that I use life satisfaction. Adopting the terminology in the cited sources makes the text easier to read.

However, much evidence has also been generated to back the "stop/having" hypothesis about life satisfaction. Conceptually, the having element of life satisfaction is clearly articulated in some of the items in the Satisfaction With Life Scale (Diener et al., 1985). For example, item four reads "So far I *have* gotten the important things I want in life" (italics added). The first two items are also tilted toward a "stop/having" interpretation, as they are worded "In most ways my life *is* close to my ideal," and "The conditions of my life *are* excellent" (italics added). These items refer to a life in stability and fulfillment, i.e., a state that occurs when an activity has successfully led to the completion of its goal and thus maintains a stable end-states (e.g., Denton, 2005; Luhmann & Hennecke, 2017; Panksepp, 1998; Walsh, 2015).

Consistent with the proposal that high life satisfaction is an indicator of stability, Luhmann and Hennecke (2017) suggest that the goals that are approached by satisfied people are oriented toward constancy, whereas those activated by dissatisfied people are oriented toward change. In the seven studies reported in their paper, Luhmann and Hennecke consistently found that participants low in life satisfaction reported a greater desire to change their life circumstances compared with participants high in life satisfaction. Individuals with low life satisfaction scores were also more oriented toward change than individuals with high life satisfaction scores were. A field experiment by Card et al. (2012) supports Luhmann and Hennecke's conclusion. Card and colleagues made a randomly selected group of employees at a US university aware of a website revealing the salaries of all workers at their university. Shortly afterward, Card's research group surveyed the university staff. Compared with colleagues with above-average salaries, those with earnings below the mean became less satisfied with their jobs as a consequence of learning about their relative low-income status. The most exciting findings appeared in a follow-up study 3 years later. Now, more employees in the below-average group had left their jobs. This effect was not found in the below-average salary control group that was not made aware of the income website. Other studies have also reported that low job satisfaction predicts quitting the job (e.g., Kaiser & Oswald, 2022). The same mechanisms operate within other kinds of domain satisfaction, such as for marriage and housing: low satisfaction predicts leaving one's spouse and finding a new house (respectively). Kaiser and Oswald refer to this tendency as "get-me-out-of-here actions."

In another investigation of motivation and satisfaction, Koo and Fishbach (2010) asked participants to complete a task. A random half were instructed to pay attention to the remaining work, in a procedure of executing stepwise subgoals before the final goal was reached. The other group was instructed to focus on the work that had been completed and not on that which remained. Participants in the latter condition were more satisfied with their accomplishments and less motivated to continue than those in the first group. These results also suggest that satisfaction is more closely associated with stability (remaining at the current task level) than with change (striving to reach a more difficult task level). Similarly, Emmons (1986) found that life satisfaction correlated positively with past fulfillment of personal projects and with projects that did not take any effort. Life satisfaction was negatively correlated with project difficulty.

The distinction between ease and difficulty constitutes a significant distinction in Oishi's wellbeing vocabulary as well (e.g., Oishi et al., 2020; Oishi & Westgate, 2022). By separating a happy life (high life satisfaction and a high positive-to-negative affect ratio) and a rich life (comprising a variety of interesting and perspective-changing experiences), Oishi and colleagues predicted and found that a happy life was associated with security, stability, comfort, extraversion, conscientiousness, and low neuroticism, while a rich life was associated with novelty, complexity, and openness to experience. "Those leading happy and/or meaningful lives tend to prefer to maintain social order and the status quo, whereas those leading psychologically rich lives seem to embrace social change" (Oishi & Westgate, 2022, p. 10).

Another chapter in the literature on cognitive ease was written by Laura King and her colleagues. For example, Scollon and King (2011) found that striving and success were typically not included in folk theories of global happiness. The authors report that US Americans typically think of a good life as an easy life. "Effort that leads to fulfillment was valued, but only if it did not compromise leisure time and was not energy depleting. Thus, in this series of studies, the people's own concepts diverged from scientific theories such as flow (Csikszentmihalyi), eudaimonia (Waterman), and competence and mastery (White)" (Scollon & King, 2011, pp. 6–7). Napa and King (2004) similarly observed that the images people presented in their narratives were typically those of an easy life. The ease associated with a happy life stands in stark contrast to the stories people tell about a mature life, which is depicted as more complex, effortful, and oriented toward change. The happy people interviewed in the studies by King and her colleagues are also more likely to tell stories with happy endings, whereas the stories that mature people tell include an active struggle toward a life change. In quantifying the difference between happy and mature lives, the correlations between the two variables range from 0.08 to 0.13. "A conclusion that has been reached in my research program over the past few years is that happiness and maturity may follow two different and independent pathways" (King, 2001, p. 54).

Baumeister has also commented on the ease of being satisfied and happy. His work will be reviewed in Chap. 6, but briefly, Baumeister finds that happiness is associated with ease, whereas meaning in life is often (although not always) associated with difficulties: "the unhappy but meaningful life is seriously involved in difficult undertakings" (Baumeister et al., 2013, p. 515). Similarly, Grzeskowiak et al. (2006) found that consumers who buy a home with the least amount of effort experience a sense of wellbeing. Another piece of evidence for the cognitive ease hypothesis comes from a study by Ditto et al. (2003). These researchers report that favorable and desirable information, "good news," is processed effortlessly and mindlessly, whereas unfavorable or undesirable information, "bad news," commands attention and more effortful processing.

Together with colleagues and students, some of my own work has also demonstrated how this "goodness bias" may operate in the context of wellbeing research. For example, in one study (Collett & Vittersø, 2016), we presented survey participants with images that had either a stability/harmony content (e.g., a child playing with flowers on a meadow; a palm beach) or a change/opportunity content (e.g., an advertisement for Amnesty International; a picture of Mother Teresa). Each image was rated in terms of (1) how good or bad it was, (2) how interesting or uninteresting it was, (3) how difficult it was to rate the image as good or bad, and (4) how difficult it was to rate the image as interesting or uninteresting. As expected, we found higher scores of goodness for the stability/harmony pictures and higher scores for interest in the change/opportunity pictures. We also observed that the stability/harmony pictures were easier to rate as good or bad, as indicated by a negative correlation ($r = -0.34$, $p < 0.001$) between the stability/harmony images and the difficulty scale—running from 1 (very easy) to 7 (very difficult). The correlation between goodness difficulty and the change/opportunity images was positive ($r = 0.40$, $p < 0.001$), indicating that these images were more difficult to evaluate as good or bad. We interpreted this result in support of the hypothesis that stimuli vary in how easy it is to rate them as good or bad. Some images will easily submit themselves to such evaluations, while others do not seem to fit the notion of a good–bad evaluation. Collett and I also found support for a second hypothesis, which suggested that satisfied people prefer images that are easy to categorize as good or bad over images that are difficult to judge as good or bad. We found that life satisfaction correlated positively with good–bad evaluations but not with interesting–uninteresting ratings. In contrast, personal growth correlated positively with interesting–uninteresting ratings but not with good–bad ratings.

The final set of arguments presented in support of the stability hypothesis about life satisfaction comes from philosophy. Martha Nussbaum discusses the concept of life satisfaction in one of her attacks on scientific wellbeing research (Nussbaum, 2008). Nussbaum talks, somewhat confusingly, about satisfaction both as a pleasant feeling state and something that represents goodness in a reflective judgment sense. She then reveals that her own conception of a good life "attaches a great deal of value to striving, longing, and working for a difficult goal. Therefore, if I ever notice myself feeling feelings of satisfaction, I blame myself and think that, insofar as I have those feelings, I am like Mill's 'pig satisfied' or Aristotle's 'dumb grazing animals,' and thus, reflectively, I report dissatisfaction with my life as a whole" (p. S87). Nussbaum then speculates that John Stuart Mill must have been satisfied with his life, despite much pain and struggle: "While judging that his life is on balance successful, he is almost certainly not experiencing feelings of satisfaction or pleasure" (p. S87). Nussbaum offers a somewhat analogous interpretations for the lives of composers such as Schiller, Beethoven, and Mahler. She even suggests that "Mahler's Resurrection Symphony revolves precisely around the contrast between the herdlike feeling of satisfaction and the more exalted judgment that one's whole life is rich and meaningful—because it is governed by an active kind of love. The former is represented by the swoopy, aimless clarinet phrases of the third movement, the latter by the passionate heartbeat that the final movement associates with the wings of the soul" (p. S88).

Another neo-Aristotelian authority, Julia Annas, describes empirical studies on life satisfaction differently than Nussbaum and more in line with the mainstream SWB literature. Annas argues that the life satisfaction approach is an improvement in the science of wellbeing "since it involves not just a positive feeling but some kind of overall judgment about one's life as a whole, and thus some kind of evaluation of how one's life as a whole is going. If you are studying happiness in the social sciences, this is the obvious item to try to study, since we can ask people what their overall evaluation of their life is and record answers, whereas asking people about their feelings or whether their desires are satisfied does not lend itself to measurement" (Annas, 2011, loc. 1866).

Life Satisfaction and Value Fulfillment

People make clear distinctions between the value of pleasure and the value of life satisfaction, with the latter being far more important than the former (e.g., Benjamin et al., 2014). Although few people consider pleasure or satisfaction to be their most important values in life (see below), the substantial difference in value ranking between them constitutes another reason why pleasure and life satisfaction should be considered distinct indicators of wellbeing.

However, the value debate goes far beyond ranking wellbeing dimensions from most to least desirable. For instance, a significant question ponders how life satisfaction is affected by pursuing different kinds of life goals, i.e., which values people strive to reach. Some refer to this issue as a question about identifying "healthy values." A different question concerns the "all things considered" myth and asks whether self-reported life satisfaction is biased in terms of including more "easy values" than "difficult values" in the overall evaluation of one's life conditions (Vittersø et al., 2009). A third question regards the role of wellbeing as a societal goal and as an aim for public policy. If we are wrong in ranking SWB as the ultimate goal in people's lives, we cannot take for granted that life satisfaction deserves a privileged place among other values a society should care about (e.g., Clark et al., 2018; Fabian & Pykett, 2021; Flanagan et al., 2023; Sim & Diener, 2018). I will survey these three questions in turn but start with a brief review of the concept of values.

As for so many concepts in the social sciences, agreement remains to be established for a definition of values (e.g., Campbell, 1963; Hecher, 1993; Rohan, 2000). Consequently, Howard (1985) argues that the term has served as "a catchall category for an enormous array of very different judgments, decisions, preferences, and orientations" (p. 25). However, a coarse approximation of the idea of a value can be obtained by examining the most common uses of the term. For example, Frankfurt (1982) observed that popular prose holds values to be things we consider important, that we care for, hold dear, admire, etc. More complex proposals, such as Kluckhohn's classic definition, suggest that values regulate "impulse satisfaction in accord with the whole array of hierarchical, enduring goals of the personality, the requirements of both personality and sociocultural system for order, the need for respecting the interest of others and of group as a whole in social living" (Kluckhohn, 1951, p. 399). Shalom Schwartz defines values as "conceptions of the desirable that guide the way social actors (e.g., organizational leaders, policy-makers, individual persons) select actions, evaluate people and events, and explain their actions and evaluations" (Schwartz, 1999, p. 24). A simpler alternative comes from Batson et al. (1992), who considers values to be relative preferences. Others discuss values as internal criteria for evaluation (Hecher, 1993), as interests (Mandler, 1984), or even as joy and happiness (Emmons, 1986). From what seems to be the essence of the pile of definitions that exist, I suggest that values can roughly be considered as something an organism likes, wants, or cares about.

Schwartz's theory of basic human values is one of the most popular value theories in psychology, and initially, it proposed that ten universal values exist and that they form a circular structure that reflects the kind of motivation each value expresses (e.g., Schwartz, 1992, 2012; Schwartz & Sortheix, 2018). An updated version of the theory suggests that 19 basic values should be considered as universal (Schwartz & Cieciuch, 2022). The values are supposed to be panhuman because they are "based on one or more of three universal requirements of human existence: needs of individuals as biological organisms, requisites of coordinated social interaction, and survival and welfare needs of groups" (Schwartz & Sortheix, 2018, p. 2). The relationships among the values can be organized hierarchically by grouping the 19 basic values into a smaller set of second-order values. For example, the two basic values of dependency and caring can be combined to reflect the second-order value entitled benevolence. The three basic values of tolerance, concern, and nature combines into the second-order values called universalism. At an even higher level, benevolence and universalism comprises a third-order value group named self-transcendence. Other third-order values are openness to change, self-enhancement, and conservation. At a fourth-order level, conservation and self-transcendence can be combined into self-focused values, whereas openness to change and self-enhancement can be combined into personal focus values. Alternatively, self-transcendence and openness to change can be added to form growth–anxiety-free values, while conservation and self-enhancement can be added to form self-protection–anxiety-avoidance values (Schwartz & Cieciuch, 2022, Fig. 1).

Healthy Values

Inspired by clinical and humanistic psychology, Bilsky and Schwartz (1994) suggested that some of the values in Schwartz's theory can be categorized as healthy because they are cognitive transformations of growth needs. Values such as stimulation, self-direction, universalism, benevolence, and achievement are considered healthy. Conversely, some values are categorized as unhealthy because they are cognitive transformations of deficiency needs. Conformity, security, and power are examples of unhealthy values. Schwartz hypothesizes that the pursuit of healthy values may lead to increased wellbeing, whereas pursuing unhealthy values may undermine wellbeing. To provide evidence, Schwartz and Sortheix (2018) presented the results of eight studies that analyzed the relationship between basic values and wellbeing. The authors conclude that the results consistently, though not perfectly, support their hypotheses. However, the presented effect sizes are very small. When I calculated the average correlation for life satisfaction and healthy values, the coefficient was a modest $r = 0.02$. The average correlation between life satisfaction and unhealthy values was $r = -0.01$.

Somewhat stronger effects have been reported by Bojanowska and Kaczmarek (2022). In their sample of Polish adults, the correlation between life satisfaction and eight aggregated values from Schwartz's "Portrait of Values Questionnaire" varied between 0.07 for self-enhancement behavior (comprising universalism and benevolence) and 0.16 for openness (comprising hedonism and self-direction).

Another thread of value research was triggered by Kasser and Ryan's (1993) study on *A Dark Side of the American Dream*. In it, the authors follow up on the idea that some values/goal/aspirations are healthy while others are harmful. In particular, values categorized as intrinsic will increase adjustment and wellbeing, whereas values categorized as extrinsic will reduce adjustment and wellbeing and rather lead to superficial satisfaction. Three kinds of values were measured and cataloged as intrinsic aspirations (self-acceptance, affiliation, and community feeling), and one kind of value was measured and cataloged as extrinsic (financial success). The authors did not include life satisfaction in their study but rather operationalized wellbeing as self-actualization and vitality. The zero-order correlations between values and wellbeing were not strong. On average, across the two studies, intrinsic values were correlated 0.19 with self-actualization and 0.16 with vitality. Financial success correlated on average −0.18 with self-actualization and −0.06 with vitality. To adjust for the relative centrality for each value, a sum score variable comprising all value importance variables was computed and included in a series of regression analyses. To control for the within-participant general importance scores, the overall importance variable was included as an independent variable together with each of the four value variables. The wellbeing indicators operated as dependent variables, and again, the most important indicator was self-actualization. The average, standardized regression coefficient for all the intrinsic aspiration variables (summarized by me) on self-actualization was $\beta = 0.25$, and for financial aspirations predicting self-actualization, it was $\beta = -0.37$. In a follow-up study, Kasser and Ryan (1996) created an intrinsic aspiration composite variable and an extrinsic aspiration variable based on the scores from measures of three intrinsic and three extrinsic values, respectively. This time, the average regression coefficient for intrinsic values predicting self-actualization across two studies was $\beta = 0.50$ (when the overall rating of importance was controlled), and for extrinsic values predicting self-actualization, it was $\beta = -0.60$.

Carver and Baird (1998) criticized these studies for not taking into account the reason why people pursue what Kasser and Ryan refer to as intrinsic and extrinsic goals/values/aspirations. There are many possible reasons for aspiring to both intrinsic and extrinsic values, Carver and Baird point out. People might aspire to financial success because it will increase their popularity or because it will make their parents proud. But people might also hold such values because more money goes with better paid jobs, which in turn are also likely to be more fun or exciting than those lower in income. Hence, the two authors designed a replication study that, in addition to the variables measured in the two Kasser and Ryan papers referred to above, also included items that assessed people's reasons for holding intrinsic and extrinsic aspirations. Adapting a self-determination theory framework for measuring reasons for engaging in a school performance, Carver and Baird created a measure that gauged "internal" and "external" reasons for having a particular aspiration (regardless of whether the aspiration itself was considered intrinsic or extrinsic by Kasser and Ryan's idiosyncratic system for naming and categorizing goals/values/aspirations as intrinsic or extrinsic[4]).

While Carver and Baird replicated the main results in the Kasser and Ryan studies, the authors also found that financial aspirations and self-actualization were negatively associated ($\beta = -0.31$) when controlling for total aspiration score. However, when analyzing the reasons why the participants endorsed financial aspirations, the association with wellbeing became positive for those with "internal" reasons for holding a financial success aspiration. That is, people who held financial aspirations for intrinsic reasons also tended to score higher on self-actualization ($\beta = 0.27$). Thus, it seems that holding "internal," or self-determined, reasons for aspiring to an extrinsic value is positively related to self-actualization.

The results of other studies also call into question the results presented by Kasser and Ryan. Referring to a large, longitudinal study by Bowen and Bok (1998), Kahneman (2011, p. 401) reports that individuals with financial aspirations when they are young turned out more satisfied with their lives 20 years later, given—importantly—that they had reached their goal. People who wanted money but did not obtain it were significantly more dissatisfied. In terms of life satisfaction later in life, the least promising goal for young students was to become "accomplished in a performing art."

Spontaneous and Reflective Values

The second question raised in this section asks whether there is a value bias inherent in self-reported life satisfaction. The humanistic theory of wellbeing suggests that there is. The argument starts with the distinction between "spontaneous values" and "reflective values." Spontaneous values are basically about good–bad evaluations; they quickly come to mind and are easy to evaluate as good. They operate in System 1 mode, and an alternative name for at least some of them could be hedonic values. In contrast, reflective values typically take time and effort to develop; they involve judgments about morality—about what is right and what is wrong—they are complex and involve System 2 thinking. An alternative name for at least some of these reflective values could be eudaimonic values. An additional assumption in the HTW

[4]Why is, for instance, the item "You will be the one in charge of your life" intrinsic, while "You will be your own boss" extrinsic? (cf. Kasser & Ryan, 1993, p. 422).

is that even when reflective values are developed and firmly established in our value system, they may not be activated in ordinary survey responses. Context effects may prevent them from immediately entering our conscious minds.

This is the structure of the argument: If responses to life satisfaction items are grounded in spontaneous good–bad evaluations (SGBE) and if these responses also carry information about the gap between one's ideal and actual lives, then the value to which the gap refers must be quickly and easily processed as well. Hence, to the extent that values are incorporated in judgments about life satisfaction, they are probably spontaneous values rather than reflective values.

If this assumption is correct, mainstream wellbeing researchers are mistaken in considering life satisfaction as a reflective appraisal of everything important in a person's life. For example, when Diener and colleagues (Diener et al., 2012, p. 334) suggest that life satisfaction can be influenced both by hedonic and eudaimonic aspects of life (cf. the "All thing Considered" section), the HTW predicts that this may be wrong. Eudaimonic, or reflective, values are important to many people, but they are not grounded on SGBE and will therefore not have an impact on survey responses to life satisfaction items.

Some evidence supports the value bias hypothesis. For example, in a series of recent studies conducted with my colleagues and students, we found that, upon reflection, individuals tend to change their value priorities (Thorsteinsen & Vittersø, 2023; Teulings et al., in preparation). In one survey experiment, we found that participants reported more reflective values in an open-ended item if they first had been asked to rank the importance of a set of both hedonic and eudaimonic values, compared with a control group that responded to these questions in the reverse order. We also found that the gap between how much participants wish for spontaneous values in their perfect life and how much they reported to actually have fulfilled those values in their real lives strongly predicts their level of life satisfaction for hedonic values but not for eudaimonic values. Admittedly frail and preliminary, these results offer some evidence for the value bias hypothesis, although more studies are certainly needed before these findings can be considered reliable.

Life Satisfaction as Public Policy

The last value-related issue to be discussed concerns the use of life satisfaction as a policy purpose (e.g., Clark et al., 2018; Diener & Biswas-Diener, 2019; Fabian et al., 2021; Frijters et al., 2020; Odermatt & Stutzer, 2018; Semple, 2021). Fabian and Pykett (2021) argue that the science of wellbeing is increasingly influencing public policy and that research on life satisfaction plays a vital role in this trend. For example, Clark et al. (2018) hold that life satisfaction is well suited for political purposes because it is "democratic." It is democratic because "it allows individuals to assess their lives on the basis of *whatever they consider important* (italics added) to themselves. It does not impose anybody else's views on what emotions or experiences are valuable" (p. 4).

As this chapter has demonstrated, however, there are reasons to believe that self-reported life satisfaction does not tap into "whatever people consider important to themselves." Measures of life satisfaction seems rather to be biased toward some valuable areas in life while ignoring others. Additionally, most people do not consider life satisfaction to be among their most important values in life. Life satisfaction can even be associated with something negative (e.g., Carlquist et al., 2016; Nussbaum, 2008; Ralph et al., 2012). Indeed, Nussbaum goes so far as to argue that researchers who ask people about their life satisfaction are actually bullying them (Nussbaum, 2008, p. S86). Hence, the utilization of life satisfaction measures in a survey is a value-based choice, which imposes the researchers' ideas about a good life upon the participants. Promoting life satisfaction as a policy purpose is therefore a normative project.

A few other reasons to doubt the democratic life satisfaction hypothesis also deserve mentioning. For instance, in the pioneering studies by Cantril (1965), almost 20,000 survey participants from 13 countries were asked about their values in life. These open response answers were classified into 145 distinct categories, and life satisfaction was not among them. In one of his 13 subsamples (the one from the USA), Cantril included an item about life satisfaction in the questionnaire. When he correlated life satisfaction with value satisfaction, defined as the degree to which people had accomplished what really matters to them, a rather moderate effect appeared ($r = 0.32$). Hence, the Cantril studies offer only modest support for the notion that life satisfaction captures the values people most eagerly want to fulfill in their lives.

Similarly, a classic study by Rokeach (1973) found that happiness only ranked as number 5 among 18 "primary" values. Pleasure came out near the bottom of the list, ranked 17th. In an even earlier study, Richards (1966) found that among 35 rated values, the highest mean scores were received for "Being a good parent," "Being a good husband or wife," "Becoming a mature and well-adjusted person," "Finding real purpose in life," and "Becoming happy and content" (presented in decreasing order). In a more recent survey including approximately 5000 US Americans, Benjamin et al. (2014) found that among 136 values, or preferences in their vocabulary, life satisfaction was ranked 16th and happy feelings 54th, slightly above the importance of the national inflation rate. Pleasure ended as the 93 "most" important value on the list, a result that must surprise hedonists, who argue that pleasure is the only true value in people's lives. The results of the Benjamin et al. study resonates well with those of other studies, such as Delle Fave et al. (2011), Higgins (2014), Huppert (2014), and Oishi and Westgate (2022).

However, some studies have reported different results. Balestra et al. (2018) found that life satisfaction was the most important life value, and when Diener et al. (1998) investigated the importance of happiness and life satisfaction among college students in 41 nations, the authors observed that both concepts were "extremely important" (p. 34). But Diener and his colleagues had a very limited repertoire of values included in their survey. Hence, when other values are added to the ranking list, happiness and satisfaction tend to be considered less important than several other values.

A related concern about life satisfaction as policy purpose comes from Fabian and Pykett (2021). The authors are critical to implementing a mental state kind of template for public policy, because they see it as a kind of "libertarian paternalism." Targeting mental states of individuals rather than societal circumstances is a value-based priority which Fabian and Pykett refer to as "wellbeing budgeting." We may also ask how efficient these interventions truly are (e.g., Folk & Dunn, 2023), but beyond such empirical questions, the implementation of wellbeing interventions also raises value dilemmas. Thus, Fabian and Pykett (2021, p. 6) argue that "happiness interventions and well-being budgeting transgress the principles of effectiveness and autonomy and that their adherence to the principle of welfare is questionable."

If a policy purpose was to be generated from the humanistic theory of wellbeing, it would have had to be directed at the foundations for a civilization: what it takes to create habitable environments that ensures all individuals a possibility to play out their humanness in a good way. Why not? The idea of having our basic humanistic values fulfilled is no more normative—or less scientific—than the idea of endorsing life satisfaction. But I believe it would contribute to a broader and more complete kind of wellbeing than would the proposal of promoting life satisfaction as public policy.

References

Allport, G. W. (1955). *Becoming: Basic considerations for a psychology of personality*. Yale University Press.

Andrews, F. M., & Withey, S. B. (1976). *Social indicators of well-being*. Plenum Press.

Anglim, J., Horwood, S., Smillie, L. D., Marrero, R. J., & Wood, J. K. (2020). Predicting psychological and subjective well-being from personality: A meta-analysis. *Psychological Bulletin, 146*, 279–323. https://doi.org/10.1037/bul0000226

Annas, J. (2011). *Intelligent virtue [Kindle]*. Oxford University Press.

Balestra, C., Boarini, R., & Tosetto, E. (2018). What matters most to people? Evidence from the OECD better life index users' responses. *Social Indicators Research, 136*(3), 907–930. https://doi.org/10.1007/s11205-016-1538-4

Barrett, L. (2015). Essentialist views of the mind. In J. Brockman (Ed.), *This idea must die: Scientific theories that are blocking progress [Kindle]* (pp. 499–501). Harper Collins.

Batson, C. D., Shaw, L. L., & Oleson, K. C. (1992). Differentiating affect, mood and emotion: Toward functionally based conceptual distinctions. In M. S. Clark (Ed.), *Review of personality and social psychology* (Vol. 13, pp. 294–326).

Baumeister, R. F., Vohs, K. D., Aaker, J. L., & Garbinsky, E. N. (2013). Some key differences between a happy life and a meaningful life. *The Journal of Positive Psychology, 8*(6), 505–516. https://doi.org/10.1080/17439760.2013.830764

Beebe-Center, J. G. (1932). *The psychology of pleasantness and unpleasantness*. Russell & Russell.

Benjamin, D. J., Kimball, M. S., Heffetz, O., & Szembrot, N. (2014). Beyond happiness and satisfaction: Toward well-being indices based on stated preference. *The American Economic Review, 104*(9), 2698–2735. https://doi.org/10.1257/aer.104.9.2698

Berns, G. (2010). *Satisfaction: Sensation seeking, novelty, and the science of finding true fulfillment [Kindle]*. Henry Holt and Company.

Bilsky, W., & Schwartz, S. H. (1994). Values and personality. *European Journal of Personality, 8*(3), 163–181. https://doi.org/10.1002/per.2410080303

Bojanowska, A., & Kaczmarek, L. D. (2022). How healthy and unhealthy values predict hedonic and eudaimonic well-being: Dissecting value-related beliefs and behaviours. *Journal of Happiness Studies, 23*(1), 211–231. https://doi.org/10.1007/s10902-021-00396-z

Borsboom, D., Mellenbergh, G. J., & van Heerden, J. (2004). The concept of validity. *Psychological Review, 111*(4), 1061–1071. https://doi.org/10.1037/0033-295X.111.4.1061

Bowen, W. G., & Bok, D. C. (1998). *The shape of the river: Long-term consequences of considering race in college and university admissions*. Princeton University Press.

Buchanan, T. W. (2007). Retrieval of emotional memories. *Psychological Bulletin, 133*(5), 761–779. https://doi.org/10.1037/0033-2909.133.5.761

Campbell, D. T. (1963). Social attitudes and other acquired behavioral dispositions. In S. Koch (Ed.), *Psychology: A study of a science* (Vol. 6, pp. 94–172). McGraw-Hill.

Campbell, A., Converse, P. E., & Rodgers, W. L. (1976). *The quality of American life*. Sage.

Cantor, N. (1990). From thought to behavior: "Having" and "doing" in the study of personality and cognition. *American Psychologist, 45*, 735–750.

Cantril, H. (1965). *The pattern of human concerns*. Rutgers University Press. http://agris.fao.org/agris-search/search.do?recordID=US201300321344

Capic, T., Weinberg, M. A., Tomyn, A. J., & Cummins, R. A. (2020). *Nomenclature for subjective wellbeing research* (ACQol open-access publications, Australian Centre on Quality of Life., Issue).

Card, D., Mas, A., Moretti, E., & Saez, E. (2012). Inequality at work: The effect of peer salaries on job satisfaction. *American Economic Review, 102*(6), 2981–3003. https://doi.org/10.1257/aer.102.6.2981

Carlquist, E., Ulleberg, P., Delle Fave, A., Nafstad, H. E., & Blakar, R. M. (2016). Everyday understandings of happiness, good life, and satisfaction: Three different facets of well-being. *Applied Research in Quality of Life, 1–25*, 481. https://doi.org/10.1007/s11482-016-9472-9

Carlquist, E., Nafstad, H. E., & Blakar, R. M. (2018). Understanding satisfaction: An analysis of the meaning potential of the word "satisfaction" in everyday Norwegian language. *Journal of Happiness Studies, 19*(4), 939–959. https://doi.org/10.1007/s10902-017-9854-1

Carver, C. S., & Baird, E. (1998). The American dream revisited: Is it what you want or why you want it that matters? *Psychological Science, 9*(4), 289–292.

Casebeer, W. D. (2003). *Natural ethical facts: Evolution, connectionism, and moral cognition [Kindle]*. Cambridge University Press.

Cheung, F., & Lucas, R. E. (2014). Assessing the validity of single-item life satisfaction measures: Results from three large samples [journal article]. *Quality of Life Research, 23*(10), 2809–2818. https://doi.org/10.1007/s11136-014-0726-4

Clark, A. E., Flèche, S., Layard, R., Powdthavee, N., & Ward, G. (2018). *The origins of happiness: The science of well-being over the life course [Kindle]*. Princeton University Press.

Collett, L. G., & Vittersø, J. (2016, August 25–27). *The unbearable lightness of life satisfaction.* The 14th International Society for Quality of Life Studies Conference, Seoul, Republic of Korea.

Corkin, S. (2014). *Permanent present tense: The man with no memory, and what he taught the world.* Basic Books.

Crisp, R. (2017). Well-being. In E. N. Zalta (Ed.), *The Stanford encyclopedia of philosophy.* Retrieved from http://plato.stanford.edu/archives/fall2011/entries/well-being/.

Cummins, R. A. (2010). Subjective wellbeing, homeostatically protected mood and depression: A synthesis. *Journal of Happiness Studies, 11*(1), 1–17.

Cummins, R. A., & Weinberg, M. K. (2015). Multi-item measurement of subjective wellbeing: Subjective approaches. In W. Glatzer, L. Camfield, V. Møller, & M. Rojas (Eds.), *Global handbook of quality of life. Exploration of well-being of nations and continents* (pp. 239–268). Springer. https://doi.org/10.1007/978-94-017-9178-6_10

Davern, M. T., Cummins, R. A., & Stokes, M. A. (2007). Subjective well-being as an affective-cognitive construct. *Journal of Happiness Studies, 8*(4), 429–449.

Davis, W. (1981). A theory of happiness. *American Philosophical Quarterly, 18*(2), 111–120.

Deci, E. L. (1975). *Intrinsic motivation*. Plenum Press.

Delle Fave, A., Brdar, I., Freire, T., Vella-Brodrick, D., & Wissing, M. (2011). The eudaimonic and hedonic components of happiness: Qualitative and quantitative findings. *Social Indicators Research, 100*(2), 185–207. https://doi.org/10.1007/s11205-010-9632-5

Denton, D. (2005). *The primordial emotions: The dawning of consciousness*. Oxford University Press.

Dictionary, E., & Lexico. *Satisfaction*. http://oxforddictionaries.com/definition/english/satisfaction?q=satisfaction

Diener, E. (1984). Subjective well-being. *Psychological Bulletin, 95*(3), 542–575. https://doi.org/10.1037/0033-2909.95.3.542

Diener, E. (2000). Subjective well-being. The science of happiness and a proposal for a national index. *American Psychologist, 55*(1), 34–43.

Diener, E. (2006). Guidelines for national indicators of subjective well-being and ill-being. *Journal of Happiness Studies, 7*(4), 397–404. https://doi.org/10.1007/s10902-006-9000-y

Diener, E. (2008). One happy autobiography. In R. Levine, A. Rodrigues, & L. Zelezny (Eds.), *Journeys in social psychology* (pp. 1–17). Psychology Press.

Diener, E. (2012). New findings and future directions for subjective well-being research. *American Psychologist, 67*(8), 590–597. https://doi.org/10.1037/a0029541

Diener, E. (2013). The remarkable changes in the science of subjective well-being. *Perspectives on Psychological Science, 8*(6), 663–666. https://doi.org/10.1177/1745691613507583

Diener, E., & Biswas-Diener, R. (2019). Well-being interventions to improve societies. In J. D. Sachs (Ed.), *Global happiness and well-being policy report* (pp. 95–110). The Global Happiness Council. Retrieved from http://www.happinesscouncil.org/. http://www.happiness-council.org/

Diener, E., & Lucas, R. E. (2000). Explaining differences in societal levels of happiness: Relative standards, need fulfillment, culture, and evaluation theory. *Journal of Happiness Studies, 1*(1), 41–78.

Diener, E., & Seligman, M. E. P. (2004). Beyond money. Toward an economy of well-being. *Psychological Science in the Public Interest, 5*(1), 1–31.

Diener, E., & Suh, E. (1997). Measuring quality of life: Economic, social, and subjective indicators. *Social Indicators Research, 40*(1/2), 189–216.

Diener, E., & Tov, W. (2012). National accounts of well-being. In K. C. Land, A. C. Michalos, & M. J. Sirgy (Eds.), *Handbook of social indicators and quality of life research* (pp. 137–157). Springer. https://doi.org/10.1007/978-94-007-2421-1_7

Diener, E., Emmons, R. A., Larsen, R. J., & Griffin, S. (1985). The satisfaction with life scale. *Journal of Personality Assessment, 49*, 71–75. https://doi.org/10.1207/s15327752jpa4901_13

Diener, E., Sapyta, J. J., & Suh, E. (1998). Subjective well-being is essential to well-being. *Psychological Inquiry, 9*(1), 33–37.

Diener, E., Scollon, C. N., & Lucas, R. E. (2009). The evolving concept of subjective well-being. The multifaceted nature of happiness. In E. Diener (Ed.), *Assessing well-being. The collected works of Ed Diener* (pp. 67–100). Springer.

Diener, E., Fujita, F., Tay, L., & Biswas-Diener, R. (2012). Purpose, mood, and pleasure in predicting satisfaction judgments. *Social Indicators Research, 105*, 333–341. https://doi.org/10.1007/s11205-011-9787-8

Diener, E., Lucas, R. E., & Oishi, S. (2018). Advances and open questions in the science of subjective well-being. *Collabra Psychology, 4*(1).

Ditto, P. H., Munro, G. D., Apanovitch, A. M., Scepansky, J. A., & Lockhart, L. K. (2003). Spontaneous skepticism: The interplay of motivation and expectation in responses to favorable and unfavorable medical diagnoses. *Personality and Social Psychology Bulletin, 29*(9), 1120–1132. https://doi.org/10.1177/0146167203254536

Duncan, S. C., & Barret, L. F. (2007). Affect is a form of cognition: A neurobiological analysis. *Cognition and Emotion, 21*(6), 1184–1211.
Eid, M., & Diener, E. (2004). Global judgments of subjective well-being: Situational variability and long-term stability. *Social Indicators Research, 65*(3), 245–277. https://doi.org/10.1023/B:SOCI.0000003801.89195.bc
Ekman, P. (2003). *Emotions revealed: Recognizing faces and feelings to improve communication and emotional life*. Henry Holt.
Emmons, R. A. (1986). Personal strivings: An approach to personality and subjective well-being. *Journal of Personality and Social Psychology, 51*(5), 1058–1068.
Fabian, M., & Pykett, J. (2021). Be happy: Navigating normative issues in behavioral and well-being public policy. *Perspectives on Psychological Science, 0*(0), 1745691620984395. https://doi.org/10.1177/1745691620984395
Fabian, M., Agarwala, M., Alexandrova, A., Coyle, D., & Felici, M. (2021). *Wellbeing public policy needs more theory* (Bennett Institute Working Paper), Issue.
Feldman, F. (2010). *What is this thing called happiness?* Oxford University Press.
Flanagan, O., LeDoux, J., Bingle, B., Haybron, D., Moody-Adams, M., Mesquita, B., Ren, S., Sun, A. X., & Wilson, Y. (2023). *Against happiness [Kindle]*. Columbia University Press.
Fodor, J. (1975). *The language of mind*. Harvard University Press.
Folk, D., & Dunn, E. (2023). A systematic review of the strength of evidence for the most commonly recommended happiness strategies in mainstream media. *Nature Human Behaviour, 7*, 1697. https://doi.org/10.1038/s41562-023-01651-4
Frankfurt, H. (1982). The importance of what we care about. *Synthese, 53*, 257–272.
Freedman, J. (1978). *Happy people: What happiness is, who has it, and why*. Harcourt Brace Jovanovich.
Frijters, P., Clark, A. E., Krekel, C., & Layard, R. (2020). A happy choice: Wellbeing as the goal of government. *Behavioural Public Policy, 4*(2), 126–165. https://doi.org/10.1017/bpp.2019.39
Gilovich, T. D., Epley, N., & Hanko, K. (2005). Shallow thoughts about the self: The automatic components of self-assessment. In M. D. Alicke, D. Dunning, & J. Krueger (Eds.), *The self in social judgment* (5th ed., pp. 67–84). Psychology Press.
Glatz, C., & Eder, A. (2020). Patterns of trust and subjective well-being across Europe: New insights from repeated cross-sectional analyses based on the European social survey 2002–2016. *Social Indicators Research, 148*(2), 417–439. https://doi.org/10.1007/s11205-019-02212-x
Glatzer, W. (1984). Life-satisfaction and alternative measures of SWB. In W. Glatzer & W. Zapf (Eds.), *Quality of life in Germany* (pp. 177–191). Campus.
Gray, J. A. (1990). Brain systems that mediate both emotion and cognition. *Cognition and Emotion, 4*(3), 269–288.
Grzeskowiak, S., Sirgy, M. J., Lee, D.-J., & Claiborne, C. B. (2006). Housing well-being: Developing and validating a measure. *Social Indicators Research, 79*(3), 503–541. https://doi.org/10.1007/s11205-005-5667-4
Gurin, G., Veroff, J., & Feld, S. (1960). *Americans view their mental health*. Basic Books.
Haybron, D. M. (2008). Philosophy and the science of subjective well-being. In M. Eid & R. J. Larsen (Eds.), *The science of subjective well-being* (pp. 17–43). Guilford Press.
Hecher, M. (1993). Value research in the social and behavioral sciences. In M. Hechter, L. Nadel, & R. E. Michod (Eds.), *The origin of values* (pp. 1–30). Aldine de Gruyter.
Heider, F. (1958). *The psychology of interpersonal relations*. Wiley.
Helliwell, J. F., Huang, H., Grover, S., & Wang, S. (2014). Good governance and national well-being: What are the linkages?.
Helliwell, J. F., Layard, R., Sachs, J. D., De Neve, J.-E., Aknin, L. B., & Wang, S. (Eds.). (2021). *World happiness report 2021*. https://worldhappiness.report/
Henrich, J., Heine, S. J., & Norenzayan, A. (2010). Most people are not WEIRD. *Nature, 466*(7302), 29–29. https://doi.org/10.1038/466029a
Higgins, E. T. (2014). *Beyond pleasure and pain: How motivation works*. Oxford University Press.

Howard, G. S. (1985). The role of values in the science of psychology. *American Psychlogist, 40*(1), 255–265.
Huppert, F. (2014). The state of wellbeing science concepts, measures, interventions, and policies. In F. Huppert & C. Cooper (Eds.), *Wellbeing: A complete reference guide, volume VI, interventions and policies to enhance wellbeing* (pp. 1–49). Wiley-Blackwell.
Johnson-Laird, P. N., Girotto, V., & Legrenzi, P. (2004). Reasoning from inconsistency to consistency. *Psychological Review, 111*(3), 640–661.
Kahneman, D. (1999). Objective happiness. In D. Kahneman, E. Diener, & N. Schwarz (Eds.), *Well-being: The foundations of hedonic psychology* (pp. 3–25). Russell Sage Foundation.
Kahneman, D. (2009). What constitutes life satisfaction? In J. E. Brockman (Ed.), *What have you changed your mind about?: Today's leading minds rethink everything*. HarperPerennial.
Kahneman, D. (2011). *Thinking, fast and slow*. Penguin Books.
Kahneman, D., & Riis, J. (2005). Living, and thinking about it: Two perspectives on life. In F. Huppert, N. Baylis, & B. Keverne (Eds.), *The science of well-being* (pp. 285–304). Oxford University Press.
Kainulainen, S., Saari, J., & Veenhoven, R. (2018). Life-satisfaction is more a matter of feeling well than having what you want. Tests of Veenhoven's theory. *International Journal of Happiness and Development, 4*(3), 209–235. https://doi.org/10.1504/ijhd.2018.093728
Kaiser, C., & Oswald, A. J. (2022). The scientific value of numerical measures of human feelings. *Proceedings of the National Academy of Sciences, 119*(42), e2210412119. https://doi.org/10.1073/pnas.2210412119
Kasser, T., & Ryan, R. M. (1993). A dark side of the American dream: Correlates of financial success as a central life aspiration. *Journal of Personality and Social Psychology, 65*(2), 410–422.
Kasser, T., & Ryan, R. M. M. (1996). Further examining the American dream: Differential correlates of intrinsic and extrinsic goals. *Personality and Social Psychology Bulletin, 22*(3), 280–287.
Katzell, R. A. (1964). Personal values, job satisfaction, and job behavior. *Man in a World of Work*, 341–363.
Kesebir, P., & Diener, E. (2008). In pursuit of happiness: Empirical answers to philosophical questions. *Perspectives on Psychological Science, 3*(2), 117–125. https://doi.org/10.1111/j.1745-6916.2008.00069.x
King, L. (2001). The hard road to the good life: The happy, mature person. *Journal of Humanistic Psychology, 41*(1), 51–72.
Klinger, E. (1975). Consequences of commitment to and disengagement from incentives. *Psychological Review, 82*(1), 1–25. https://doi.org/10.1037/h0076171
Kluckhohn, C. K. M. (1951). Values and value orientation in the theory of action: An exploration in definition and classification. In T. Parson & E. A. Shils (Eds.), *Toward a general theory of action*. Harvard University Press.
Koo, M., & Fishbach, A. (2010). Climbing the goal ladder. *Journal of Personality and Social Psychology, 99*(1), 1–13.
Krasko, J., Intelisano, S., & Luhmann, M. (2022). When happiness is both joy and purpose: The complexity of the pursuit of happiness and well-being is related to actual well-being. *Journal of Happiness Studies, 23*(7), 3233–3261. https://doi.org/10.1007/s10902-022-00541-2
Kruger, J. (1999). Lake Wobegon be gone! The "below-average effect" and the egocentric nature of comparative ability judgments. *Journal of Personality and Social Psychology, 77*(2), 221–232. https://doi.org/10.1037/0022-3514.77.2.221
Kushlev, K., Drummond, D. M., Heintzelman, S. J., & Diener, E. (2020). Do happy people care about society's problems? *The Journal of Positive Psychology, 15*(4), 467–477. https://doi.org/10.1080/17439760.2019.1639797
LeDoux, J. (1998). *The emotional brain. The mysterious underpinnings of emotional life*. Phoenix.
Locke, E. A. (1969). What is job satisfaction? *Organizational Behavior and Human Performance, 4*(4), 309–336. https://doi.org/10.1016/0030-5073(69)90013-0

Lomas, T., Case, B., Cratty, F. J., & VanderWheele, T. (2021). A global history of happiness. *International Journal of Wellbeing, 11*(4), 68.

Lucas, R. E. (2018). Reevaluating the strengths and weaknesses of self-report measures of subjective well-being. In E. Diener, S. Oishi, & L. Tay (Eds.), *Handbook of subjective well-being. Noba scholar handbook series: Subjective well-being*. DEF publishers. nobascholar.com. https://doi.org/nobascholar.com

Lucas, R. E., Diener, E., & Suh, E. (1996). Discriminant validity of well-being measures. *Journal of Personality and Social Psychology, 71*(3), 616–628.

Luhmann, M., & Hennecke, M. (2017). The motivational consequences of life satisfaction. *Motivation Science, 3*(1), 51–75. https://doi.org/10.1037/mot0000048

Luhmann, M., Hawkley, L. C., Eid, M., & Cacioppo, J. T. (2012). Time frames and the distinction between affective and cognitive well-being. *Journal of Research in Personality, 46*(4), 431–441. https://doi.org/10.1016/j.jrp.2012.04.004

Lyubomirsky, S., & Ross, L. (1999). Changes in attractiveness of elected, rejected, and precluded alternatives: A comparison of happy and unhappy individuals. *Journal of Personality and Social Psychology, 76*(6), 988–1007.

Mandler, G. (1984). *Mind and body. Psychology of emotion and stress*. W.W. Norton & Company.

McDowell, I. (2006). *Measuring health: A guide to rating scales and questionnaires* (Third ed.). Oxford University Press.

McLean, C. P., Thomas, S., Lau, A. L. D., Weinberg, M. K., & Cummins, R. A. (2020). Normative ranges for multiple regression: GLS vs PWI domains. In R. A. Cummins (Ed.), *Personal well-being index manual* (6th ed.). Melbourne ACQol Open-Access Publications, Australian Centre on Quality of Life. http://www.acqol.com.au/publications#Open-access

Mercier, H., & Sperber, D. (2017). *The enigma of reason. A new theory of understanding*. Pinguin.

Michalos, A. C. (1980). Satisfaction and happiness. *Social Indicators Research, 8*, 385–422.

Michalos, A. C. (1985). Multiple discrepancies theory (MDT). *Social Indicators Research, 16*, 347–413.

Millingen, J. G. (2022). *The history of duelling*. DigiCat.

Mischel, W., & Shoda, Y. (1995). A cognitive-affective system theory of personality: Reconceptualizing situations, dispositions, dynamics, and invariance in personality structure. *Psychological Review, 102*, 246–268.

Montague, R. (2007). *Your brain is (almost) perfect: How we make decisions [Kindle]*. Dutton.

Myers, D. G., & Diener, E. (1995). Who is happy? *Psychological Science, 6*(1), 10–19.

Napa, C., & King, L. A. (2004). Is the good life the easy life? *Social Indicators Research, 68*, 127–162.

Neisser, U. (1967). *Cognitive psychology*. Appleton-Century-Crofts.

Nussbaum, M. C. (2008). Who is the happy warrior? Philosophy poses questions to psychology. *The Journal of Legal Studies, 37*(S2), s81–s113. https://doi.org/10.1086/587438

Odermatt, R., & Stutzer, A. (2018). Subjective well-being and public policy. In E. Diener, S. Oishi, & L. Tay (Eds.), *Handbook of subjective well-being. Noba scholar handbook series: Subjective well-being*. DEF publishers. nobascholar.com. https://doi.org/nobascholar.com

OECD. (2013). *OECD Guidelines on measuring subjective well-being*. https://doi.org/10.1787/9789264191655-en

Oishi, S. (2012). *The psychological wealth of nations. Do happy people make a happy society?* Wiley-Blackwell.

Oishi, S., & Westgate, E. C. (2022). A psychologically rich life: Beyond happiness and meaning. *Psychological Review, 129*(4), 790–811. https://doi.org/10.1037/rev0000317

Oishi, S., Choi, H., Koo, M., Galinha, I., Ishii, K., Komiya, A., Luhmann, M., Scollon, C., Shin, J.-E., Lee, H., Suh, E. M., Vittersø, J., Heintzelman, S. J., Kushlev, K., Westgate, E. C., Buttrick, N., Tucker, J., Ebersole, C. R., Axt, J., Besser, L. L., et al. (2020). Happiness, meaning, and psychological richness. *Affective Science, 1*(2), 107–115. https://doi.org/10.1007/s42761-020-00011-z

Okon-Singer, H., Hendler, T., Pessoa, L., & Shackman, A. J. (2015). The neurobiology of emotion–cognition interactions: Fundamental questions and strategies for future research [review]. *Frontiers in Human Neuroscience, 9*. https://doi.org/10.3389/fnhum.2015.00058

Okon-Singer, H., Stout, D. M., Stockbridge, M. D., Gamer, M., Fox, A. S., & Shackman, A. J. (2018). The interplay of emotion and cognition. In A. S. Fox, R. C. Lapate, A. J. Shackman, & R. J. Davidson (Eds.), *The nature of emotion. Fundamental questions* (pp. 181–185). Oxford University Press.

Pagán-Rodrıguez, R. (2012). Longitudinal analysis of the domains of satisfaction before and after disability: Evidence from the German socio-economic panel. *Social Indicators Research, 108*(3), 365–385.

Palys, T. S., & Little, B. R. (1983). Perceived life satisfaction and organization of personal project system. *Journal of Personality and Social Psychology, 44*, 1221–1230.

Panksepp, J. (1998). *Affective neuroscience*. Oxford University Press.

Panksepp, J., & Biven, L. (2012). *The archaeology of mind*. Norton.

Pavot, W., & Diener, E. (1993). Review of the satisfaction with life scale. *Psychological Assessment, 5*(2), 164–172.

Payne, J. W. (1982). Contingent decision behavior. *Psychological Bulletin, 92*(2), 382–402. https://doi.org/10.1037/0033-2909.92.2.382

Phelps, E. A. (2006). Emotion and cognition: Insights from studies of the human amygdala. *Annual Review of Psychology, 57*, 27–53.

Prati, A., & Senik, C. (2022). Feeling good is feeling better. *Psychological Science, 33*(11), 1828–1841. https://doi.org/10.1177/09567976221096158

Putnam, H. (2004). *The collapse of the fact/value dichotomy and other essays*. Harvard University Press.

Ralph, K., Palmer, K., & Olney, J. (2012). *Subjective well-being: A qualitative investigation of subjective well-being questions* (Office For National Statistics working paper, Issue.

Ramachandran, V. S. (2011). *The tell-tale brain. Unlocking the mystery of human nature*. Wiliam Heinemann.

Ramachandran, V. S., & Hirstein, W. (1999). The science of art: A neurological theory of aesthetic experience. *Journal of Consciousness Studies, 6*(6–7), 15–51.

Richards, J. M. J. (1966). Life goals of American college freshmen. *Journal of Counseling Psychology, 13*(1), 12–20. https://doi.org/10.1037/h0023049

Robinson, M. D., & Clore, G. L. (2002). Belief and feeling: Evidence for an accessibility model of emotional self-report. *Psychological Bulletin, 128*(6), 934–960.

Rohan, M. J. (2000). A rose by any name? The values construct. *Personality and Social Psychology Review, 4*(3), 255–277. https://doi.org/10.1207/s15327957pspr0403_4

Rokeach, M. (1973). *The nature of human values*. Free Press.

Rolls, E. T. (2018). Emotional vs. rational systems, and decisions between them. In A. S. Fox, R. C. Lapate, A. J. Shackman, & R. J. Davidson (Eds.), *The nature of emotion. Fundamental questions* (pp. 206–207). Oxford University Press.

Ross, M., Eyman, A., & Kishchuck, N. (1986). Determinants of subjective well-being. In J. M. Olson, C. P. Herman, & M. Zanna (Eds.), *Relative deprivation and social comparison*. Erlbaum.

Røysamb, E., Nes, R. B., Czajkowski, N. O., & Vassend, O. (2018). Genetics, personality and wellbeing. A twin study of traits, facets and life satisfaction. *Scientific Reports, 8*(1), 12298. https://doi.org/10.1038/s41598-018-29881-x

Ryan, R. M., & Deci, E. L. (2017). Self-determination theory: Basic psychological needs in motivation, development, and wellness [Kindle]. *Guilford*. Publications.

Sacks, O. (1998). *The man who mistook his wife for a hat: And other clinical tales*. Simon and Schuster.

Schimmack, U., & Oishi, S. (2005). The influence of chronically and temporarily accessible information on life satisfaction judgments. *Journal of Personality and Social Psychology, 89*(3), 395–406.

Schimmack, U., Diener, E., & Oishi, S. (2002). Life-satisfaction is a momentary judgment and a stable personality characteristic: The use of chronically accessible and stable sources. *Journal of Personality, 70*(3), 345–384.
Schimmack, U., Schupp, J., & Wagner, G. G. (2008). The influence of environment and personality on the affective and cognitive component of subjective well-being. *Social Indicators Research, 89*(1), 41–60.
Schkade, D., & Kahneman, D. (1998). Does living in California make people happy? A focusing illusion in judgements of life satisfaction. *Psychological Science, 9*(5), 340–346.
Schwartz, S. H. (1992). Universals in the content and structure of values: Theoretical advances and empirical tests in 20 countries. In M. P. Zanna (Ed.), *Advances in experimental social psychology* (Vol. 25, pp. 1–65). Academic Press. https://doi.org/10.1016/S0065-2601(08)60281-6
Schwartz, S. H. (1999). A theory of cultural values and some implications for work. *Applied Psychology, 48*(1), 23–47.
Schwartz, S. H. (2012). An overview of the Schwartz theory of basic values. *Psychol Cult, 2*(1), 11.
Schwartz, S. H., & Cieciuch, J. (2022). Measuring the refined theory of individual values in 49 cultural groups: Psychometrics of the revised portrait value questionnaire. *Assessment, 29*(5), 1005–1019. https://doi.org/10.1177/1073191121998760
Schwartz, S. H., & Sortheix, F. M. (2018). Values and subjective well-being. In E. Diener, S. Oishi, & L. Tay (Eds.), *Handbook of subjective well-being. Noba scholar handbook series: Subjective well-being*. DEF publishers. nobascholar.com. https://doi.org/nobascholar.com
Schwarz, N., & Clore, G. L. (1983). Mood, misattribution and judgments of well-being: Information and directive functions of affective states. *Journal of Personality and Social Psychology, 45*, 513–523.
Schwarz, N., & Clore, G. L. (1988). How do I feel about it? The informative function of affective states. In K. Fiedler & J. P. Forgas (Eds.), *Affect, cognition and social behavior* (pp. 44–62). C.J. Hogrefe.
Schwarz, N., & Strack, F. (1991). Evaluating one's life: A judgement model of subjective well-being. In F. Strack, M. Argyle, & N. Schwarz (Eds.), *Subjective well-being. An interdisciplinary perspective* (pp. 27–48). Pergamon Press.
Schwarz, N., & Strack, F. (1999). Reports of subjective well-being: Judgmental processes and their methodological implications. In D. Kahneman, E. Diener, & N. Schwarz (Eds.), *Well-being: The foundations of hedonic psychology* (pp. 61–84). Russell Sage Foundation.
Schwarz, N., Strack, F., Kommer, D., & Wagner, D. (1987). Soccer, rooms, and the quality of your life: Mood effects on judgments of satisfaction with life in general and with specific domains. *European Journal of Social Psychology, 17*(1), 69–79. https://doi.org/10.1002/ejsp.2420170107
Scollon, C. N., & King, L. (2011). What people really want in life and why it matters: Contributions from research on folk theories of the good life. In R. Biswas-Diener (Ed.), *Positive psychology as social change* (pp. 1–14). Springer. http://www.springer.com/psychology/book/978-90-481-9937-2
Scott, W. A., Osgood, D. W., & Peterson, C. (1979). *Cognitive structure: Theory and measurement of individual differences*. Wiley.
Seligman, M. E. P. (2002). *Authentic happiness. Using the new positive psychology to realize your potential for deep fulfillment*. Nicholas Brealey Publishing.
Seligman, M. E. P. (2011). *Flourish. A visionary new understanding of happiness and well-being [Kindle]*. Free Press.
Semple, N. (2021). Good enough for government work? Life-evaluation and public policy. *Journal of Happiness Studies, 22*(3), 1119–1140. https://doi.org/10.1007/s10902-020-00266-0
Shackman, A. J., & Lapate, R. C. (2018). Afterword: How do emotion and cognition interact? In A. S. Fox, R. C. Lapate, A. J. Shackman, & R. J. Davidson (Eds.), *The nature of emotion. Fundamental questions* (pp. 209–211). Oxford University Press.
Sharot, T., Korn, C. W., & Dolan, R. J. (2011). How unrealistic optimism is maintained in the face of reality. *Nature Neuroscience, 14*(11), 1475–1485.

Sherman, S. J., & Corty, E. (1984). Cognitive heuristics. In R. S. Wyer & T. Srull (Eds.), *Handbook of social cognition* (Vol. 3). Erlbaum.

Shizgal, P. (1999). On the neural computation of utility: Implications from studies of brain stimulation reward. In D. Kahneman, E. Diener, & N. Schwarz (Eds.), *Well-being: The foundations of hedonic psychology* (pp. 502–526). Russell Sage Foundation. http://cogprints.org/740/1/Well-Being_v4_15.html

Sim, B., & Diener, E. (2018). Accounts of psychological and emotional well-being for policy purposes. In E. Diener, S. Oishi, & L. Tay (Eds.), *Handbook of subjective well-being. Noba scholar handbook series: Subjective well-being*. DEF publishers. nobascholar.com. https://doi.org/nobascholar.com

Sirgy, J. M. (2012). *The psychology of quality of life. Hedonic well-being, life satisfaction, and eudaimonia* (2nd ed.). Springer. https://doi.org/10.1007/978-94-007-4405-9

Slovic, P., & Lichtenstein, S. (1971). Comparison of Bayesian and regression approaches to the study of information processing in judgment. *Organizational Behavior and Human Performance, 6*(5), 649–744.

Steel, P., Schmidt, J., & Shultz, J. (2008). Refining the relationship between personality and subjective well-being. *Psychological Bulletin, 134*(1), 138–161.

Steptoe, A., Deaton, A., & Stone, A. A. (2015). Subjective wellbeing, health, and ageing. *The Lancet, 385*(9968), 640–648. https://doi.org/10.1016/S0140-6736(13)61489-0

Stiglitz, J. E., Sen, A., & Fitoussi, J.-P. (2009). *Report by the Commission on the measurement of economic performance and social progress*. http://www.stiglitz-sen-fitoussi.fr/en/index.htm

Stouffer, S. A., Suchman, E., DeVinney, L., Star, S., & Williams, R. (1949). *The American soldier. Adjustment during army life*. Princeton University Press.

Strack, F., Argyle, M., & Schwarz, N. (Eds.). (1991). *Subjective well-being*. Pergamon Press.

Suh, E., Diener, E., Oishi, S., & Triandis, H. C. (1998). The shifting basis of life satisfaction judgements across cultures: Emotions versus norms. *Journal of Personality and Social Psychology, 74*(2), 482–493.

Sumner, L. W. (1996). *Welfare, happiness, and ethics*. Clarendon Press.

Taylor, J. B. (2008). *My stroke of insight [Kindle]*. Hodder & Stoughton.

Tetlock, P. E. (1992). The impact of accountability on judgment and choice: Toward a social contingency model. In *Advances in experimental social psychology,* Vol. 25 (pp. 331–376). Academic Press. https://doi.org/10.1016/S0065-2601(08)60287-7

Thorndike, E. L. (1927). The law of effect. *The American Journal of Psychology, 39*(1/4), 212–222. https://doi.org/10.2307/1415413

Thorsteinsen, K., & Vittersø, J. (2023, August, 21–25). Subjective wellbeing as life values. How important are pleasure and life satisfaction in people's lives? The 21th annual conference for The International Society for Quality of Life Studies Rotterdam, The Netherlands.

Tiberius, V. (2014). Life satisfaction judgments. In A. C. Michalos (Ed.), *Encyclopedia of quality of life and well-being research* (pp. 3591–3593). Springer.

Tomyn, A. J., & Cummins, R. A. (2011). The subjective wellbeing of high-school students: Validating the personal wellbeing index—School children [journal article]. *Social Indicators Research, 101*(3), 405–418. https://doi.org/10.1007/s11205-010-9668-6

Tononi, G. (2004). An information integration theory of consciousness. *BMC Neuroscience, 5*(1), 42. https://doi.org/10.1186/1471-2202-5-42

Trope, Y. (1986). Self-enhancement and self-assessment in achievement behavior. In *Handbook of motivation and cognition: Foundations of social behavior* (pp. 350–378). Guilford Press.

Tsurumi, T., Yamaguchi, R., Kagohashi, K., & Managi, S. (2021). Are cognitive, affective, and eudaimonic dimensions of subjective well-being differently related to consumption? Evidence from Japan. *Journal of Happiness Studies, 22*(6), 2499–2522. https://doi.org/10.1007/s10902-020-00327-4

Veenhoven, R. (1984). *Conditions of happiness*. Kluwer Academic.

Veenhoven, R. (1988). The utility of happiness. *Social Indicators Research, 22*, 333–354.

Veenhoven, R. (2013). The four qualities of life ordering concepts and measures of the good life. In A. Delle Fave (Ed.), *The exploration of happiness: Present and future perspectives*. Springer Science.
Vittersø, J. (2018). Do it! Activity theories and the good life. In E. Diener, S. Oishi, & L. Tay (Eds.), *Handbook of well-being*. DEF Publishers. https://doi.org/nobascholar.com
Vittersø, J., & Nilsen, F. (2002). The conceptual and relational structure of subjective well-being, neuroticism, and extraversion: Neuroticism is again found to be the important predictor of happiness. *Social Indicators Research, 57*(1), 89–118.
Vittersø, J., Oelmann, H., & Wang, A. L. (2009). Life satisfaction is not a balanced estimator of the good life. Evidence from reaction time measures and self-reported emotions. *Journal of Happiness Studies, 10*(1), 1–17. https://doi.org/10.1007/s10902-007-9058-1
Walsh, D. M. (2015). *Organisms, agency, and evolution*. Cambridge University Press. https://doi.org/10.1017/CBO9781316402719
Watson, D. (2002). Positive affectivity: The disposition to experience pleasurable emotional states. In *Handbook of positive psychology* (pp. 106–119). Oxford University Press.
Weiss, H. M. (2002). Deconstructing job satisfaction. Separating evaluations, beliefs and affective experiences. *Human Resource Management Review, 12*(2), 173–194.
Yap, S. C. Y., Wortman, J., Anusic, I., Baker, S. G., Scherer, L. D., Donnellan, M. B., & Lucas, R. E. (2016). The effect of mood on judgments of subjective well-being: Nine tests of the judgment model. *Journal of Personality and Social Psychology*, No Pagination Specified. https://doi.org/10.1037/pspp0000115

Chapter 5
Hedonia

Introduction

> All happy families are alike, each unhappy family is unhappy in its own way. (Tolstoy, 2014)

Lev Tolstoy's masterpiece of an opening line in *Anna Karenina* reflects an existential tension between simplicity and complexity. It therefore speaks to the idea of hedonia. In both "the high literature and the popular culture," as the influential literary critic Gary Saul Morson (2014) puts it, Tolstoy's first sentence is taken to mean that happy families resemble one another because their lives are simple—without drama. And without tension, there can be no story. Unhappy families, by contrast, suffer much drama, and each is complicated in its own way.

Privately, Tolstoy was attracted to ease and simplicity. What he wanted to say in *Anna Karenina* has therefore gone unnoticed by most commentators. That is at least what Morson argues. What matters to Tolstoy is "the countless ordinary events" in life. The moral heroine in the novel is therefore not Anna, but Dolly Oblonsky. Dolly is a modest and ordinary character who faithfully serves her husband Stiva and stands in contrast to Anna (Morson, 2014, pp. xi–xvi). Interestingly, and completely detached from Morson's analyses, the personality psychologist Gordon Allport has also carefully examined Tolstoy's writing. Allport's conclusions agree with those of Morson. Allport was convinced that Tolstoy must have been attracted to an ideal about "the utmost possible simplification of life" and that he equalized happiness with simplicity (Allport, 1961, p. 197). Everything in the world should be reduced to "this great fundamental Tolstoyan principle," the simplification of life. This is how Allport interprets the Russian novelist's world view, given that pleasure, still according to Tolstoy, can only be found "by reducing the complexities of life" (p. 199). Tolstoy's passion for the simplification of life was his cardinal disposition, Allport says, his way of maintaining unity and homeostatic balance (pp. 377–378). This puts Tolstoy's ideas about a good life at the center of the tension reduction motive, which is vital in a modern account of pleasure.

J. Vittersø, *Humanistic Wellbeing*, https://doi.org/10.1007/978-3-031-69292-5_5

Pleasure

The study of pleasure has a long and rich history. Philosophers, biologists, neuroscientists, psychologists, economists, sociologists, and anthropologists are among those who have contributed knowledge about pleasure and how it should be comprehended. For example, in the early days of modern biology, Darwin pondered pleasure and its role in evolution. He was convinced that it had evolved for a reason and argued that pleasure can cause animals to "pursue that course of action which is the most beneficial to the species" (McMahon, 2006, p. 422). Similarly, William James (1890) pointed out that pleasure facilitates life-enhancing activities and that we would not have had these feelings had they not served some useful purpose in our evolutionary history (cited in Denton, 2005, p. 8). The evolutionary roots of pleasure go way back in time. Berridge and Kringelbach (2015) suggested, for instance, that pleasure can be thought of as "evolution's boldest trick" (p. 646), and biologists speculate that even the tiny roundworm *Caenorhabditis elegans*, with its modest number of 302 neurons, might have some basic, neurological "pleasure" circuitry. "These worms typically feed on bacteria and are very good at following odor cues to find clumps of them. However, when a group of eight key neurons containing dopamine are silenced, the worms are mostly indifferent to this favorite food source (even though they can still detect odors)" (Linden, 2012, Chap. 1). As summarized by Skov (2019), "the key idea is that biological organisms have evolved a neurobiological system for tagging stimuli with an affective 'gloss' that can aid the organism in deciding how to interact with it." Following Damasio, pleasure also signalizes "whether the underlying 'global' state of the body is generally conducive to the continuation of life and to survival, and to how strong or weak that life trend happens to be at a given moment" (Damasio, 2018, p. 105). Pleasure is therefore a signal of wellbeing, Damasio says, because it is the feeling that follows "when the organism is functioning with a good balance between what it requires to operate well and what it gets" (Damasio, 2021, p. 104).

The study of pleasure was central when psychology became a science in the late nineteenth century. This was partly due to its close association with sensations—a very hot topic at that time. As reviewed in Chap. 1, pleasure was a core mental element in Wundt's theory of subjective experiences, and it has been central in psychological research more generally ever since. An early and comprehensive theory was offered by Beebe-Center (1932). Based on exhaustive empirical experimentation, he rejected the idea that pleasure is a sensational attribute and rather considered it to be a basic element, a "natural kind," in itself. As such, pleasantness has its own phenomenology, intensity, and duration and cannot be a subdimension or an attribute of another basic element. Beebe-Center proposed that the term hedonic tone would be a proper name for such basic feelings, the things we experience along a bipolar dimension running from unpleasantness to pleasantness. Beebe-Center was, however, not interested in the phenomenology of pleasantness, what pleasure feels like, since he considered that question to be a metaphysical one.

Fortunately, the metaphysical stigma of phenomenological studies waned with the hegemony of behaviorism, and psychologists became more willing to study what it feels like to have a pleasant experience. Arnold (1960) was an early bird who regarded pleasantness and unpleasantness as rudimentary evaluations (p. 171). Arnold argued that pleasure never stands alone but is always a "gloss" to some other experience. As such, pleasure is not a "quale," i.e., a specific irreducible feeling quality. Pleasure is something that comes on top of the feeling quality (cited in Frijda, 2010, p. 100).

What pleasure adds to the quality of a feeling, Frijda maintains, is information about how well we are doing in the current situation. Pleasure is a message about harmony, a signal telling us that nothing needs to be changed right now—everything is fine as they are (Frijda, 2010). Pleasure is not qualia in the sense of reflecting a particular feeling tone but rather "a specific irreducible experience. It does not even have a characteristic phenomenology, as has the color red or the experience of bright pressure" (Frijda, 2010, p. 100). This idea is worked out in more detail by Cabanac, who was briefly introduced in Chap. 3.

Michel Cabanac

A physiologist by education, Michel Cabanac developed a thought-provoking theory of pleasure that neatly combines its structural and functional elements. For approximately half a century, Cabanac conducted experimental research at the crossroad between biology and psychology. Based on these studies, he elaborated some radical ideas about the concept of pleasure. For instance, Cabanac suggested that pleasure is a motivating mechanism powerful enough to be compared with the four major forces in physics: gravity, electromagnetism, strong nuclear, and weak nuclear. Pleasure, he says, acts on conscious brains much as the forces of physics influence masses and particles (Cabanac, 2009, p. 25).

To recapitulate Cabanac's four attributes of a feeling state, valence is a quantitative dimension that runs from pleasant to unpleasant and contains a zero point (indifferent), whereas quality is a categorical dimension reflecting a particular phenomenology ("quale"). The quality of a feeling can be classified as a typical sensation, such as a sweet taste, a cold room, or seeing the color red. It also includes mental feelings, such as fear, sadness, happiness, and interest. Intensity and duration are quantitative attributes that vary from weak to strong (intensity) and from short to long (duration).

In terms of functioning, the valence of a feeling provides information about usefulness or value. The pleasantness (or unpleasantness) of a situation enables us to prioritize alternative states. Our ability to discriminate is thus contingent on our ability to feel pleasure. The principle is simple: When people must choose among competing behaviors, they need a cue to make their priorities, and that is exactly what pleasure gives us. Hence, the valence dimension solves a fundamental challenge faced by all living organisms: How can biological needs be assessed against the opportunities, or threats, presented by the environment? The answer, Cabanac says, is that the organism must have an idea about the difference between an unfavorable state and a favorable state. "For this to happen, the required resource must first exhibit a gradient in the external environment. Otherwise, there will be nowhere better to move to" (Cabanac, 2009, p. 47).

The role of the quality dimension is different. The information provided by a feeling quality regard the nature of the environment and how it can be separated into qualitatively distinct entities. Hence, feeling qualities critically assist us in the process of categorizing, or give meaning to, our inner and outer environments. The third attribute of a feeling's state, intensity, expresses the quantity of a stimulus, whereas duration indicates how long the stimulus is present.

Cabanac has found support for these ideas in several intriguing experiments, spanning from video games, grammatical and mathematical problem solving, and judgments of ethical dilemmas to evaluating the aesthetics of poetry. One of these studies demonstrated how different levels of pleasure and displeasure are negotiated to maximize the experience of pleasure (Cabanac, 1992). The design involved regulating a comfortable body temperature and minimizing the displeasure of physical exercise. The experiment followed a three-step procedure. On the first day, participants were exposed to varying temperatures in a room, and they rated the degree of pleasantness experienced as the temperature increased or sunk. On the second day, the participants were asked to walk on a treadmill while maintaining a constant speed. The slope of the treadmill varied, and steeper slopes obviously required more effort. The participants rated the pleasantness experienced at various levels of effort. On the final day, the participants completed ten separate sessions of walking the treadmill. In five sessions, they could regulate the slope of the treadmill while the room temperature was kept constant (although at varying temperatures for each session). In the remaining five sessions, they could regulate the temperature, whereas the slopes were held constant throughout each session. When the room was cold, the subjects could increase their body temperature by increasing the steepness of the treadmill slope. In a warm room, the body temperature was lowered by choosing a flatter slope. Similarly, when the treadmill slope was fixed, body temperature could be kept optimally pleasant by increasing (for flat slopes) or decreasing (for steep slopes) the room temperature. The outcome of these experiments showed an amazing coherence with the theoretical prediction, i.e., that maximal pleasure follows the rule of adding different sources of pleasure and displeasure. Participants consistently chose to maximize pleasure by regulating temperature or treadmill slopes to balance their body temperature and energy expenditure within the narrow but optimal range of comfort. The maximization of pleasure in this context coincides perfectly with optimal physiological thermoregulation. This study supports the assumption that when given a free choice, humans will contribute to the effort needed to maintain their physiology in homeostatic balance, but not more.

More detailed analyses revealed that pleasure maximization was also optimal from the point of view of energy consumption. The pleasure-regulated behavior maintained muscle circulation and respiration at an optimal power output. In other words, when everything else is removed, pleasure guides the organism toward optimal functioning. Studies such as this have inspired Cabanac to conclude that pleasure acts as an indicator of good behavior and that displeasure acts as an indicator of bad behavior. The hedonic dimension of an experience is thus a mechanism that regulates optimal functioning.

There is a small anomaly in some of Cabanac's results, however, suggesting that the hedonic model cannot sufficiently account for optimal functioning the way he has proposed. In one study, Cabanac found a delay in the response to increased unpleasantness, which means that participants continued their activity even if their experiences were more unpleasant than pleasant. The extended activity violates the principle of pleasure maximization. I suggest that this delay can be interpreted as a kind of engagement in an ongoing activity: An opportunity feeling kicks in and overrules the homeostatic pull toward stability. My suggestion speaks to the idea that not only pleasure but also the feeling qualities in themselves can be valuable. According to this interpretation, engagement in an activity can overrule the priority function typically ascribed to the valence dimension. This would fit the functional assumption that the humanistic theory ascribes to opportunity feelings, i.e., that they encourage us to pursue an activity toward an important goal, even in states of increasing homeostatic imbalance. We can be interested and engaged in an activity even if it feels unpleasant and is not directed toward an immediate regain of homeostatic equilibrium.

Allen Parducci

Parducci published a provocative paper in 1968, launching the idea that happiness was a blend of the range and frequency of pleasant events (Parducci, 1968). In this and later work (e.g., Parducci, 1995), he defended the view that happiness equals pleasure and that pleasure is an attitude or a judgment. To say that something is pleasant is to say that it compares favorably with other events in the context with which it is experienced (Parducci, 1995, p. 23). Like Cabanac, Frijda, and others, Parducci does not consider the concept of pleasure to be a referent of a particular feeling quality, such as the saltiness of a peanut or the loudness of music. Sometimes loud music can be preferred, such as when it is part of a rock concert, and it will thus be judged as pleasant. Other times, loud music is not preferred, such as when it comes from a neighbor's late-at-night party, and then it will be judged as unpleasant.

What makes Parducci's theory special is first its constructivist stance (happiness is completely relative) and second its conceptualization of pleasure. As for the relativism, Parducci argues that happiness is not a matter of how intense your pleasantness is; rather, it compares to the total amount of pleasant moments you have over a lifetime. More precisely, your total happiness is defined by the range and the frequency of pleasant experiences. Note that pleasure is not a feeling quality, but it is nevertheless related to an experience in the sense that it is the target for judgments of preferences of that experience. In contrast to the quality dimension of an experience, which we typically are aware of, the judgmental nature of pleasure is often not conscious.

Parducci grounded his theory on a solid body of research, demonstrating that ratings of pleasure can be predicted from the stimulus context. It also builds on other empirical studies, such as those presented by Beebe-Center (1932). Among other things, Beebe-Center showed how a neutral odor can be reported as either pleasant or unpleasant depending on the context within which it is presented to the participants. To Parducci, such findings illustrate how we evaluate an event as either pleasant or unpleasant depending on the other events in the context, and this calls for a constructivist explanation. Pleasure is only experienced as pleasant because it compares favorably with other events that vary on a scale of preferences, and no feeling quality is needed to make that judgment.

Pleasure and displeasure, i.e., judgments of favorability and unfavorability, are created along a one-dimensional scale of preferences, which Parducci refers to as hedonic judgments. The purpose of hedonic judgments is to locate different experiences within a given context along a hierarchy of goodness and badness. Hedonic judgments are, in other words, a valuation mechanism. The hedonic element of an experience is simply the rank order of that experience relative to the other relevant experiences. Hence, all experiences that hold similar rank orders are equally pleasant.

In more detail, the rank order in a hedonic judgment is defined as a compromise between two factors: the range (the distance between the best and worst experience) and the frequency (how often the experience takes place). The compromise between the range and the frequency is articulated in the range–frequency theory and algebraically formulated as the claim that the mean of all judgments about pleasure (JMean) is equal to the difference between the mean and the midpoint of the contextual stimuli, divided by their range: JMean = (Mean—Midpoint)/Range (e.g., Parducci, 1968, 1995).

In one of Parducci's experiments (reported in Parducci, 1995, pp. 71–72), college students were invited to play a game in which they were given the opportunity to win small amounts of money by repeatedly picking one out three cards from a table in front of them. The payoff for each card was specified on the hidden side, and after each trial, the participant stated how satisfied he or she was with the profit. Unknown to the players, they all won the same amount of money. However, the windfalls occurred at different rates. In one group, the profit varied from 1 to 21 cent, and the players were made aware of this range. The members of the other group were made aware that their possible winnings varied from 7 to 29 cent for each card. To make the profit equal in the two groups, members of the first group had to frequently win money close to the upper end of the range, while members of the second group had to win relatively more money from cards of low amounts. By this move, the first group was experimentally given a negatively skewed distribution of profits, and the second group was given a positively skewed distribution. According to the range–frequency theory, "happiness is a negatively skewed distribution," which implies that players in the first group should be more pleased (satisfied) with their monetary reward than players in the second and positively skewed group. That was exactly what Parducci and his team found. Even if all players won the same amount of money in the end, those in the "1 to 21 cents" group (with a negatively skewed distribution of monetary payoffs) were significantly more satisfied (which means pleased in Parducci's vocabulary) with their winnings than players from the "7 to 29 cents" group (with a positively skewed distribution). The satisfied group had more wins close to the upper range of their distributions, which should make them more satisfied. Not only were 15 of the 20 players in the positive skew condition less satisfied than any of the 20 players in the negative skew condition, but their mean ratings were also very close to the theoretical prediction of the range frequency theory. The theoretical predictions were 4.5 and 3.5 for the negative skew and the positive skew groups, respectively, and the observed means were 4.6 and 3.4, respectively.

Parducci takes the lessons learned from this and similar experiments as principles representative of real-life events and consequently argues that overall, happiness is nothing more than the theoretical algebraic sum of all hedonic judgments divided by the total period in question (Parducci, 1995, p. 203). This assumption makes Parducci a kind of hedonist, in the sense that he defends the idea that happiness is nothing more than the summation of separate moments of pleasure and pain (Parducci, 1995, p. 11). It should be noted, however, that the hedonic approach taken by Parducci does not imply moral hedonism (i.e., that we ought to seek pleasure) or psychological hedonism (our only motive in life is to seek pleasure and avoid pain). Neither is he a hedonist in the sense of arguing that the good life is juxtaposed with a feeling. Pleasure is a comparison, a judgment about the favorability and unfavorability of a situation, and it can even operate unconsciously. Hence, Parducci's concept of pleasure is closer to the common usage of terms such as preference or satisfaction, and his theory is not consistent with the idea that happiness is the same as flourishing, eudaimonia, or the ultimate good. Very clearly, Parducci announces that he rather sees that "people are good than that they are happy" (Parducci, 1995, p. 14). When Parducci defines happiness as the sum of momentary pleasures, he does not aim at defining a good life in a complete sense, and his is thus not a theory of hedonism.

Jaak Panksepp

Pleasure is not a basic emotion in Panksepp's taxonomy but rather a feeling that helps regulate our universal need for stability (Burgdorf & Panksepp, 2006; Panksepp, 1998; Panksepp & Biven, 2012). According to his neuropsychological nomenclature, Panksepp describes pleasure as something that reflects the capacity of certain stimuli to return the body to homeostatic equilibrium when it has deviated from its biologically dictated "setpoint" level (Panksepp, 1998, p. 182).

The pleasure system, i.e., the pleasure–displeasure valence dimension, sustains the regulation of bodily processes, including feeding, drinking, and temperature regulation. Panksepp therefore argues that the pleasure system is a valuation mechanism or a value-coding device in our brains (Panksepp, 1998, p. 165). The system translates stimuli that promote a return to the homeostatic set point into a pleasant feeling and those impairing homeostasis into an unpleasant one. Rather than feeling exited and curious, as was the case in the *SEEKING* system, or feeling joyful, as in the *PLAY* system, the state of pleasure is dominated by a feeling of satisfaction. Panksepp therefore suggests that pleasure provides us with information about something that is biologically useful. It is a feeling that "takes us in the right direction" (Panksepp, 1998, p. 182). An important neurochemical ingredient in the pleasure system is endogenous opioids and drugs that typically stimulate the system are narcotics such as morphine and heroin. Pleasure is typically linked to a reduction in the LH dopamine system (Panksepp, 1998, p. 147). However, it has been difficult to mechanistically conceptualize how such feelings might actually participate in the causal control of animal behavior.

Kent Berridge and Wanting Versus Liking

As a neuroscientist specializing in pleasure and rewards, Kent Berridge has contributed convincing evidence that, somewhat counterintuitively, wanting and liking are separable mental conditions. Even though we commonly think of wanting and liking as synonyms, we can sometimes want things without liking them and vice versa. In the vocabulary of Berridge, wanting therefore refers to the motivational aspect of reward and is often linked to the anticipation of the pleasure one expects to feel when something is consumed, when a need is fulfilled, or when a goal is achieved. Liking, by contrast, refers to the hedonic or pleasurable experience itself and is not produced by the active approach of something we want. Liking is the feeling that accompanies consumption and is the result of need fulfillment or goal achievement. Both wanting and liking can be conscious, as a feeling, and unconscious, as a non-felt motivation (e.g., Berridge & Winkielman, 2003; Winkielman et al., 2005).

Wanting and liking typically interact with each other as different phases in what Berridge refers to as a pleasure cycle. The process starts with an appetitive phase dominated by wanting, a motivation to seek reward, and proceeds into a consummatory phase dominated by liking, which translates to the hedonic experience of pleasure. The cycle ends in a satiety phase dominated by a learning process. Since Pavlov and Thorndike, learning theorists have known that experiencing a sensory object as pleasurable makes an animal crave it when it is encountered again at a later occasion (Skov, 2019). Hence, positive hedonic values are said to reward or reinforce behavior, which is why learning processes are included in the pleasure cycle together with wanting (Berridge, 2004; Kringelbach & Berridge, 2017). Thus, the basic idea of a pleasure cycle is framed in the context of motivation and reward and considers wanting to be our motivation for reward, liking to be the actual pleasure component or hedonic impact of a reward, and learning to be the associations, representations, and predictions about future rewards based on past experiences (Berridge & Kringelbach, 2016, pp. 136–137). Wanting, but not liking, is furthermore associated with addiction. People might become addicted to drugs, social media, or other things that are strongly wanted but not necessarily liked (Berridge, 1999).

By introducing the term pleasure cycle, Berridge and Kringelbach seem to operate with two slightly different conceptualizations of pleasure. On the one hand, the concept of a pleasure cycle covers a psychological composite state of three distinct but interacting elements of a motivational cycle. On the other hand, pleasure also refers to one of the elements in the cycle. Pleasure is in other words a kind of pleasure. In the latter sense, pleasure is defined as "positive hedonic valence, which can occur as either an objective 'liking' reaction or a subjective liking reaction to the hedonic impact of a stimulus—and usually both together" (Kringelbach & Berridge, 2017, p. 192). According to this meaning, pleasure is generated by a hedonic brain system—a valuation mechanism—which incorporates the simpler mechanism of liking.

Overall, the hedonic brain system comprises a series of "hot spots" distributed in both subcortical regions of the brain, such as the nucleus accumbens, and in cortical regions such as the lateral orbitofrontal cortex. These neural liking circuits are different from the neural wanting circuits. They are, for instance, regulated by opioid stimulation rather than dopamine stimulation, which is the typical neurological correlate for wanting. There is also strong evidence that a characteristic facial expression for liking exists in humans, monkeys, and rats. These facial expressions are not found for wanting. Wanting also feels different from liking and is related to an appetitive rather than a consummatory phase of behavior. Wanting motivations range from gambling to shopping, pornography, hobbies, addictive drugs, or taking excessive medication in an addictive fashion. However, these behaviors are not typically reported as "intense pleasure" (Berridge & Kringelbach, 2015, p. 656). Berridge therefore proposed that hedonic happiness can be conceived "as 'liking' without 'wanting'" (Berridge & Kringelbach, 2016, p. 142).

The Functions of Pleasure

Aristotle considered emotions to be functional, although he did not always think of pleasure as very useful (see the section on Hedonism below). However, later philosophers, such as Spinoza, who thought that pleasure brought us closer to our human nature, became more explicit about the positive effects of pleasure (Frijda, 1986, p.244). To Spinoza, pleasure is associated with a transition from a lesser state of perfection to a greater one, where perfection is the completeness of which an individual has realized her desires (Kringelbach & Berridge, 2010, p. 11). Darwin also had a functional perspective on pleasure and wrote about it in *The Expression of the Emotions in Man and Animals* (Darwin, 1872). Although not a core topic in the book, Darwin understood pleasure through the lens of natural selection and adaptation. He considered it useful for survival and reproduction because pleasure motivates the kind of behavior that secures the fulfillment of basic needs and mating. Darwin further observed how pleasure, during play, stimulated the exercise of muscular movements and facilitated the development of skills. Importantly, Darwin also elaborated on the social benefits of pleasure.

Inspired by Darwin, the developmental psychologist Charlotte Bühler was an early proponent of the idea that pleasure was a highly functional psychological state. As briefly mentioned in Chap. 1, she even gave it the name "Funktionslust," or "Function Pleasure." Funktionslust referred to the idea that movements in themselves are endowed with pleasure, given that the movements proceed superbly and smoothly (Bühler, 1928). Somewhat later, Hebb (1955) included mental growth on the list of the functions that pleasure can have, specifying the role of pleasure as the encouragement for "growth or development in cerebral organization" (cited in Feibleman, 1964, p. 255). Pleasure has also been proposed to be the inspirator for virtuous activities (Kubovy, 1999). However, the kind of mental pleasure Kubovy speaks about is different from the experience of valence that is typically discussed in the literature on pleasure. Kubovy defines pleasure more broadly as the feeling we have when we are doing something well (p. 147).

Somewhat differently perceived, Fredrickson has suggested that momentary or bodily pleasures are functional in that they draw healthy people to do what their bodies need at that moment. Yet, by serving this role, Fredrickson holds that pleasure should be excluded from the real function of positivity as laid out in the broaden-and-build theory. As noted in Chap. 1, the theory suggests that positive emotions broaden our minds and build psychological resources further down the road (Fredrickson, 2009). When biologists such as Cabanac argue that pleasure is functional because they guide organisms toward optimal functioning, this does not seem to be the kind of functioning Fredrickson's theory is concerned with. However, pleasure may play a role in stimulating social interaction, which in turn could lead to psychological resource-building, as Fredrickson writes about.

From an information processing point of view, the ability to feel pleasure saves our mental system from creating and storing an enormously large database of potential benefits and dangers. Because we feel pleasure and displeasure, our survival does not depend on detailed knowledge about, for example, the relation between a foul odor and bacterial contamination, between sweet tastes and nutrient-rich food, or between sex and the reproductive mechanisms of DNA (Johnston, 2003). Finally, in formulating a general summary of its functions, Frijda maintains that pleasant feelings are responses that signal that an individual's competences are functioning well, "the positive outcome of constantly monitoring one's functioning, and competences are doing what they are for" (Frijda, 2007, p. 82).

Common Currency

One function often attributed to pleasure is that of a common currency. An organism cannot function properly without a mechanism that allows different motivations to talk to one another. Without such a functioning, it would be impossible to rank priorities. Aristotle showed concern for this problem and was "puzzled over how a pig and a bed, which both contribute to the good life in very different ways, could nonetheless be valued on a single scale" (Skidelsky & Skidelsky, 2013, p. 90). Economists turned to the concept of utility to solve the problem of comparing the "noncomparable," whereas biologists and psychologists prefer the concept of pleasure. As we have seen, Cabanac suggests that a living organism needs a comparison stick that enables it to compare the utility of each alternative confronting it. Pleasure is that common currency (Cabanac, 1992).

If the common currency is represented as a feeling in the human mind, it cannot be one among many equally valuable feeling qualities. Rather, such a feeling must be able to transcend the entire spectrum of different feeling qualities into one dimension. This is what Cabanac proposed by nominating pleasure as the common currency. Empirical studies have corroborated these ideas, as in Levy and Glimcher (2011), who repeatedly found that people are remarkably good at mapping apples and oranges onto a single scale and "select the option with the highest value on that scale" (p. 14693). Even if separate brain networks exist for different valuation objects such as money and food, "distinct representations converge on a common representation in the vmPFC[1] that is appropriate for choice" (Levy & Glimcher, 2011, p. 146703).

Human neuroimaging studies indicate that a surprisingly similar circuitry is activated across the board of very diverse feeling states, suggesting that some kind of communality is formed by a network of interacting brain regions (e.g., Berridge & Kringelbach, 2015). Hence, the variety of feeling qualities generated by food, sex, addictive drugs, friendship, music, art, and even sustained states of happiness can produce strikingly similar patterns of brain activity—an activity that the mind experiences as pleasure. These mechanisms suggest that some kind of a common currency exists in the sense "that there is a shared underlying 'neural currency' or mesocorticolimbic mechanism for generating the pleasure of all those psychologically diverse experiences and emotions" (Berridge & Kringelbach, 2016, p. 135).

Others have argued along similar lines without using the term "common currency" (e.g., Chikazoe et al., 2014; Kobayashi & Hsu, 2019; Parducci, 1995). Damasio (2010) writes that to work well, "the brain required a representation of (1) the *current* state of the living tissue, (2) the *desirable* state of the living tissue corresponding to the homeostatic goal, and (3) a simple comparison" (Damasio, 2010, loc. 884, italics in original). Such a comparison is made possible by some kind of a common currency, and pleasure is a strong candidate to take that role. Berridge and Kringelbach (2015) write, for instance, that "An implication of the common currency hypothesis is that insights into brain hedonic substrates gained by experiments using one kind of pleasure, such as food 'liking', may apply to many other pleasures too" (p. 649).

However, a single common currency is not the only valuation mechanism at our disposal. As detailed in Chaps. 1 and 3, several evaluative channels must sometimes operate in parallel to establish a preference. Even though pleasure can organize a

[1] Ventromedial prefrontal cortex.

value hierarchy based on a variety of different, momentary experiences, the utility function of pleasure seems to break down in regard to more complex mental states, such as life goals, morality, and cultural value systems. Hence, in regard to complex mental states, Thagard (2010) argues that there is nothing in the brain to suggest that values can be reduced to a "common currency" (p. 197). For example, studies show that people spontaneously donate more money to a single victim of natural disasters or a famine than they give to several victims (Slovic, 2007). However, upon deliberative reflection, this irrational tendency changes, and people stop favoring a single victim over a larger group of victims (Small et al., 2007). Slovic and his colleagues attributed the first decision to a spontaneous, affective heuristic, the result of a System 1 way of thinking. The more thoughtful decision made in the deliberative context is likely endorsed by System 2 (Slovic et al., 2007). Hence, competing valuation mechanisms exist. Some are driven by System 1 processing, such as the pleasure-generated common currency principle. Others are more reflective and operated by System 2 evaluations.

The reductionism of a common currency is useful in some situations but not in others. As Kagan (2009) noted, insisting on the rule of a common currency would make us unable to see the difference between spending a thousand dollars for a birthday gift for a loved one and paying a similar amount for a washer and dryer. The take-home message must therefore be that pleasure is a valuable feeling because it provides an spontaneous online suggestion as to what we should prioritize in concrete situations, but more complex valuations depend on decisions that are too heavy for pleasure to carry. Our lives are too long and complex to be managed by a one-dimensional spontaneous good–bad evaluation system alone, and pleasure therefore fails to be the ultimate value compass in human life.

Is Pleasure a Go Signal or a Stop Signal?

One debate in the literature on the functions of pleasure concerns approach and avoidance behavior. Approach or appetitive motivation is often associated with positivity, while avoidance or defensive motivation is directed by negativity (e.g., Huntsinger et al., 2014; Lang & Bradley, 2013). Bentham's idea about the two sovereign masters of human motivation, pleasure and pain, is, for instance, an ally of this perspective (Elliot & Covington, 2001, p. 74). The dichotomy and its relevance for wellbeing were also pointed out by Veenhoven (1984), who writes that pleasure plays a signaling and amplifying motivational role in human behavior. Much empirical evidence supports the notion that pleasure is a major driver of approach behavior, whereas displeasure is the major driver of avoidance (e.g., Monni et al., 2020).

A wellbeing authority such as Kahneman defends this view and argues that pleasure is a go signal that "guides the organism to continue important activities such as foreplay or consuming sweet, energy-rich food" (Kahneman et al., 1997, p. 379). Moreover, Diener et al. (2002) reported that survey participants with a cheerful mood at college entry achieved things such as higher income, better job satisfaction, and less unemployment 20 years later. Similarly, an experimental study by Oswald et al. (2009) reported that participants who were primed into a positive mood had an approximately 11% greater quantity of work output, without any loss in quality, compared with participants who were primed into a negative mood.

On the other hand, a study by Schueller and Seligman (2010) found that orientation toward pleasure was weakly but negatively correlated with educational and occupational achievements. A learning style experiment showed that participants in the active condition learned more than participants allocated to a passive condition. However, passive learning was perceived as more joyful and easier than active learning (Deslauriers et al., 2019). Somewhat similar results were reported by Higgins (2014).

The mixed results from these and many other studies on positivity and approach motivation may to some extent be attributed to conceptual confusions. For instance, many studies do not properly distinguish between the quality dimension and the valence dimension of a feeling state. A positive feeling quality may well be a go signal and motivate approach activity even if pleasure is a stop signal. To see how this duality operates, a further look at the function of pleasure and displeasure in the process of homeostasis may be helpful.

According to Denton (2005), the first important mechanism of a pleasure–displeasure–controlled homeostasis evolved to regulate the system of thirst. It developed when early versions of vertebrate species migrated from water to dry land, a move that required a more complex mechanism for regulating biochemical balances in the body. While living in seawater, the salt balance in the blood could be taken care of by a reflex. But later in evolution, when water was not part of the immediate external milieu, the salt balance had to be regulated more actively. The intention to seek, find, and drink water, what we call thirst, was thus invented as the response to the new demands that followed when reflexes were replaced by more sophisticated ways of regulating physical needs. Therefore, the function of thirst is to inform an organism about an imbalance in the salt concentration in the body and that drinking is needed to reestablish the salt balance. However, the feeling also includes an unpleasant valence signal that motivates the organism to do something. Displeasure is, in other words, a go signal, whereas the feeling quality, i.e., thirst, tells us where to go and what to do.

Along with the go signal broadcasted throughout the brain as the feeling of displeasure, another feeling system also evolved in our distant past, one that could stop drinking when the water supply was secured. Water holes are dangerous places, and there is an enormous survival advantage for the animals to stop drinking and move away from them as quickly as possible. Thus, a message must be generated to tell the brain that an imbalance has been mended and that the homeostatic equilibrium has been restored. Feeling satiated conveys such a message.

Feeling pleased in the sense of being satiated is a stop signal. This idea is not new, and Young argued many years ago that "pleasantness is felt when one relaxes, or simply 'does nothing'" (cited in Ruckmick, 1925, p. 376). Similarly, McDougall claimed that pleasure results when a goal is successfully achieved or "when the striving attains its natural goal, or progresses toward it" (cited in Duncker, 1941, p. 393). The stop hypothesis continues to receive theoretical and empirical support, as when Frijda (2010) maintains that pleasure promotes stability and acceptance of the current state of affairs and reflects the absence of a need to change. Pleasure, he says, "is a pointer to stability and actual acceptance" and can be seen as the "absence of need to change" (Frijda, 2010, p. 102). Pleasure has therefore been characterized as signal to "do nothing" (Lazarus, 1991, p. 824). That is also why Baumeister (2018) considers a happy life to be one of "ease and enjoyment, focused on taking pleasures in the present." A meaningful life, by contrast, may involve complex activities and "inevitably, involvement in such activities will bring some stress and struggle" (p. 32).

The thesis that pleasure is a stop signal, or at least a "slow down" signal, has also been defended by Carver (2003) and his "coasting hypothesis." This thesis suggests that pleasure is a stability regulator that occurs when a goal is completed. Pleasure signalizes that you are done with what was previously a pressing goal but which no longer is. It therefore stimulates the breakup from effortful behavior and await opportunities to pursue alternative goals and say that you are free to "coast" on the current goal while preparing to embark on another and eventually more important goal. Several studies have supported this effect empirically (e.g., Fulford et al., 2010; Louro et al., 2007).

Hedonic Markers

When we see or hear something, a latent experience of whether it is easy or difficult to understand is instantaneously produced in our minds. If the cognitive process runs fluently, the flow of information is perceived as easy, and that makes us pleased, at least according to the hedonic fluency model (HFM), which was introduced by Winkielman and Cacioppo (2001). The HFM suggests that fast and effortless processing of information may signal positive states of the environment and of one's own cognitive processes.

This idea came from two studies that experimentally induced processing fluency in participants who later reported enhanced liking and smiling. These findings were the origin of the idea that processing fluency is inherently positive and triggers (mildly) positive affect (Landwehr & Eckmann, 2020). Because easily processed information is typically pleasant, the experience of cognitive fluency has been called a hedonic marker. Winkielman et al. (2003) presented several reasons to support this notion, one of which is that high fluency is indicative of familiarity, which is known to be processed faster than novel stimuli. Thus, high fluency may be positive because it is a cue that a stimulus has been encountered before or is in some way familiar. Familiarity can be pleasant because it allows for greater predictability, which means a reduction in anxiety (e.g., Churchland, 2018). Being in a familiar environment is pleasant, Churchland says, because it exploits the neural circuitry for feelings of safety and comfort in a "rest and digest conditions" (Churchland, 2018, p. 46).

Fluency may also be a hedonic marker because it is linked with the observation of symmetrical stimuli, which are typically associated with faster and less complex information processing. Symmetrical stimuli are generally liked better than non-symmetrical stimuli. Fluency may ultimately trigger a pleasant response because it provides positive feedback about the ongoing cognitive operations. Fast, easy, and coherent processing suggests a speedy progress toward a goal, which is typically experienced as rewarding. Hence, the fluency-as-progress notion suggests to Winkielman and his colleagues that preference for familiarity, symmetry, and prototypicality is a byproduct of their influence on speed, effort, and coherence of processing, and several studies have provided empirical support for these assumptions (e.g., Reber et al., 2004; Winkielman & Schwarz, 2001; Winkielman et al., 1998, 2003, 2005). Gilovich and Griffin (2010, p. 550) also reported that the feeling of fluency or difficulty has the same effect as being in a good or bad mood.

To summarize the science of pleasure, a consensus seems to be established about its evolutionary origin. Most likely, pleasure developed in tandem with displeasure to advance the regulation of homeostasis as organisms evolved to become more complex. As an evolutionary achievement, the importance of valenced feelings—the experience of pleasure and displeasure—can hardly be overstated. As noted in Chap. 1, Claude Bernard argued that homeostatic regulation is conditional for the freedom and independence we enjoy as human beings (cited in Denton, 2005, p. 81).

Pleasure has come to be included as an element in most feeling states, and in humans, it operates in a variety of situations that extend far beyond its original domain of homeostatic regulation. Pleasure can therefore be seen more generally as a positive update about needs and goals, a signal that tells us that our physiological, psychological, and social parameters are currently in a favorable state. Pleasure is one of several elements of a feeling state, and it represents the endpoint of a bidirectional dimension running from pleasure via neutral to displeasure. This dimension is often referred to as valence or hedonicity. In contrast to wanting, which is a motivational go signal that stimulates appetitive behavior, pleasure is typically felt when needs and goals have been or are about to be fulfilled. Pleasure is also associated with the effortless, familiar, and simple aspects of a stimulus or situation. According to the hedonic fluency model, pleasure is therefore a signal of the ease of mental information processing.

Hedonism

Hedonism has been a robust pillar in the history of philosophy, and an early version appeared in the Cārvāka, an Indian philosophical tradition. It began about 600 B.C.E. and has persisted for 2000 years (Weijers, 2021). The term hedonia, however, comes from the ancient Greek hêdonê (ἡδονή), their word for pleasure. A nearby dictionary will define hedonic as "an adjective relating to, or characterized by pleasure" (Merriam-Webster) or as "connected with feelings of pleasure" (Cambridge Dictionary). von Wright (1963, p. 63) writes that "Our term 'hedonic goodness' is supposed to cover roughly the same ground as the word 'pleasure' in ordinary language."

As briefly mentioned in Chap. 2, hedonism is a philosophical doctrine proposing that pleasure is the only thing that truly makes people's lives go better for them. However, and acknowledging the varieties of hedonistic theories, Feldman (2004, p. 27) argues that to understand the idea, it is useful to operate with "default hedonism," which he defines as follows:

1. Every episode of pleasure is intrinsically good; every episode of pain is intrinsically bad.
2. The intrinsic value of an episode of pleasure is equal to the number of hedons[2] of pleasure contained in that episode, the intrinsic value if an episode of pain is equal to the number of dolors[3] of pain contained in that episode.
3. The intrinsic value of life is entirely determined by the intrinsic values of the episodes of pleasure and pain contained in that life, in such a way that one life is intrinsically better than another if and only if the net amount of pleasure in the one is greater than the net amount of pleasure in the other.

A variant of these theses is formulated by Fletcher (2016): "(1) All and only pleasure is (noninstrumentally) good for us; (2) All and only pain is (noninstrumentally) bad for us; and (3) A person's overall level of wellbeing is determined solely by the balance of pleasure and pain they experience" (p. 8). If hedonism is true, Fletcher explains that a person's hedonic level, i.e., their overall balance of pleasure and pain, must be perfectly correlated with wellbeing (p. 10). The following claims will therefore apply:

1. If someone's hedonic level increases (they experience more pleasure and/or less pain), then it must be the case that their level of wellbeing increases.
2. If someone's hedonic level decreases, then it must be the case that their level of wellbeing decreases.
3. If someone's wellbeing increases, then it must be the case that their hedonic level increases (they experience more pleasure and/or less pain).
4. If someone's wellbeing decreases, then it must be the case that their hedonic level decreases.

The narrative of hedonism suffers from widespread disagreement about the meaning of pleasure, as testified with the examples provided in Table 5.1.

The table reveals that pleasure can be taken to mean anything from a simple sensation to a complex attitude or a grab bag term that covers anything that is experienced as positive or favorable. According to one of these understandings, pleasure is a particular feeling tone. This perspective is sometimes referred to as internalism in the philosophical literature (e.g., Sumner, 1996). The internalist approach sees

---

[2] Feldman (2004, p. 25) imagines that there is a standard unit of measurement for the amount of pleasure a person experiences. It is called a hedon and is operationalized as combination of duration and intensity. More concretely, pleasant experiences come in episodes, each with a certain *duration* (lasting from the pleasure starts through it stops) and an *intensity* (calculated as the average strength of the experienced pleasure during the episode).

[3] Dolors are the pain equivalent to hedons.

Table 5.1 Some philosophical definitions of pleasure

Definition	Source
1. Pleasures are bodily states	Aristippus (cited in Feldman, 2004, p. 30)
2. Pleasures are mental states	Epicurus (cited in McMahon, 2006, p. 55)
3. Pleasure is generated from the restoration of harmony by "the passage and return of all things to their nature"	Socrates (cited in Feibleman, 1964, p. 251)
4. Pleasure is an awareness of an activity	Aristotle (cited in Casebeer, 2003, loc. 552)
5. Pleasure is a feeling which, when experienced by thinking beings, is at least implicitly taken to be desirable or (in cases of comparison) preferable	Sidgwick (1907, p. 58)
6. Pleasure refers to whatsoever delight is felt by us	Locke (cited in Moen, 2013, p. 529)
7. Pleasure involves passing to state of greater perfection, that is, to greater power	Spinoza (cited in Schmitter, 2021, p. 116)
8. Pleasure is the object, duty, and goal of all rational beings	Voltaire (cited in Cabanac, 2009, p. 17)
9. I'll use the term "pleasure" for the whole class of good feelings and "pain" for all the bad ones	Hurka (2011, p. 9)
10. Pleasure and pain designate any kind of positive or negative type of sensation, perception, feeling, mood, or attitude. It comprises simple pleasures like munching a juicy apple, but also complex ones such as the enjoyment	Frede (2006, p. 258)

pleasure as having a unique phenomenology that makes it different from other positive feelings. Another approach considers pleasure to be an overarching term that covers positive affect defined in its broadest sense, which is clearly inconsistent with a definition of pleasure as particular feeling tone. Seen as a homogenous experiential quality, pleasure is a particular kind of positive affect. Seen as an overarching grab bag concept, a synonym for what most scientists refer to as positive affect, pleasure reflects a multitude of different feeling states.

A yet third meaning of pleasure is attitudinal, sometimes referred to as externalism (e.g., Sumner, 1996). According to this perspective, pleasure is homogeneous in the sense of referring to something we like, prefer, favor, and so on. Such a conceptualization bears some resemblance to the common currency approach and was early articulated by James Mill (John Stuart's father):

> I have one sensation, then another, and then another. The first is of such a kind, that I care not whether it is long or short; the second is of such a kind that I would put an end to it instantly if I could; the third is of such a kind that I like it prolonged. To distinguish these

> feelings I give them names. I call the first Indifferent; the second, Painful; the third, Pleasurable; very often, for shortness, I call the second, Pain, the third, Pleasure. (Cited in Sumner, 1996, p. 90)

A version of this approach is offered by Feldman (2004, 2010), who considers pleasure to be a cognitive or reflective phenomenon. Such perceived pleasure is not felt but rather appears as a perception, attitude, imagination, or judgment, resembling Parducci's conceptualization of pleasure presented above. For example, a person may, after having thought about it for a second, be pleased about the fact that he lives in Massachusetts. He is in some sense "in favor of it" (Feldman, 2010, p. 111). As we have discussed in previous chapters, however, it is difficult to specify how somethings can be evaluated as favorable without referring to something affective.

All the dissimilar conceptualizations of pleasure pave the way for a multitude of different hedonisms. To see these variations in more detail, a few of the many philosophical perspectives on pleasure will be presented next, starting with the Ancient Greeks.

Pleasure in Ancient Greek Philosophy

Plato had apparently several different ideas about pleasure, and Michalos and Robinson (2012) identified at least five distinct meanings to which Plato applied the concept: a desire satisfaction theory, a needs satisfaction theory, a harmony theory, a true pleasure theory, and a class theory of pleasure. According to Katz (2016), however, Plato's view gravitated toward a tradition referred to as the "improvement indicator view." This means that Plato basically saw pleasure as the satisfaction generated when a need is fulfilled. Such a need could stem from biological disequilibrium (belonging to the body) or from imperfect knowledge (belonging to the soul) and implies that pleasure is a feeling that signals that the body has moved from "a state of deficiency to a naturally healthy state." In this conception, Plato's pleasure bears a resemblance to a modern view that relates pleasure to the process of homeostasis (e.g., Damasio, 2018; Panksepp, 1998). However, for Plato, pleasure only had a role to play in the physical world. According to his dualistic philosophy, which divides reality into a physical world and a world of ideas, physical bodies are regarded as imperfect and transient. Since the function of pleasure is to regulate physical needs, the feeling is redundant in a perfect, nonphysical world of eternal and unchanging ideas. Hence, "the absolutely best life would be a divine one of permanent perfect knowing without the possibility of further learning or any other improvement, and in which there would therefore be no pleasure at all" (Katz, 2016, p. 15).

Aristippus was a follower of Socrates and, like his teacher, concerned himself with ethical issues and the questions of "summum bonum" or final ends. What is such an ultimate goal of our actions, and what is valuable for its own sake? To Aristippus, the answer was pleasure. As shown in Table 5.1, he argued that "physical, bodily pleasures are more valuable than mental, intellectual pleasures" (Feldman, 2004, p. 30). According to Aristippus, "only one's own physical, positive, momentary pleasure is a good, and it is so regardless of its cause" (Tatarkiewicz, 1976, p. 317). Thus, Aristippus' recipe for a good life includes advice such as "snatch the pleasure of the passing moment" (Watson, 1895, p. 33) and "excluding all reflection, and making the most of the present moment" (Watson, 1895, p. 41). Aristippus's philosophy is close to a kind of "vulgar hedonism," what Steger et al. (2013, p. 164) refers to as "doing whatever the hell I want to."

The thinking of Epicurus reflects a different perspective on hedonism, as he strongly warned against careless living. Epicurus saw pleasure as a mental feeling, a valuation of certain preferences and considered no life pleasant, unless it is wise, moral, and just (Nussbaum, 2001; Tatarkiewicz, 1976). In contrast to Aristippus, Epicurus regarded the pleasure of tranquility as the highest of all pleasures.

> When we say that pleasure is the goal, we are not talking about the pleasure of profligates or that which lies in sensuality, as some ignorant persons think…; rather it is freedom from bodily pain and mental anguish. For it is not continuous drinking and revels, nor the enjoyment of women and young boys, not of fish and other viands that a luxurious table holds, which makes for a pleasant life, but sober reasoning, which examines the motives for every choice and avoidance, and which drives away those opinions resulting in the greatest disturbance to the soul. (Cited in McMahon, 2006, pp. 55–56)

Aristotle

Aristotle could be vague and inconsistent in his opinions about pleasure. He typically considered it as something more than mere gustatory or tactile pleasure and rather thought of it as an awareness of an activity (Casebeer, 2003). Aristotle could, for instance, describe pleasure as "the actions of the present, the hope of the future and the remembrance of things past" (cited in Warburton, 1996, p. 1). He could also be inconsistent about how pleasure relates to happiness, although his writing is basically interpreted as not identifying pleasure with happiness. This position is illustrated in his well-known saying that "living for pleasure only would be to choose the life of dumb grazing animals" (cited in Nussbaum, 2004, p. 64).

Chapter 6 will examine Aristotle's theory of happiness in more detail, but in brief, his *Nicomachean Ethics* presents two rather different conceptions of pleasure. Book VII offers a relatively short explanation of it, whereas Book X provides a fuller and, according to Nussbaum (2008), probably better account. It has been argued that Aristotle's treatment of pleasure in Book VII comes dangerously close to hedonism by, for instance, calling pleasures "ends in themselves" and saying that they are "necessary parts of a good life" (Moen, 2015, pp. 6–7). Similarly, Broadie (1991, p. 313) argues that "Aristotle maintains that the highest good is necessarily pleasant." In Book VII, Aristotle also identifies pleasure with "the unimpeded performance of the activities that constitute happiness" (Nussbaum, 2004, p. 61). In Book X, in contrast, pleasure is associated with behavior of a certain kind, something one gets "by doing the relevant activity in a certain, apparently unimpeded or complete way" (Nussbaum, 2004, p. 64). Here, Aristotle builds on the thesis that "pleasure cannot be our ultimate target, because what counts as pleasant must be judged by some standard other than pleasure itself, namely, the judgment of the virtuous person" (Kraut, 2022, p. 44). According to one of Aristotle's accounts, pleasure therefore is

> something that comes along with, supervenes on, activity, 'like the bloom on the cheek of youth.' In other words, it is so closely linked to the relevant activities that it cannot be pursued on its own, any more than bloom can be adequately cultivated by cosmetics. To get that bloom you have to pursue health. Similarly, one gets the pleasure associated with an activity by doing that activity in a certain way, apparently a way that is not impeded or is complete. It would seem that what Aristotle has in mind is that pleasure is a kind of awareness of one's own activity, varying in quality with the activity to which it is so closely linked. In any case, pleasure is not a single thing, varying only in intensity and duration (the Eudoxan position). It contains qualitative differences, related to the differences of the activities to which it attaches. (Nussbaum, 2008, pp. s84–s85).

Utilitarian Hedonism

The birth of utilitarian hedonism is attributed to Bentham, John Stuart Mill, and Sidgwick, although the core ideas and terminology of utilitarianism were formulated 100 years earlier. They were published by the neo-Aristotelian Scotsman Francis Hutcheson in 1725, articulated as the greatest happiness principle, i.e., the greatest happiness for the greatest numbers' (Thin, 2012, p. 3). Yet, it is Bentham who became the iconic hedonist.

Jeremy Bentham

Bentham is well known for the opening of the *Introduction to the Principles of Morals and Legislation* (Bentham, 1789/1948). As mentioned in Chap. 2, Bentham smugly suggested that both moral theory and motivational psychology are under the governance of pleasure and pain (Bentham, 1789/1948, p. 7). From this condensed notion, Bentham developed the simplest form of hedonism on offer (e.g., Crisp, 2017; Sumner, 1996), which merely claims that the more pleasantness one can pack into one's life, the better it will be. It follows that the more pain one encounters, the worse it will be. Pleasure is in itself the only good in life, and pain is in itself the only evil in life. That is why Bentham identified pleasure (net of pain) with happiness.

What did Bentham mean by the term pleasure? Philosophical literature typically tells us that Bentham held a homogenous view, which means that he saw pleasures as a unitary phenomenon, fluctuating only along a single, quantitative dimension that varies in intensity and duration.[4] What pleasures have in common, Bentham argued, is "their positive feeling tone: an intrinsic, unanalysable quality of pleasantness which is present to a greater or lesser degree in all of them" (Sumner, 1996, p. 88). Homogeneity is the essence of hedonism since it enables a value ranking of stimuli and situations. This unidimensionality of Benthamian pleasure makes it a common currency. The quantitative element of pleasure is always the same regardless of how it is obtained (Edwards, 1979), and this attribute explains why Bentham could hold pushpin[5] to be as good as poetry (McMahon, 2006, p. 221).

The common currency quality of pleasure also makes it possible to summarize pleasures across situations and people by means of a "felicific calculus," an algorithm Bentham formulated—without using the term himself—to quantify happiness. According to Crimmins (2023), Bentham suggested that the value of pleasure could be estimated as a function of its intensity, duration, certainty, and degree of remoteness. However, Bentham did realize that this idea was just an approximation, an ideal that no one could strictly follow over time. However, the felicific (or hedonic) calculus resembles the procedure Kahneman developed to measure experienced utility instantly in his early work on wellbeing (Chap. 2).

John Stuart Mill

Mill's hedonism is confusing. On the one hand, he defended Bentham's program by sharply declaring that "By happiness is intended pleasure, and the absence of pain" (Mill, 2001, p. 6). He went on to say that "pleasure, and freedom from pain, are the only things desirable as ends; and…all desirable tings…are desirable either for the pleasure inherent in themselves, or as means to the promotion of pleasure and the prevention of pain" (Mill, 2001, pp. 6–7). Mill also defended moral hedonism, arguing that "as a matter of lawful fact about human beings, we must seek pleasure, it is unreasonable to suggest that anything else could be morally demanded of us" (cited in Wilson, 2014, p. 60). Wilson notes that Mill's argument rests on a logical deduction from is to ought: we ought to seek pleasure because that is just the way human beings are. In Mill's world, it is impossible not to aim for pleasure, "and any action attempting the impossible is bound to be pointless" (Wilson, 2014, p. 60). Mill further argued that since each person aims to maximize their own happiness, the overall effect will be to maximize the pleasure of all. But Mill did not believe that people seek to maximize happiness in others. Only in a perfect world would that be the case. In our current state of affairs, individuals seldom seek such a general happiness (Wilson, 2014, pp. 63–64).

At some point, Mill decided that some pleasures are sensual pleasures, while others are mental. He referred to the two kinds as lower pleasures and higher

[4] Attributes such as certainty or uncertainty and propinquity or remoteness are sometimes added to Benthamian pleasure, but as far as I understand, Bentham did not believe that these aspects altered the unidimensional quality of his pleasure concept.

[5] Pushpin is a very simple, nineteenth century children's game.

pleasures. Neither pains nor pleasures are homogenous; he now wants us to believe and argues that by their very nature, some pleasures are more valuable than others. This is not consistent with Benthamian hedonism, of course, but Mill came to realize that for him, personally, it is better to read William Wordsworth's poetry than to play pushpin. To distinguish Mill's elevated elements of pleasure from Bentham's quantitative approach, Mill therefore adds a fourth dimension to his conception of pleasure. He calls this "quality" (Crisp, 2017). The distinction between lower and higher pleasures makes it possible for Mill to prefer being "Socrates dissatisfied than a pig satisfied" (Mill, 2001, p. 9).

Mill's distinction between lower and higher pleasures is not consistent with default hedonism. Different feeling qualities cannot enter Bentham's felicific calculus because only quantities belonging to a single dimension can be mathematically aggregated (e.g., Michell, 1999). A certain amount of higher pleasures cannot be traded against any number of lower pleasures (Alexandrova, 2017, Chap. 2, p. 4). This problem, as we will see in the next section, has caused much confusion in the literature on hedonism.

Hedonism According to Crisp

Roger Crisp (2006b) favors hedonism about wellbeing. If you ask him about the life good, he will answer that enjoyable feelings are "the only 'good-for-making' property there is" (Crisp, 2006a, p. 623).

Crisp tells us that the term enjoyment is a better word than pleasure because the latter is strongly associated with sensualism. "To avoid such difficulties, let me use 'enjoyment' instead of 'pleasure,' and 'suffering' instead of 'pain'" (Crisp, 2006a, p. 622). Crisp then goes on to give his concept of enjoyment two different meanings. The argument is complicated and starts by referring to a particular taxonomic rationality. The rationality draws on logical rules about relations between properties, centering around the terms determinable and determinates. According to Wilson (2021), determinable and determinates are type-level properties that stand in a distinctive specification relation. For example, color is a determinable having red, green, yellow, and blue and other specific shades of color as determinates. We experience the determinates red, or blue as different, yet we still see them as colors. According to Crisp's theory, and analogous to seeing a "color," enjoyment is a determinable when it feels enjoyable. However, an enjoyable feeling can comprise a variety of different feeling qualities, analogous to seeing red, green, yellow, blue, and so on. That makes enjoyable experiences a determinate. A determinate experience is phenomenologically heterogeneous, i.e., it consists of different feelings and qualities. Crisp explains that enjoyable experiences differ from one another in the same way that colors differ from each other. Feelings of sweetness, warmth, beauty, work, drinking, eating, and nobility are other examples of heterogeneous experiences mentioned by Crisp, who explains that when we introspect such feelings, "we can find nothing common to the experiences we enjoy that might be characterized as 'enjoyment'" (Crisp, 2006a, p. 627). Despite their diverging feeling qualities, however, there is an additional, common phenomenological quality among these determinates. That is the homogeneous feeling of enjoyment, a kind of feeling that cannot be described or defined. Enjoyable feelings have no intensity and can only be known through experience.

The distinction between enjoyable feelings as heterogeneous and enjoyable feelings as homogenous is not easy to understand, and the color analogy has been criticized for being too far apart to be useful (e.g., Alston, 1969). To defend himself, Crisp surprisingly leaves the arena of philosophical debate and turns to affective neuroscience. Here, he finds that "some physical correlates for some forms of enjoyment have already been discovered" (Crisp, 2006a, p. 630). With reference to "hedonic hot spots" in the brain, Crisp seeks to link his concept of enjoyment to Berridge's concept of liking. However, as surveyed above, liking is one of several distinguishable components in a "pleasure cycle." Crisp can, in other words, not receive the scientific support he needs to preserve the idea that homogeneous enjoyment relates to phenomenological variability, the way color relates to the variability of color perceptions. If Crisp connects his concept of enjoyment with the neuroscientific valuation mechanism of liking, his theory has not identified a plausible candidate for a psychological entity that represents the only "good-for-making" property there is.

Against Hedonism

Hedonism is a smug idea that claims that pleasure (net of pain) is the only true value in a good life, and this doctrine has been abandoned by many current philosophers (see Griffin, 1986). According to Crisp, hedonism can be rejected for at least three reasons. First, Mill's distinction between higher and lower pleasures is provoking because the divide undermines the elegance of the theory, either by removing its one-dimensional core or by being incoherent. Crisp refers to this as the "philosophy of swine" problem. Second, G.E. Moore delivered serious criticism against hedonism in Chap. 3 of his influential *Principia Ethica*. Finally, Nozick's so-called experience machine was a "near-fatal blow" to hedonism (Crisp, 2006a, p. 620). Crisp's hunch is that Moore's objection has lost its bite, since Moore, in the preface to a revised version of *Principia*, admits that the book "is full of mistakes and confusions." That leaves hedonism with two major challenges. I will discuss them in turn and then add a third concern the doctrine should worry about. We may call this final criticism for the scientific objections to hedonism.

The Philosophy of Swine

A one-dimensional pleasure concept is important for default hedonism because it makes the intensity and duration of pleasure the only factors along which wellbeing can vary. As illustrated in Kahneman's use of a temporal integral to test the peak–end rule (Chap. 2), the amount of a feeling state—how much we have of it—can be fully quantified as a combination of its intensity and duration. According to the logic of hedonism, a large pleasure integral results in a better life than a small pleasure integral. Indeed, the core of hedonistic utilitarianism is that the total amount of experienced pleasure in the universe should be included in the integral, and then it is our moral duty to maximize that amount. However, the mathematics breaks down if we have to include other feelings qualities, or other values, as constituents of a good life. This is the problem of higher and lower pleasures, and that is the essence of the philosophy of swine debate.

The problem goes back at least to Plato, who pointed out that if pleasure is all you have, then "your life would be the life, not of a man, but of an oyster" (cited in Moore, 2019, p. 29). John Stuart Mill shared Plato's concern and thought that if pleasurable intensity is the only valuable difference between, say, reading poetry and playing pushpin, hedonism is reduced to a "doctrine worthy only of swine" (Mill, 2001, p. 7). Crisp (2006a) uses a thought experiment to illustrate this dilemma.

> You are a soul in heaven waiting to be allocated a life on Earth. It is late Friday afternoon, and you watch anxiously as the supply of available lives dwindles. When your turn comes, the angel in charge offers you a choice between two lives, that of the composer Joseph Haydn and that of an oyster. Besides composing some wonderful music and influencing the evolution of the symphony, Haydn will meet with success and honour in his own lifetime, be cheerful and popular, travel and gain much enjoyment from field sports. The oyster's life is far less exciting. Though this is rather a sophisticated oyster, its life will consist only of mild sensual pleasure, rather like that experienced by humans when floating very drunk in a warm bath. When you request the life of Haydn, the angel sighs, 'I'll never get rid of this oyster life. It's been hanging around for ages. Look, I'll offer you a special deal. Haydn will die at the age of seventy-seven. But I'll make the oyster life as long as you like. (Crisp, 2006a, pp. 630–631)

The problem for strict hedonism is that adding up the mild pleasure of a long oyster life amounts to more goodness than the intense pleasure of a short Haydn life. Mill tried to solve the puzzle by separating higher and lower pleasures, but it is unclear how that move avoids the abandonment of hedonism (which he defended). If higher pleasures are qualitatively different than lower pleasures, Mill has invited non-hedonic values into his theory.

Crisp believes that his rephrasing of pleasure into enjoyment may get hedonism off the philosophy of the swine hook. Imagine, he says, that a person who drinks a glass of lemonade also completes her first reading of Jane Austen's *Pride and Prejudice*. In this situation, there is nothing to prevent this person from thinking that she would never enjoy a glass of lemonade as much as she enjoyed the novel, "no matter how long the experience of enjoyable drinking could be prolonged" (Crisp, 2006a, p. 633). To quarrel, one could imagine Crisp's protagonist, located in the

Sahara Desert, on the brink of perishing from thirst. In that situation, there is nothing to prevent her from declaring a willingness to give up all future readings of Jane Austen in exchange for a glass of lemonade.

The point is that within the realm of thought experiments, we can imagine all kinds of trade-offs people might be willing to do, some in favor of hedonism and some against hedonism. However, thought experiments tend to be never-ending games unable to solve serious challenges such as the philosophy of the swine puzzle. Crisp is aware of this limitation and again turns to neuropsychology to solve his philosophical problem. Recently, he could therefore announce that "neuroscientific evidence for the higher/lower thesis is currently lacking" (Crisp & Kringelbach, 2018, p. 215). In other words, the monist hypothesis of hedonism has not yet been empirically falsified, and the doctrine is therefore preserved. However, with the abandonment of Mill's higher and lower pleasures, the oyster problem is unsolved, and hedonism remains a philosophy of swine.

The Experience Machine

Hedonism was famously attacked by Nozick and his telling illustration of the "experience machine." This thought experiment offers you an opportunity to be hooked up to a devise that gives you complete control over your experiences—at the cost of not being able to return to your original and authentic life. Here are the details of the proposal:

> Suppose there were an experience machine that would give you any experience you desired. Superduper neuropsychologists could stimulate your brain so that you would think and feel you were writing a great novel, or making a friend, or reading an interesting book. All the time you would be floating in a tank, with electrodes attached to your brain. Should you plug into this machine for life, preprogramming your life's experiences?... Of course, while in the tank you won't know that you're there; you'll think it's all actually happening. Others can also plug in to have the experiences they want, so there's no need to stay unplugged to serve them... Would you plug in? (Nozick, 1974, pp. 42–43)

By introducing the idea of an experience machine, Nozick wanted to convince us that values other than pleasure matter. Although the gimmick is celebrated, it has, against Nozick's prediction, not ended hedonism. When confronted with the fantasy of being plugged in to the machine, some people agree, and others refuse. Thus, as noted by Sumner (1996, p. 94), it is not clear just what lesson we should draw from Nozick's thought experiment. The debate triggered by Nozick again suggests that there is no end to the ways in which a thought experiment can be interpreted and twisted. Some argue, for instance, that Nozick has demonstrated nothing but a well-established "status quo" bias: those refusing to plug in do so because they hesitate dramatic changes in their lives. They don't refuse because values other than pleasure are important to them. Some have pointed to uncertainties about the machine itself: what happens if the machine breaks down, etc. For all we know, we might already be in the machine, as vividly suggested in films such as *The Matrix* trilogy.

In other words, those in favor of hedonism continue to be so regardless of Nozick's contribution. Fletcher (2016) and Prinzing (2021) provide nice overviews for readers interested in further details about the experience machine debate.

Scientific Objections to Hedonism

Criticizing hedonism, Griffin (1986) tells a story about Sigmund Freud. Toward the end of his life, ill and in pain, the funder of psychoanalysis is said to have refused any drugs except aspirin. Rather than not being able to reason clearly, the old thinker "preferred to work in torment" (Griffin, 1986, p. 8). Allport presented similar arguments in his work on personal growth and maintained that the idea of hedonism is inconsistent with an adult's principal goals in life (Allport, 1961, p. 201). Indeed, much of Allport's writing is devoted to showing why psychological hedonism must be wrong, using, among others, the life of the Arctic explorer Roald Amundsen as an example. Amundsen sat himself extremely ambitious life goals and was willing to sacrifice much pleasure to reach them.

Another example is Bertrand Russell, a philosopher who was generally sympathetic to hedonism. Nevertheless, he turned away from the idea that everything he sought was motivated by a desire to maximize pleasure. In his *Autobiography* (2014/1967), Russell remarks how often he has found himself drawn to activities that he never believed would bring him happiness. Elsewhere, Russell declared that he rarely desires something because of the pleasure that it would give him (cited in Overskeid, 2002, pp. 81–82). Even the biblical story of the Garden of Eden seems to suggest that a life of unlimited pleasure and no pain are not fully satisfying for humans. Adam and Eve fell pray for the temptation to eat the fruits of the tree of knowledge and had to leave paradise and their lives of endless pleasure and become moral human beings (Greenblatt, 2017).

But the most devastating critique of hedonism comes from science and, most brutally, from studies of pain. Evolutionary speaking, pain did not evolve to be intrinsically bad for us. To the contrary, if we could not feel pain, we would not survive, neither as a species nor as individuals. The so-called congenital insensitivity to pain with anhidrosis (CIPA) illustrates this point. CIPA is a rare, inherited disease with symptoms such as inability to feel pain and temperature. The symptoms dramatically increase the risk of accidental self-injury and drastically reduce patients' wellbeing. Without intensive care, most CIPA patients die prematurely (e.g., Eregowda et al., 2016; Linton, 2005; Melzack & Wall, 1996; Paul et al., 2022).

Generically, pain is a mental state generated by a local dysfunction or damage somewhere in our body. As such, pain is a signal of ill-being. Not good in itself and if turned into a pathological and chronic condition, pain can cause unbearable suffering. However, under normal circumstances, pain is valuable because it promotes avoidance learning and protection. The British writer and theologian C. S. Lewis describes, for instance, pain as something that "insists upon being attended to" and as a megaphone God used "to rouse a deaf world" (Lewis, 1940, p. 52). A less divine metaphor is offered by Damasio, who used to think of pain as putting a good lock on the door after a house has been robbed. However, the neurophysiologist Pierre Rainville convinced Damasio that putting a bodyguard in front of the house while repairing the broken window is a better metaphor. "After all, pain does not result in preventing yet another injury, at least not immediately, but rather in protecting the injured tissue, facilitating tissue repair, and avoiding infections if the wound" (Damasio, 1999, p. 78). Under some circumstances, small doses of pain can even be something we want and value. Examples cover everything from picking a sore tooth to painful participation in painful, religious rituals (Bloom, 2021).

To say that pain is functional and necessary for survival is not to say that pain is all good. Being in pain is normally not a good feeling, and chronic pain causes many serious consequences. The point I am trying to make is that pain is not all bad, which is what hedonism argues.

For the pleasure part of hedonism, scientific reasoning also speaks against the idea that pleasure is the only intrinsic value in a human's life. The previous "Pleasure" section provided strong arguments against the monist notion of pleasure and the doctrine that a good life comes with the maximization of pleasure. In the research group I am affiliated with, we have started to ask survey participants to estimate how much positive and negative affect they would prefer to have in a perfect life. Nothing has been published from these studies yet, but only rarely do we see participants who think of the good life as one in which they experience nothing but pleasure. The average amount of desirable pleasure in one of these studies was to experience it 85% of the time. Very few wanted a life without negative experiences either; on average, participants wanted to experience negative emotions between 5% and 15% of the time (Liu, 2024). Hence, most of us value the experience of negative feelings in some situations, such as the horror from watching a movie, the fear of riding a roller coaster, or the painful mourning one can and wants to feel with respect to someone who has passed away.

Another argument against hedonism comes from Kagan (1998), who explains that "children build sandcastles and adults climbs rugged mountains because implementing actions that are guided by an idea of perfection is as much a biologically prepared disposition as are the pursuit of sweet tastes and the avoidance of bodily pain. After we have protected ourselves from actual or possible harm, the affirmation of virtues takes precedence over the search for sensory pleasure most of every day" (p. 153). Thus, we can appreciate unpleasant feelings, and we can value the richness of phenomenological variety in itself (e.g., Vittersø, 2016). Reducing feeling qualities to a single element will by itself spoil an important "good-for-making" property of human affects because a variety of feelings are valuable by themselves. Or, to return to the color metaphor, we may like some colors better than others, but that doesn't mean we don't value the others (e.g., Strauss et al., 2013).

Despite the overwhelming evidence against hedonism, Crisp and other hedonists hang on to their doctrine. "Maybe the time will come for us to bury hedonism for good," Crisp says before adding "but that time is not now" (Crisp, 2006a, p. 640). This is just as predicted by Chalmers (2015), who was cited in Chap. 3 on critiquing the lack of progress among philosophers: "philosophical arguments typically lead not to agreement but to sophisticated disagreement" (Chalmers, 2015, p. 19). An analogy to Freud's psychoanalytic theory seems appropriate. Freud's theory was criticized by Popper (2005) for being dogmatic and formulated in a non-falsifiable terminology. Hedonism is like that. It defends a prescientific idea about pleasure or enjoyment as the only true value in human life. Hence, despite the massive body of empirical studies showing that people's behavior, thinking, and feelings are inconsistent with the assumptions of the doctrine, hedonists continue to bite the bullet, as Alexandrova (2017) puts it. Despite overwhelming scientific evidence that pleasure is but one of several valuation mechanisms that aid humans in navigating their lives, and even if most people do not regard pleasure as particularly important, hedonists remain faithful to the doctrine that a unidimensional pleasure-like, or enjoyment-like, or attitude-like state exists and comprises the only true value in human lives. Despite irresistible scientific evidence that pain is useful, hedonists continue to insist that pain is the only thing that is truly bad. However, if pain is necessary for survival, how is it possible to keep arguing that pain is the evilest thing in the universe? Disregarding all the evidence just mentioned and faced with solid knowledge about what pain and pleasure do in our lives, some holdouts cling to the notion that pleasure must be the only "good-for-making" property there is and pain must be the only "bad-for-making" property there is.

Hedonic Wellbeing

The term hedonic is older than the hills but the phrase hedonic wellbeing (HWB) is a newcomer. To my knowledge, it was introduced by Ryan and Deci (2001) as a companion to the phrase eudaimonic wellbeing (EWB). This dual taxonomy was partly proposed as a response to the hedonic bias the authors observed as inherent in traditional research on subjective wellbeing, exemplified in the authoritative *Well-Being: The Foundations of Hedonic Psychology* (Kahneman et al., 1999b).[6] Ryan and Deci's intention with respect to the HWB versus EWB dichotomy was to let the former replace the term subjective wellbeing, as testified in statements such as "The hedonic viewpoint focuses on subjective wellbeing, which is frequently equated with happiness and is formally defined as more positive affect, less negative affect, and greater life satisfaction" (Ryan & Deci, 2001, p. 161). With their tendency to define concepts in a variety of ways, however (see Chap. 6), Ryan and Deci also refer to hedonic as "pleasure or happiness" (p. 143) and as "pleasure attainment and pain avoidance" (p. 141). The authors further consider Ed Diener to be one of the most prominent advocates of hedonic wellbeing, although Diener was ambivalent about the term hedonic and warned against using HWB as a synonym for SWB. The notion of hedonic wellbeing has some roots in Greek hedonism, Diener writes, but even if pleasure is included as one aspect of SWB, that concept "is much

---

[6] Richard Ryan, personal communication, July 2, 2022.

broader in that it includes purpose, meaning, and feelings of fulfillment" (Diener & Tov, 2012, p. 139).

Hedonia comes as we have seen from the ancient Greek hêdonê and is etymology speaking only about pleasure and not about pain (Cabanac, 2009). However, philosophical hedonism includes both pleasure and pain, so the positive affect and negative affect elements in Ryan and Deci's taxonomy do not diverge strongly from the established idea of hedonism. Ryan and Deci are therefore close to default hedonism later in their article, when they describe the hedonic idea as "pleasure attainment and pain avoidance" (Ryan & Deci, 2001, p. 141).

The categorization of life satisfaction as hedonic is more questionable, however, and Haybron (2016) has deemed it "deeply misguided." He maintains that "life satisfaction measures are not hedonic in any plausible sense of the word" (Haybron, 2016, p. 41). Haybron even considers it dubious to call positive and negative affect a hedonic matter, "since our emotional conditions run much deeper than the hedonic quality of our experience" (p. 41). Thus, Ryan and Deci have come to change their minds about life satisfaction and HWB, and they write in a later publication that "a more precise interpretation of hedonic well-being would, however, use just positive affect and negative affect to index happiness, because life satisfaction is not strictly a hedonic concept. Rather, it involves a cognitive evaluation of the conditions of one's life" (Deci & Ryan, 2008, p. 2). This latter formulation is also more in line with the APA Dictionary of Psychology, which defines hedonic wellbeing as "the type of happiness or contentment that is achieved when pleasure is obtained and pain is avoided."

However, some researchers hold that life satisfaction should be regarded as an element of hedonia. Kashdan et al. (2008) explicitly consider life satisfaction an element of hedonic happiness, together with high frequencies of positive affect and low frequencies of negative affect (p. 219). A similar position is held by what seems like a growing number of researchers who use HWB and SWB as synonyms (e.g., Chen et al., 2013; Cooke et al., 2016; Dagenais-Desmarais & Savoie, 2012; Gallagher et al., 2009; Jayawickreme et al., 2012; Joseph & Heferon, 2013; Lambert et al., 2020; Oishi & Westgate, 2022; Schueller & Seligman, 2010; Stone & Mackie, 2013; Tov & Lee, 2016). Opposing these views, van de Weijer et al. (2018) argue that the use of the term hedonic wellbeing is becoming increasingly less frequent.

Other attempts to define hedonic wellbeing complicate things further. In a review of the concept, Tov and Lee (2016, p. 586) unsurprisingly found that "HWB has also been inconsistently operationalized." Some researchers assess the affective component only (Baumeister et al., 2013; Hofmann et al., 2014; Waterman, 1993), whereas others combine measures of both affect and satisfaction (Fredrickson et al., 2013; McGregor & Little, 1998). More names could also be added to the list of researchers who disagree about HWB, such as Parducci (1995, p. 14), who holds that the notion of hedonia only has to do with pleasure, whereas Scollon and King (2011, p. 4) describe it more generally as "how an individual feels about his or her life." Slightly more limited, Steptoe et al. (2015) suggest that "hedonic wellbeing refers to everyday feelings or moods such as experienced happiness (the mood, not the evaluation of life), sadness, anger, and stress" (p. 641). Seligman suggests that hedonics has to do with "how we feel from moment to moment" (Seligman, 2002, p. 16). Huta and Ryan (2010) define hedonic as pleasure, enjoyment, and comfort, whereas Keyes (2007) equals the term with "positive emotions towards one's life" (p. 98). Shizgal (1999) refers to hedonia as a good/bad dimension (p. 504). Berridge and Kringelbach find that most psychologists "generally agree that hedonia at least corresponds psychologically to a state of pleasure. Thus, a particularly important topic for hedonic psychology and affective neuroscience is to understand how pleasure is generated by brain mechanisms so as to contribute to well-being" (Berridge & Kringelbach, 2011, p. 1).

However, other scholars define hedonic psychology broader, such as Kahneman, Diener, and Schwarz, who write that "Although the adjective 'hedonic' is often used to refer solely to pleasure, hedonic psychology covers the full spectrum from the pleasant to the unpleasant" (Kahneman et al., 1999a, p. iv). What the full spectrum covers is not entirely clear, but according to these authors, it does include feelings "of interest and boredom, of joy and sorrow, and of satisfaction and dissatisfaction. It is also concerned with the whole range of circumstances, from the biological to the societal, that occasion suffering and enjoyment" (Kahneman et al., 1999a, p. iv).

The HTW uses the term hedonic wellbeing as a common name for two subdimensions referred to as harmony feelings (tranquility, contentment, happiness, and high pleasure) and spontaneous judgments (life satisfaction, domain satisfactions, and presence of meaning in life). According to the HTW, hedonic wellbeing is about stability regulation and indicates how well we are performing in terms of need fulfillment and goal achievement, i.e., the constant task of rebalancing disequilibria throughout life. The other major dimension of wellbeing is called eudaimonic, and the details of these dimensions will be examined in Chap. 7.

On a final note, it is important to realize that none of the above conceptualizations of hedonic wellbeing are associated with the kind of vulgar connotations held by Steger and his associates, who, as mentioned above, see hedonia as equivalent to "doing whatever the hell I want to" (Steger et al. 2013, p. 164). Neither is hedonic wellbeing restricted to the meaning given to it by a scale with "hedonic" items such as "having sex purely to get pleasure," "masturbating," or "keep eating more than I intended of something because it tastes so good" (Steger et al., 2008). Not surprisingly, items such as these are not highly correlated with pleasant experiences in everyday life (e.g., Grimm et al., 2015; Steger et al., 2013, p. 162), although they may be somewhat related to variables more specifically tailored to measuring desires (Krasko et al., 2022). Contrast these "vulgar" ideas about HWB with the association triggered in the Danish science writer Lone Frank, as she reflects on the meaning of hedonia. "There is something about this word. It rolls across the tongue like walking on a red carpet and leaves a pleasant sensation behind. Hedonia might well have been the name of the Garden of Eden before the serpent made its malicious offer of wisdom and insight" (Frank, 2018, p. 97). No coincidence, perhaps, that Denmark is among the happiest countries in the world.

References

Alexandrova, A. (2017). *A philosophy for the science of well-being*. Oxford University Press.

Allport, G. W. (1961). *Pattern and growth in personality*. Holt, Rinehart and Winston.

Alston, W. P. (1969). Feelings. *The Philosophical Review, 78*(1), 3–34.

Arnold, M. (1960). *Emotion and personality*. Columbia University Press.

Baumeister, R. F. (2018). Happiness and meaningfulness as two different and not entirely compatible versions of the good life. In J. P. Forgas & R. E. Baumeister (Eds.), *The social psychology of living well* (pp. 21–33). Routledge.

Baumeister, R. F., Vohs, K. D., Aaker, J. L., & Garbinsky, E. N. (2013). Some key differences between a happy life and a meaningful life. *The Journal of Positive Psychology, 8*(6), 505–516. https://doi.org/10.1080/17439760.2013.830764

Beebe-Center, J. G. (1932). *The psychology of pleasantness and unpleasantness*. Russell & Russell.

Bentham, J. (1789/1948). *An introduction to the principles of moral and legislation* [Kindle]. Hafner. Retrieved from http://www.econlib.org/library/Bentham/bnthPML1.html

Berridge, K. C. (1999). Pleasure, pain, desire and dread: Hidden core processes of emotion. In D. Kahneman, E. Diener, & N. Schwarz (Eds.), *Well-being: The foundations of hedonic psychology* (pp. 527–559). Russell Sage Foundation.

Berridge, K. C. (2004). Motivation concepts in behavioral neuroscience. *Physiology & Behavior, 81*(2), 179–209.

Berridge, K. C., & Kringelbach, M. L. (2011). Building a neuroscience of pleasure and well-being. *Psychology of Well-Being, 1*(1), 1–26, Article 3. https://doi.org/10.1186/2211-1522-1-3

Berridge, K. C., & Kringelbach, M. L. (2015). Pleasure systems in the brain. *Neuron, 86*(3), 646–664. https://doi.org/10.1016/j.neuron.2015.02.018

Berridge, K. C., & Kringelbach, M. L. (2016). From pleasure to happiness. "Liking" and "wanting" in mind and brain. In L. F. Barrett, M. Lewis, & J. M. Haviland-Jones (Eds.), *Handbook of emotions* (pp. 133–145). Guilford Publications.

Berridge, K. C., & Winkielman, P. (2003). What is an unconscious emotion? (The case for unconscious "liking"). *Cognition and Emotion, 17*(2), 181–211.

Bloom, P. (2021). *The sweet spot. The pleasures of suffering and the search for meaning [Kindle]*. Random House.

Broadie, S. (1991). *Ethics with Aristotle*. Oxford University Press.

Bühler, C. (1928). Displeasure and pleasure in relation to activity. In M. L. Reymert (Ed.), *Feelings and emotions: The Wittenberg symposium* (pp. 195–199). Clark University Press.

Burgdorf, J., & Panksepp, J. (2006). The neurobiology of positive emotions. *Neuroscience & Biobehavioral Reviews, 30*(2), 173–187. https://doi.org/10.1016/j.neubiorev.2005.06.001

Cabanac, M. (1992). Pleasure: The common currency. *Journal of Theoretical Biology, 155*(2), 173–200. https://doi.org/10.1016/S0022-5193(05)80594-6

Cabanac, M. (2009). The fifth influence. *The dialectics of pleasure*. iUniverse.

Carver, C. S. (2003). Pleasure as a sign you can attend to something else: Placing positive feelings within a general model of affect. *Cognition and Emotion, 17*(2), 241–261.

Casebeer, W. D. (2003). *Natural ethical facts: Evolution, connectionism, and moral cognition [Kindle]*. Cambridge University Press.

Chalmers, D. J. (2015). Why isn't there more progress in philosophy? *Philosophy, 90*(1), 3–31. https://doi.org/10.1017/S0031819114000436

Chen, F. F., Jing, Y., Hayes, A., & Lee, J. (2013). Two concepts or two approaches? A bifactor analysis of psychological and subjective well-being. *Journal of Happiness Studies, 14*(3), 1033–1068. https://doi.org/10.1007/s10902-012-9367-x

Chikazoe, J., Lee, D. H., Kriegeskorte, N., & Anderson, A. K. (2014). Population coding of affect across stimuli, modalities and individuals [Article]. *Nature Neuroscience, 17*(8), 1114–1122. https://doi.org/10.1038/nn.3749

Churchland, P. S. (2018). *Braintrust: What neuroscience tells us about morality [Kindle]*. Princeton Science Library.

Cooke, P. J., Melchert, T. P., & Connor, K. (2016). Measuring wellbeing: A review of instruments. *The Counseling Psychologist, 44*, 730–757.
Crimmins, J. E. (2023). Jeremy Bentham. In E. N. Zalta (Ed.), *The Stanford encyclopedia of philosophy* (Winter 2021 ed.). Retrieved from https://plato.stanford.edu/archives/fall2023/entries/bentham/
Crisp, R. (2006a). Hedonism reconsidered. *Philosophy and Phenomenological Research, 73*(3), 619–645. https://doi.org/10.1111/j.1933-1592.2006.tb00551.x
Crisp, R. (2006b). *Reasons and the good*. Clarendon Press.
Crisp, R. (2017). Well-being. In E. N. Zalta (Ed.), *The Stanford encyclopedia of philosophy*. Retrieved from http://plato.stanford.edu/archives/fall2011/entries/well-being/
Crisp, R., & Kringelbach, M. (2018). Higher and lower pleasures revisited: Evidence from neuroscience. *Neuroethics, 11*(2), 211–215. https://doi.org/10.1007/s12152-017-9339-2
Dagenais-Desmarais, V., & Savoie, A. (2012). What is psychological well-being, really? A grassroots approach from the organizational sciences. *Journal of Happiness Studies, 13*(4), 659–684. https://doi.org/10.1007/s10902-011-9285-3
Damasio, A. (1999). *The feeling of what happens: Body and emotion in the making of consciousness*. Avon Books.
Damasio, A. (2010). *Self comes to mind: Constructing the conscious brain [Kindle]*. Pantheon Books.
Damasio, A. (2018). *The strange order of things: Life, feeling, and the making of culture [Kindle]*. Pantheon Books.
Damasio, A. (2021). *Feeling & knowing: Making minds conscious [Kindle]* (Vol. 12, p. 65). Pantheon.
Darwin, C. (1872). *The expression of the emotions in man and animals*. University of Chicago Press. http://www.gutenberg.org/files/1227/1227-h/1227-h.htm
Deci, E. L., & Ryan, R. M. M. (2008). Hedonia, eudaimonia, and well-being: An introduction. *Journal of Happiness Studies, 9*(1), 1–11. https://doi.org/10.1007/s10902-006-9018-1
Denton, D. (2005). *The primordial emotions: The dawning of consciousness*. Oxford University Press.
Deslauriers, L., McCarty, L. S., Miller, K., Callaghan, K., & Kestin, G. (2019). Measuring actual learning versus feeling of learning in response to being actively engaged in the classroom. *Proceedings of the National Academy of Sciences, 116*(39), 19251–19257. https://doi.org/10.1073/pnas.1821936116
Diener, E., & Tov, W. (2012). National accounts of well-being. In K. C. Land, A. C. Michalos, & M. J. Sirgy (Eds.), *Handbook of social indicators and quality of life research* (pp. 137–157). Springer. https://doi.org/10.1007/978-94-007-2421-1_7
Diener, E., Nickerson, C., Lucas, R., & Sandvik, E. (2002). Dispositional affect and job outcomes. *Social Indicators Research, 59*(3), 229–259.
Duncker, K. (1941). On pleasure, emotion, and striving. *Philosophy and Phenomenological Research, 1*(4), 391–430. https://doi.org/10.2307/2103143
Edwards, R. B. (1979). *Pleasures and pains: A theory of qualitative hedonism*. Cornell University Press.
Elliot, A., & Covington, M. (2001). Approach and avoidance motivation. *Educational Psychology Review, 13*(2), 73–92. https://doi.org/10.1023/a:1009009018235
Eregowda, N. I., Yadav, S., Parameshwarappa, P., & Basavraj, R. K. (2016). A girl with no pain: Congenital insensitivity to pain and anhidrosis (HSAN) type IV-A case report. *Journal of Clinical and Diagnostic Research: JCDR, 10*(2), ZL01.
Feibleman, J. K. (1964). A philosophic analysis of pleasure. In R. G. Heath (Ed.), *The role of pleasure in behavior. A symposium by 22 authors* (pp. 251–256). Harper & Row Publishers.
Feldman, F. (2004). *Pleasure and the good life. Concerning the nature, varieties, and plausibility of hedonism*. Clarendon Press.
Feldman, F. (2010). *What is this thing called happiness?* Oxford University Press.
Fletcher, G. (2016). *The philosophy of well-being: An introduction*. Routledge.

Frank, L. (2018). *The pleasure shock: The rise of deep brain stimulation and its forgotten inventor [Kndle]*. Penguin.
Frede, D. (2006). Pleasure and pain in Aristotle's ethics. In R. Kraut (Ed.), *The Blackwell guide to Aristotle's Nicomachean ethics* (pp. 255–275). Blackwell.
Fredrickson, B. L. (2009). *Positivity: Groundbreaking research to release your inner optimism and thrive [Kindle]*. Crown Publishers.
Fredrickson, B. L., Grewen, K. M., Coffey, K. A., Algoe, S. B., Firestine, A. M., Arevalo, J. M. G., Ma, J., & Cole, S. W. (2013). A functional genomic perspective on human well-being. *Proceedings of the National Academy of Sciences, 110*(33), 13684–13689. https://doi.org/10.1073/pnas.1305419110
Frijda, N. H. (1986). *The emotions*. Cambridge University Press.
Frijda, N. H. (2007). *The laws of emotions*. Lawrende Erlbaum Associates.
Frijda, N. H. (2010). On the nature and function of pleasure. In M. L. Kringelbach & K. C. Berridge (Eds.), *Pleasures of the brain* (pp. 99–112). Oxford University Press.
Fulford, D., Johnson, S. L., Llabre, M. M., & Carver, C. S. (2010). Pushing and coasting in dynamic goal pursuit : Coasting is attenuated in bipolar disorder. *Psychological Science, 21*(7), 1021–1027.
Gallagher, M. W., Lopez, S. J., & Preacher, K. J. (2009). The hierarchical structure of well-being. *Journal of Personality, 77*(4), 1025–1049.
Gilovich, T. D., & Griffin, D. W. (2010). Judgment and decision making. In S. T. Fiske, D. T. Gilbert, & G. Lindzey (Eds.), *Handbook of social psychology* (5th ed., pp. 542–588). Wiley.
Greenblatt, S. (2017). *The rise and fall of Adam and Eve*. WW Norton & Company.
Griffin, J. (1986). *Well-being. Its meaning, measurement, and moral importance*. Clarendon Press.
Grimm, C., Kemp, S., & Jose, P. E. (2015). Orientations to happiness and the experience of everyday activities. *The Journal of Positive Psychology, 10*(3), 207–218. https://doi.org/10.1080/17439760.2014.941382
Haybron, D. M. (2016). The philosophical basis of eudaimonic psychology. In J. Vittersø (Ed.), *Handbook of Eudaimonic well-being* (pp. 27–53). Springer International Publishing. https://doi.org/10.1007/978-3-319-42445-3_2
Hebb, O. D. (1955). Drives and the C. N. S. (conceptual nervous system). *Psychological Review, 62*(4), 243–254. https://doi.org/10.1037/h0041823
Higgins, E. T. (2014). *Beyond pleasure and pain: How motivation works*. Oxford University Press.
Hofmann, W., Luhmann, M., Fisher, R. R., Vohs, K. D., & Baumeister, R. F. (2014). Yes but are they happy? Effects of trait selfcontrol on affective well-being and life satisfaction. *Journal of Personality, 82*(4), 265–277. https://doi.org/10.1111/jopy.2014.82.issue-4 10.1111/jopy.12050
Huntsinger, J. R., Isbell, L. M., & Clore, G. L. (2014). The affective control of thought: Malleable, not fixed. *Psychological Review, 121*(4), 600–618. https://doi.org/10.1037/a0037669
Hurka, T. (2011). *The best things in life. A guide to what really matters [Kindle]*. Oxford University Press.
Huta, V., & Ryan, R. M. (2010). Pursuing pleasure or virtue: The differential and overlapping well-being benefits of hedonic and eudaimonic motives. *Journal of Happiness Studies, 11*, 735–762. https://doi.org/10.1007/s10902-009-9171-4
James, W. (1890). *Principles of psychology*. Great books of the Western world Chicago.
Jayawickreme, E., Forgeard, M. J. C., & Seligman, M. E. P. (2012). The engine of well-being. *Review of General Psychology, 16*(4), 327–342. https://doi.org/10.1037/a0027990
Johnston, V. S. (2003). The origin and function of pleasure. *Cognition and Emotion, 17*(2), 169–179.
Joseph, S., & Heferon, K. (2013). Post-traumatic growth: Eudaimonic happiness in the aftermath of adversity. In S. David, I. Boniwell, & A. C. Ayers (Eds.), *The Oxford handbook of happiness* (pp. 926–940). Oxford University Press.
Kagan, J. (1998). *Three seductive ideas*. Harvard University Press.
Kagan, J. (2009). *The three cultures. Natural sciences, social sciences, and the humanities in the 21st century*. Cambridge University Press.

Kahneman, D., Wakker, P. P., & Sarin, R. (1997). Back to Bentham? Explorations of experienced utility. *Quarterly Journal of Economics, 112*(2), 375–405.

Kahneman, D., Diener, E., & Schwarz, N. (1999a). Preface. In D. Kahneman, E. Diener, & N. Schwarz (Eds.), *Well-being: The foundations of hedonic psychology*. Russel-Sage.

Kahneman, D., Diener, E., & Schwarz, N. (Eds.). (1999b). *Well-being: The foundations of hedonic psychology*. Russel-Sage.

Kashdan, T. B., Biswas-Diener, R., & King, L. A. (2008). Reconsidering happiness: The costs of distinguishing between hedonics and eudaimonia. *The Journal of Positive Psychology, 3*(4), 219–233. https://doi.org/10.1080/17439760802303044

Katz, L. D. (2016). Pleasure. In E. N. Zalta (Ed.), *The Stanford encyclopedia of philosophy* (Winter 2016 ed.). Retreived from https://plato.stanford.edu/archives/win2016/entries/pleasure/

Keyes, C. L. M. (2007). Subjective well-being in mental health and human development research worldwide: An introduction. *Social Indicators Research, 77*, 1–10.

Kobayashi, K., & Hsu, M. (2019). Common neural code for reward and information value. *Proceedings of the National Academy of Sciences, 116*(26), 13061–13066. https://doi.org/10.1073/pnas.1820145116

Krasko, J., Intelisano, S., & Luhmann, M. (2022). When happiness is both joy and purpose: The complexity of the pursuit of happiness and well-being is related to actual well-being. *Journal of Happiness Studies, 23*(7), 3233–3261. https://doi.org/10.1007/s10902-022-00541-2

Kraut, R. (2022). Aristotle's ethics. In E. N. Zalta (Ed.), *The Stanford encyclopedia of philosophy* (Spring 2022 ed.). Retrieved from https://plato.stanford.edu/archives/fall2022/entries/aristotle-ethics/

Kringelbach, M. L., & Berridge, K. C. (2010). Fundamental pleasure questions. In M. L. Kringelbach & K. C. Berridge (Eds.), *Pleasures of the brain* (pp. 7–23). Oxford University Press.

Kringelbach, M. L., & Berridge, K. C. (2017). The affective core of emotion: Linking pleasure, subjective well-being, and optimal metastability in the brain. *Emotion Review, 9*(3), 191–199. https://doi.org/10.1177/1754073916684558

Kubovy, M. (1999). On the pleasures of the mind. In D. Kahneman, E. Diener, & N. Schwarz (Eds.), *Well-being: The foundations of hedonic psychology* (pp. 135–154). Russell Sage Foundation.

Lambert, L., Lomas, T., van de Weijer, M. P., Passmore, H. A., Joshanloo, M., Harter, J., Ishikawa, Y., Lai, A., Kitagawa, T., & Chen, D. (2020). Towards a greater global understanding of well-being: A proposal for a more inclusive measure. *International Journal of Wellbeing, 10*(2), 1.

Landwehr, J. R., & Eckmann, L. (2020). The nature of processing fluency: Amplification versus hedonic marking. *Journal of Experimental Social Psychology, 90*, 103997. https://doi.org/10.1016/j.jesp.2020.103997

Lang, P. J., & Bradley, M. M. (2013). Appetitive and defensive motivation: Goal-directed or goal-determined? *Emotion Review, 5*(3), 230–234. https://doi.org/10.1177/1754073913477511

Lazarus, R. S. (1991). Progress on a cognitive-motivational-relational theory of emotion. *American Psychologist, 46*(8), 819–834.

Levy, D. J., & Glimcher, P. W. (2011). Comparing apples and oranges: Using reward-specific and reward-general subjective value representation in the brain. *The Journal of Neuroscience, 31*(41), 14693–14707. https://doi.org/10.1523/jneurosci.2218-11.2011

Lewis, C. S. (1940). *The problem of pain*. Centenary.

Linden, D. J. (2012). *The compass of pleasure: How our brains make fatty foods, orgasm, exercise, marijuana, generosity, vodka, learning, and gambling feel so good [Kindle]*. Penguin.

Linton, S. J. (2005). *Understanding pain for better clinical practice: A psychological perspective*.

Liu, J. (2024). We want negative affect, and some is good for us. *Paper presented at The Second ModHap Conference*, May 30–31, Oslo, Norway.

Louro, M. J., Pieters, R., & Zeelenberg, M. (2007). Dynamics of multiple-goal pursuit. *Journal of Personality and Social Psychology, 93*(2), 174–193. https://doi.org/10.1037/0022-3514.93.2.174

McGregor, I., & Little, B. (1998). Personal projects, happiness, and meaning: On doing well and being yourself. *Journal of Personality and Social Psychology, 74*(2), 494–512. https://doi.org/10.1037/0022-3514.74.2.494
McMahon, D. (2006). *The pursuit of happiness. A history from the Greeks to the present.* Allen Lane.
Melzack, R., & Wall, P. D. (1996). *The challenge of pain* (3rd ed.). Penguin.
Michalos, A. C., & Robinson, S. R. (2012). The good life: Eighth century to third century BCE. In K. C. Land, A. C. Michalos, & M. J. Sirgy (Eds.), *Handbook of social indicators and quality of life research* (pp. 23–61). Springer. https://doi.org/10.1007/978-94-007-2421-1_2
Michell, J. (1999). *Measurement in psychology: Critical history of a methodological concept.* Cambridge University Press.
Mill, J. S. (2001). *Utilitarianism [Kindle].* Hackett Publishing (Original work published 1863). (1863).
Moen, O. M. (2013). The unity and commensurability of pleasures and pains [journal article]. *Philosophia, 41*(2), 527–543. https://doi.org/10.1007/s11406-012-9383-4
Moen, O. M. (2015). Hedonism before Bentham. *Journal of Bentham Studies, 17*(1), 1–18. https://doi.org/10.14324/111.2045-757X.007
Monni, A., Olivier, E., Morin, A. J. S., Olivetti Belardinelli, M., Mulvihill, K., & Scalas, L. F. (2020). Approach and avoidance in Gray's, Higgins', and Elliot's perspectives: A theoretical comparison and integration of approach-avoidance in motivated behavior. *Personality and Individual Differences, 166*, 110163. https://doi.org/10.1016/j.paid.2020.110163
Moore, A. (2019). Hedonism. In E. N. Zalta (Ed.), *The Stanford encyclopedia of philosophy* (Winter 2019 ed.). Retrieved from http://plato.stanford.edu/entries/hedonism/
Morson, G. S. (2014). *Introduction to Anna Karenina* (M. Schwartz, Trans.). Yale University Press. (Original work published 1878).
Nozick, R. (1974). *Anarchy, state, and utopia.* Basic Books.
Nussbaum, M. C. (2001). *Upheavals of thought. The intelligence of emotions.* Cambridge University Press.
Nussbaum, M. C. (2004). Mill between Aristotle & Bentham. *Daedalus, 133*(2), 60–68. https://doi.org/10.1162/001152604323049406
Nussbaum, M. C. (2008). Who is the happy warrior? Philosophy poses questions to psychology. *The Journal of Legal Studies, 37*(S2), s81–s113. https://doi.org/10.1086/587438
Oishi, S., & Westgate, E. C. (2022). A psychologically rich life: Beyond happiness and meaning. *Psychological Review, 129*(4), 790–811. https://doi.org/10.1037/rev0000317
Oswald, A. J., Proto, E., & Sgroi, D. (2009). *Happiness and productivity* (IZA discussion paper no. 4645), issue.
Overskeid, G. (2002). Psychological hedonism and the nature of motivation: Bertrand Russell's adhedonic desires. *Philosophical Psychology, 15*(1), 77–93.
Panksepp, J. (1998). *Affective neuroscience.* Oxford University Press.
Panksepp, J., & Biven, L. (2012). *The archaeology of mind.* Norton.
Parducci, A. (1968). The relativism of absolute judgments. *Scientific American, 219*, 84–90.
Parducci, A. (1995). *Happiness, pleasure, and judgment: The contextual theory and its applications.* Lawrence Erlbaum.
Paul, M., Bamba, C., Chugh, V., Ravikumar, N., & Jayaram, S. (2022). A boy who knows no pain: Anaesthetic management of congenital insensitivity to pain with anhidrosis. *Cureus, 14*(10).
Popper, K. (2005). *The logic of scientific discovery.* Routledge.
Prinzing, M. (2021). How to study well-being: A proposal for the integration of philosophy with science. *Review of General Psychology, 25*(2), 152–162. https://doi.org/10.1177/10892680211002443
Reber, R., Schwarz, N., & Winkielman, P. (2004). Processing fluency and aesthetic pleasure. *Personality and Social Psychology Review, 8*, 364–382. https://doi.org/10.1207/s15327957pspr0804_3
Ruckmick, C. A. (1925). The psychology of pleasantness. *Psychological Review, 32*(5), 362–383.

Russell, B. (2014/1967). *The autobiography of Bertrand Russell*. Routledge. (Original work published 1967).
Ryan, R. M. M., & Deci, E. L. D. (2001). On happiness and human potentials: A review of research on hedonic and eudaimonic well-being. *Annual Review of Psychology, 52*, 141–166. http://psych.AnnualReviews.org/cgi/reprint/52/1/141.pdf
Schmitter, A. M. (2021). 17th and 18th century theories of emotions. In E. N. Zalta (Ed.), *The Stanford encyclopedia of philosophy* (Summer 2021 ed.). Retrieved from https://plato.stanford.edu/archives/sum2021/entries/emotions-17th18th/
Schueller, S. P., & Seligman, M. E. P. (2010). Pursuit of pleasure, engagement, and meaning: Relationships to subjective and objective measures of well-being. *Journal of Positive Psychology, 5*(4), 253–263.
Scollon, C. N., & King, L. (2011). What people really want in life and why it matters: Contributions from research on folk theories of the good life. In R. Biswas-Diener (Ed.), *Positive psychology as social change* (pp. 1–14). Springer. http://www.springer.com/psychology/book/978-90-481-9937-2
Seligman, M. E. P. (2002). *Authentic happiness. Using the new positive psychology to realize your potential for deep fulfillment*. Nicholas Brealey Publishing.
Shizgal, P. (1999). On the neural computation of utility: Implications from studies of brain stimulation reward. In D. Kahneman, E. Diener, & N. Schwarz (Eds.), *Well-being: The foundations of hedonic psychology* (pp. 502–526). Russell Sage Foundation. http://cogprints.org/740/1/Well-Being_v4_15.html
Sidgwick, H. (1907). *The methods of ethics* [Kindle] (7th ed.). Hackett Publishing. http://www.earlymoderntexts.com/assets/pdfs/sidgwick1874.pdf
Skidelsky, R., & Skidelsky, E. (2013). *How much is enough: The love of money and the case for the good life [Kindle]* (2nd ed.). Penguin Books.
Skov, M. (2019). The neurobiology of sensory valuation. In M. Nadal & O. Vartanian (Eds.), *The Oxford handbook of empirical aesthetics*. Oxford University Press. https://doi.org/10.1093/oxfordhb/9780198824350.013.7
Slovic, P. (2007). "If I look at the mass I will never act": Psychic numbing and genocide. *Judgment and Decision making, 2*(2), 79.
Slovic, P., Finucane, M. L., Peters, E., & MacGregor, D. G. (2007). The affect heuristic. *European Journal of Operational Research, 177*(3), 1333–1352. https://doi.org/10.1016/j.ejor.2005.04.006
Small, D. A., Loewenstein, G., & Slovic, P. (2007). Sympathy and callousness: The impact of deliberative thought on donations to identifiable and statistical victims. *Organizational Behavior and Human Decision Processes, 102*(2), 143–153. https://doi.org/10.1016/j.obhdp.2006.01.005
Steger, M. F., Kashdan, T. B., & Oishi, S. (2008). Being good by doing good: Daily eudaimonic activity and well-being. *Journal of Research in Personality, 42*(1), 22–42. https://doi.org/10.1016/j.jrp.2007.03.004
Steger, M. F., Shin, J. Y., Shim, Y., & Fitch-Martin, A. (2013). Is meaning in life a flagship indicator of well-being? In A. Waterman (Ed.), *The best within us: Positive psychology perspectives on eudaimonia* (pp. 159–182). American Psychological Association. https://doi.org/10.1037/14092-009
Steptoe, A., Deaton, A., & Stone, A. A. (2015). Subjective wellbeing, health, and ageing. *The Lancet, 385*(9968), 640–648. https://doi.org/10.1016/S0140-6736(13)61489-0
Stone, A. A., & Mackie, C. (2013). *Subjective well-being: Measuring happiness, suffering, and other dimensions of experience*. National Academies Press.
Strauss, E. D., Schloss, K. B., & Palmer, S. E. (2013). Color preferences change after experience with liked/disliked colored objects. *Psychonomic Bulletin & Review, 20*(5), 935–943. https://doi.org/10.3758/s13423-013-0423-2
Sumner, L. W. (1996). *Welfare, happiness, and ethics*. Clarendon Press.
Tatarkiewicz, W. (1976). *Analysis of happiness*. Nijhoff.
Thagard, P. (2010). *The brain and the meaning of life [Kindle]*. Princeton University Press.

Thin, N. (2012). *Social happiness. Theory into policy and practice*. The Policy Press.
Tolstoy, L. (2014). *Anna Karenina* (Rosamund Bartlett, Trans.). Oxford University Press. (Original work published 1878).
Tov, W., & Lee, H. W. (2016). A closer look at the hedonics of everyday meaning and satisfaction. *Journal of Personality and Social Psychology, 111*(4), 585–609. https://doi.org/10.1037/pspp0000081
van de Weijer, M., Baselmans, B., van der Deijl, W., & Bartels, M. (2018). A growing sense of well-being: A literature review on the complex framework well-being. https://doi.org/10.31234/osf.io/3rmx9
Veenhoven, R. (1984). *Conditions of happiness*. Kluwer Academic.
Vittersø, J. (2016). The feeling of excellent functioning: Hedonic and eudaimonic emotions. In J. Vittersø (Ed.), *Handbook of eudaimonic well-being* (pp. 253–276). Springer International Publishing. https://doi.org/10.1007/978-3-319-42445-3_17
von Wright, G. H. (1963). *The varieties of goodness*. Routledge.
Warburton, D. M. (1996). The function of pleasure. In D. M. Warburton & N. Sherwood (Eds.), *Pleasure and quality of life* (pp. 1–10). Wiley.
Waterman, A. S. (1993). Two conceptions of happiness: Contrasts of personal expressiveness (eudaimonia) and hedonic enjoyment. *Journal of Personality and Social Psychology 64*(4), 678–691. https://doi.org/678-691.10.1037/0022-3514.64.4.678
Watson, J. (1895). *Hedonistic theories. From Aristippus to Spencer*. Macmillan.
Weijers, D. (2021). *Hedonism*. Internet Encyclopedia of Philosophy. https://iep.utm.edu/hedonism/
Wilson, F. L. (2014). John Stuart Mill. In E. N. Zalta (Ed.), *The Stanford encyclopedia of philosophy* (Spring 2014 ed.). Available from: http://plato.stanford.edu/archives/spr2014/entries/mill/
Wilson, J. (2021). Determinables and determinates. In E. N. Zalta (Ed.), *The Stanford encyclopedia of philosophy* (Spring 2021 ed.). Available from: https://plato.stanford.edu/archives/spr2021/entries/determinate-determinables/
Winkielman, P., & Cacioppo, J. T. (2001). Mind at ease puts a smile on the face: Psychophysiological evidence that processing facilitation elicits positive affect. *Journal of Personality and Social Psychology, 81*(6), 989–1000.
Winkielman, P., & Schwarz, N. (2001). How pleasant was your childhood? Beliefs about memory shape inferences from experienced difficulty of recall. *Psychological Science, 12*(2), 176–179.
Winkielman, P., Schwarz, N., & Belli, R. F. (1998). The role of ease of retrieval and attribution in memory judgments: Judging your memory as worse despite recalling more events. *Psychological Science, 9*(2), 124–126.
Winkielman, P., Schwarz, N., Fazendeiro, T. A., & Reber, R. (2003). The hedonic marking of processing fluency: Implications for evaluative judgment. In J. Musch & K. C. Klauer (Eds.), *The psychology of evaluation. Affective processes in cognition and emotion* (pp. 189–217). Lawrence Erlbaum.
Winkielman, P., Berridge, K. C., & Wilbarger, J. L. (2005). Unconscious affective reactions to masked happy versus angry faces influence consumption behavior and judgments of value. *Personality and Social Psychology Bulletin, 31*(1), 121–135. https://doi.org/10.1177/0146167204271309

Chapter 6
Eudaimonia

Introduction

To be mature you have to realize what you value most. (Roosevelt, 1983, p. 72)

Ever since systematic thinking about happiness began, objections have been raised against the notion that pleasant feelings or individualized desire fulfillment are the only true values in human life. Critical voices have deemed these goals unworthy for human beings and more suitable for swine or "dumb grazing animals" (e.g., Nussbaum, 2004). Hence, the third category in the philosophical classification scheme of wellbeing theories, named "Aristotelian happiness" or "objective list theories," offers an alternative to the default theories of hedonism and satisfactionism, or their scientific offspring, which is often referred to as subjective wellbeing (Chap. 2).

Aristotelian happiness is often named eudaimonism and is the prototype and dominating approach among objective wellbeing theories (Annas, 1993; MacIntyre, 2007; Michalos & Robinson, 2012; Sumner, 1996). However, Aristotle did not coin the term eudaimonia,[1] and his was certainly not the only eudaimonic theory in the classic era of Greek philosophy (e.g., Keyes & Annas, 2009). Yet, the Aristotelian version will be central to the analysis of eudaimonism in this chapter. Aristotle is after all one of the greatest philosophers of all time (Shields, 2022), and his major treatises in ethics, the *Nicomachean Ethics* and the *Eudemian Ethics*, are foundational in the history of ethical thinking.

Translating eudaimonia[2] (εὐδαιμονία) from Greek to English is easier said than done. A series of attempts have been proposed, and more are coming in. A common proposal is to have the prefix "eu" translated into the English good or well and to

[1] The word eudaimonia was employed in Greek texts more than a hundred years before Aristotle was born (e.g., Haybron, 2016).

[2] The Latinized versions "eudaemonia" (or "eudemonia") is no longer recommended (e.g., Nussbaum, 2001).

J. Vittersø, *Humanistic Wellbeing*, https://doi.org/10.1007/978-3-031-69292-5_6

replace "daimon" with divinity or guardian spirit. To be eudaimon is accordingly to have a good spirit guarding you or to be living in a way that is well favored by a god (Kraut, 2015, 2022). Getting more technical about "daimon," a debate has been raised about the mortal and immortal dimensions of a person. In classic Greek, the term "eidolon" refers to the earthly part of a person, whereas "daimon" is the spiritual and immortal part. Thus, being eudaimon means being fortunate enough to lead a life that is blessed in a spiritual way, and having a good daimon on your side means being "lucky" (McMahon, 2006, pp. 3–4). As Kraut prefers to formulate it, "To be eudaimon, then, is to have, as it were, a guardian angel who is doing well in guiding one's life. Or, as we might put it, it is to be smiled upon by Lady Luck" (Kraut, 2015, p. 24).

The connotation of a good fortune is one reason why the term eudaimonia, almost as a philosophical paradigm, was translated into English as happiness (Jost, 2002, p. xxi). The term happiness has historically been defined as good luck and favorable external conditions (e.g., McMahon, 2006; Oishi, 2018; Oishi et al., 2013). After all, happiness comes from the old English usage of "happenstance," meaning "a lucky break" (Bok, 2010). More recently, however, happiness has been redefined to mean either a feeling state or subjective wellbeing (Chaps. 2 and 3), and commentators now propose that eudaimonia should be translated as wellbeing, flourishing, or welfare rather than happiness (e.g., Crisp, 2017; Fowers, 2016; Jost & Shiner, 2002; Nussbaum, 2001; Sumner, 2002). Following this trend, as we saw in Chap. 2, it can be argued that Aristotelian eudaimonism is not a theory of happiness but rather a theory about wellbeing (Haybron, 2008, p. 32).

Not all experts on ancient philosophy agree with the new translations of eudaimonia. For instance, Gregory Vlastos insists that we should continue translating eudaimonia into happiness, partly because wellbeing has no adjectival or adverbial forms. This may seem a small matter to armchair translators, philosophers dogmatizing on how others should do their jobs. Not so, Vlastos suggests, if one is struggling with its nitty-gritty, trying for clause-by-clause English counterparts that might be faithful to the sentence structure, no less than the sentence, of the Greek original. In addition, well being is a stiff bookish phrase bereft of the ease and grace with which the living words of a natural language perform in a wide diversity of contexts. By contrast, eudaimonia fits perfectly street-Greek and Aristophanic slapstick, yet also, no less perfectly, the most exalted passage of tragedy (cited in Jost, 2002, p. xxii).

I shall not have much to say about street-Greek and Aristophanic slapstick jargon but will make a distinction between philosophical and scientific approaches to eudaimonia. As for the first, I shall mainly use the terms eudaimonia and eudaimonism. When it comes to science, I prefer the terms eudaimonia and eudaimonic wellbeing (EWB).

Eudaimonism

Like hedonism and satisfactionism, eudaimonism is an "-ism" and is thus more tightly connected to philosophy and metaphysics than to science. The term eudaimonism refers to a cluster of theories and not one single theory. According to Annas (2003), these theories share the idea that "the agent has a final end to which all her actions are, in one or another way, directed" (p. 28). To Aristotle, this end was virtue activities; to Epicurus, it was being in a state of pleasure. Epicurus therefore had a hedonic theory of eudaimonism, whereas Aristotle did not (Keyes & Annas, 2009).

A different version of a "one-liner" explanation of the eudaimonic riddle comes from Sumner (1996), who sees eudaimonia as "a complete state of being and doing well" (p. 69). MacIntyre (2007) suggested that eudaimonia could be defined as "being well and doing well in being well" or as "man-as-he-could-be-if-he-realized-his-essential-nature" (p. 52). In her summary, Besser-Jones (2015) stresses that our lives are eudaimon when we make optimal use of our capacities, i.e., when we are functioning optimally, or according to the best of our nature. Other definitions and approaches are easily available in the philosophical literature. Michalos and Robinson (2012) give, for instance, a nice summary of 12 ancient perspectives of the good life, including advice such as trusting and law-abiding good human relations, living in peace, and enjoying the fruits of one's labor.

Aristotelian Eudaimonism

Aristotle's impact on Western thinking can hardly be overrated, and a proper study of wellbeing cannot afford to ignore his teaching. However, Aristotle's life and ideas were embedded in a prescientific rationality and submerged in an ancient, patriarchic, and elitist culture that is inconsistent with central ideas in modern ethical thinking. Clearly, Neo-Aristotelians must repudiate many of his views, such as the belief that only wealthy, slave-owning men could lead good lives. Other parts of Aristotle's theory should be abandoned because of their inconsistency with scientific knowledge. The unavoidable question about Aristotle is therefore how useful his thinking really is today. The answer, Annas (2011) suggests, is that most of the main structure of Aristotelian eudaimonism will survive a modern examination. She claims that Aristotle's elitist morale "does not determine the way he thinks of happiness, and virtue, in terms of living your life, which is why his ethical theory has been found relevant by both women and men in a wide variety of different historical and cultural circumstances" (Annas, 2011, loc. 2721). As we shall see, other answers to the question of how relevant Aristotelian thinking is for a modern life are also conceivable.

Everything Has a Goal

Aristotle developed his notion of telos after carefully observing "the goal-directedness of all things." That idea was mentioned in Chap. 1 as a milestone in the history of ideas, and it changed biological thinking forever.[3] According to Mayr (2004), it might even be "the most characteristic feature of the world of living organisms" (p. 52). Book I of *Nicomachean Ethics* is devoted to investigating the concept of telos, and the principle has since been recognized as the very process by which life is generated and maintained. In at least some respects, modern biology has adapted Aristotle's thinking about the purposeful nature of living organisms (Mayr, 1982). Biologists refer to this feature of life as "teleonomy," and as recalled from Chap. 1, Aristotelian teleonomy is considered "remarkably modern" (Mayr, 2004). It has even been referred to as "empirically irrefutable" (Pross, 2016, p. 9).[4] Despite Aristotle's lack of an evolutionary perspective, Darwin respected and admired him "to the point that he said privately that the intellectual heroes of his own time 'were mere schoolboys compared to old Aristotle'" (Romero, 2012, p. 6).

Identifying the Good

People diverge in their views on the human good, but Aristotle suggests that some agreement might be achieved by employing an evaluative rationality known as the functioning argument. The basic principle of the functioning argument is deceptively simple: something is good when it fulfills its telos well. The purpose of a knife is to cut; thus, a knife is good when it cuts well. Similarly, an eye that sees properly is a good eye and so on. The crux of this seemingly simple idea is both sophisticated and elegant: if you understand what something is meant to do, it's telos, you will also understand its function. When you know what the function of something is, there is a small step to determine its goodness. "For all things that have a function or activity, the good and the 'well' is thought to reside in the function" (Aristotle, trans. 1908, p. 14).

This is important because it provides a logical connection between something factual (i.e., proper functioning) and something normative (i.e., a valuable goal). Aristotle suggests that this principle also can be applied to human wellbeing, because, he argues, a human being stands to a good human as a knife stands to a good knife. By implication, this logic overrules Hume's law that no ought can be concluded from an is (MacIntyre, 2007, p. 58).

However, for the argument to work, factual human functioning must be convincingly determined. Here, Aristotle put his money on rationality. Rational activity, he reasoned, is our "characteristic activity," and humans are the only species that have

[3] As clarified in Chap. 1, we no longer attribute a telos to nonliving things.

[4] Teleonomy is controversial, but Mayr (1982, pp. 47–51) gives a very informative analyses of the various forms a telos can take in modern science. Interested readers are referred to the useful reviews by Walsh (2015) and Haig (2020).

a rational soul (Kraut, 2022, p. 6). By juxtaposing the idea that a knife is good when it cuts well with the idea that a human is good when it reasons excellently, Aristotle had the argument he needed to claim that the good life "depends on performing rational activities well" (Korsgaard, 2008, p. 144). Aristotle was now ready to say that "human good turns out to be activity of soul in accordance with virtue, and if there are more than one virtue, in accordance with the best and most complete" (Aristotle, trans. 1908, p. 14).

> So when Aristotle says that the function of a human being is the activity of the rational part of the soul, he does not mean simply that reasoning is the purpose of a human being. (…) He means rather that rational activity is how we human beings do what we do, and in particular, how we lead our specific form of life. (Korsgaard, 2008, p. 141)

Humans' characteristic activity, then, is rational behavior. This, in turn, can excel only by being virtuous. Virtues are, briefly explained, dispositions to do the right thing. In more detail, being virtuous means that we must "think, feel, and act at the right time, about the right things, toward the right people, for the right end, and in the right way" (Badhwar, 2014, p. 143).

According to Annas (1993), we can obtain a good understanding of ancient virtues by analyzing them according to three main dimensions. These are the dispositional, affective, and intellectual elements of a virtue. These dispositions further involve two things. "One is the ability to reason reflectively in the morally right way. (…) The other thing involved in virtue is a developed habit of feeling and reacting in the right way, that is, the way that accords with the correct reasoning" (Annas, 1998, p. 40). Being virtuous thus involves an interaction between reasoning and feeling that is embedded in morality and which result is appropriate behavior. Annas uses the example of spending money wisely to illustrate the mechanism. "Only the virtuous person properly knows how to put money to use and do the right things with it; and thus only in the virtuous person's life does money make a contribution to happiness" (Annas, 1998, p. 49).

Aristotle on Pleasure

Aristotle thinking about pleasure was introduced in Chap. 5 as vague and inconsistent. One confusion regards the role he allocated to pleasure in his theory of eudaimonism. According to one interpretation, Aristotle basically argued that being virtuous means finding virtuous activities pleasant. "Virtues are dispositions not only to act in particular ways but also to feel in particular ways" (MacIntyre, 2007, p. 149). Thus, happiness in eudaimonist thinking does not exclude pleasure, "but it excludes the idea that happiness could just be pleasure (Annas, 2011, loc. 1947). However, Annas reminds us "that if happiness is construed as feelings of pleasure, we have produced a conception of happiness which is not only radically different from the eudaimonist one, but strikingly trivialized" (loc. 1817).

A useful review of the role of pleasure in Aristotelian thinking is provided by Frede (2006). She agrees that "virtuous actions must be in themselves pleasant" and goes on to argue that "pleasure and the activity of the soul are no longer rival candidates for the summum bonum; they are, in a way, mutual complements (...) [Aristotle] thereby confirms the close connection between pleasure and action: an activity in the full sense must contain its end in itself" (pp. 260–263). Frede then wraps up her review by treasuring Aristotle's "contention that certain pleasures are an integral part of the human life that finds its fulfillment in morally and intellectually worthy activities" (p. 273).

Another interpretation is given by Katz (2016), who explains that to Aristotle, pleasantness and value vary together. In this, Katz argues, Aristotelian ideas are quite like Csikszentmihalyi's theory of flow. Flow experiences are intense feelings characterized by a state of total involvement that occurs during activities in which there is a balance between challenges and skills (e.g., Nakamura & Csikszentmihalyi, 2014). Annas (2008) reached a similar conclusion. She explains that it is "when we are most engaged in skillful complex activity that the activity is experienced as 'unimpeded', in Aristotle's terms, or as 'flow'" (p. 21).

Weiss (1979) claims that Aristotle "comes dangerously close to committing himself to the position that pleasure is indeed the supreme good" (p. 214), whereas others have noted how Aristotle also argues against hedonism (e.g., Moen, 2015). In this regard, Nussbaum (2008) explains that Aristotle offers

> two very different conceptions of pleasure, one in book VII and one in book X of the *Nicomachean Ethics*. The first identifies pleasure with unimpeded activity (not so odd if we remember that we speak of "my pleasures" and "enjoyments"). The second, and probably better, account holds that pleasure is something that comes along with, supervenes on, activity, "like the bloom on the cheek of youth." In other words, it is so closely linked to the relevant activities that it cannot be pursued on its own, any more than bloom can be adequately cultivated by cosmetics. (Nussbaum, 2008, pp. s84–s85)

Finally, in his introduction to the *Nicomachean Ethics*, Ross tells us that for Aristotle, "Happiness is not to be equated with pleasure, but, for all that, he will (in Book X) solve the ancient question of the relation between pleasure and the highest good by finding that the truly happy life will indeed be the most pleasant, even though the source of its being the highest good is not its pleasantness" (Ross, 2009, p. xi).

Aristotle on Meaning

In the science of wellbeing, meaning in life has become a core characteristic of eudaimonia (e.g., Bauer, 2016; Dolan, 2015; Heintzelman, 2018; Huta & Waterman, 2014; OECD, 2013; Oishi & Westgate, 2022; Tov, 2018). However, meaning in the sense of finding a purpose in life was never a central part of Aristotle's philosophy about the good life (Gotthelf, 1976; Grene, 1972). The only possible interpretation of Aristotelian eudaimonism as meaning in life is by interpreting his idea of telos as having to do with some kind of meaning (Megone, 1994; Russell, 2013). For example, Megone (1994) suggests that meaning and purpose in life can be related to Aristotle's functioning argument. He argues that if something has a function or purpose, "then that thing will be achieving its goal, in the best state (so a good example if its kind), when it completely achieves that function or purpose" (p. 36). From this, it follows that "if a human being has a function, or purpose (simply as a human being), then he will be in the best state when that purpose is achieved" (Megone, 1994, p. 36).

But most philosophers will probably consider this a far-fetched interpretation, at least in the sense of modern conceptualizations of meaning and purpose in life. According to Grene, for example, the Aristotelian telos has nothing to do with purpose "either Man's or God's." It was the Judaeo-Christian tradition that, with the help of neo-Platonism, imposed the dominance of cosmic teleology upon Aristotelian nature (Grene, 1972, p. 398). Russell (2013) further explains that in Aristotle's teaching, the purpose of life is the same for all of us, and "there is exactly one final end per person, and what's more, it is the same final end for each of us" (Russell, 2013, p. 9). Hence, when Smith (2017) analyzed answers to the question of life's meaning provided by famous US Americans, she found that each of the responses was distinct, reflecting the unique values, experiences, and personalities of the respondents.

As will be discussed later in this chapter, there are some commonalities in the answers presented in Smith's book on *The Power of Meaning*, yet the idea that each of us is free to create our own list of life meanings is certainly not Aristotelian. To the contrary, such a sweeping purpose is the opposite of Aristotelian thinking (Grene, 1972, p. 398). To Aristotle, telos was not about purpose or a "feeling of meaning" but about ontogeny and adaptation in living organisms.

Against Aristotle

A core idea in Aristotle's theory of wellbeing is that rational activity in accordance with virtues constitutes the good life (e.g., Kraut, 2022, p. 6). Such a conceptualization can, however, not be easily translated to modern science. For example, Aristotle overstated the role of human rationality and used it too exclusively as an argument for his way of ordering the universe: "This approach meant that species were rigid elements of the world and, thus, he never contemplated mutability or anything close to evolution" (Romero, 2012, p. 5). Aristotle also held women to be defective in their ability to reason, and he tried to convince his readers that whereas "the nature or function of man is to reason in ways that are distinctively human, the nature and function of woman is to reproduce, like other animals" (Held, 2006, p. 59).

As a pre-Darwinian, Aristotle was also unaware of the role played by variation in natural selection. This ignorance helps explain some of his exaggerated distinctions between species. Equally important, Aristotle underestimated within-species variations, a position that might be attributed to his half-mythological and premodern understanding of biology (Gelman & Rhodes, 2012; Thagard, 2010). By downplaying within-species variations, the concepts of personality traits and individual differences were excluded from the Aristotelian worldview (Lewin, 1931). Lewin points out that Aristotle's idea of an essential human nature forced him to consider individual variations as "erroneous" deviations from a homogenous and true human template. He thus defended the idea that all humans have the same potential and the same ultimate goal. Rather than striving to become "the best version of yourself," Aristotelian striving is toward "the best version of a human being that we can be" (Bradford, 2015, p. 127).

Another weakness in Aristotelian thinking is its mythical elements. Aristotle described, for instance, the motion of objects in terms of higher forms and lower forms, with circular motions representing the highest form occurring only in "heavenly" movements (Lewin, 1931, p. 142). The mythical element in Aristotelian thinking also creates a problem for his eudaimonic theory. Aristotle believed that all objects had a natural tendency to move toward their telos, i.e., the place appropriate to their nature. To Aristotle, this striving toward perfection resides within the objects. The objects themselves caused this movement. "The kind and direction of the physical vector in Aristotelian dynamics are completely determined in advance by the nature of the object concerned" (Lewin, 1931, p. 164). In other words, whatever influences a situation has on an object is nothing but a disturbing force. This view is inconsistent with modern thinking, including the strong impact that interactions play in biology (Mayr, 2004) and psychology (Lewin, 1936). Indeed, Lewin famously proposed that behavior (B) should be understood as an interaction between a person (P) and an environment (E), articulated in the formula B = f(P, E); i.e., behavior is a function of the person and his or her environment.

To provide just one empirical example of the interactionist nature of human behavior, consider the following experiment by Liberman et al. (2004). Study participants were invited to play a game, the prisoner's dilemma, but were introduced to it under different names. Half of the participants were invited to play something called the "Wall Street Game," the other half were invited to play the "Community Game." When playing the Wall Street Game, 33% of the participants preferred to cooperate. In contrast, when playing the Community Game, approximately 70% of the participants preferred to cooperate. By merely manipulating the name of the game, the researchers demonstrated that the likelihood of cooperation can change dramatically.

Referring to this interaction effect, one might say that humans are both cooperators and defectors by nature. To Aristotle, however, this process is not straightforward. Following Lewin, such a change in situation appears to Aristotle "as something fortuitous that disturbs and obscures the essential nature. It was therefore valid and customary to exclude the 'influence of the situation' as far as possible to "abstract" from the situation, in order to understand the essential nature of the object and the direction of its goal" (Lewin, 1931, p. 165).

A more recent achievement in the person and situation debate was initiated by Mischel's (1973) thoughtful commentary about how personal dispositions could be altered by context. Milgram's obedience studies (Milgram, 1963), Zimbardo's prison experiment (Haney et al., 1973), and Batson's Good Samaritan study (Darley & Batson, 1973) illustrate Michel's argument by showing how important a situation can be in determining behavior. A fine review of the debate can be found in Ross and Nisbett (2011). Philosophers have also passionately debated the implications of the person and the situation literature, (e.g., Doris, 1998; Harman, 2000; Merritt, 2000; Van Zyl, 2018). A critical part of this literature focuses on whether Aristotle's strict criteria for virtuous behavior stand up against scientific knowledge about persons and situations.

Prinz (2009) adds a cross-cultural argument to the virtues and person–situation debate. If virtues are culturally constructed, he suggests, "then the standard strategy for grounding the normativity of virtue ethics in human nature is undermined" (p. 117). Cultural variation "poses a serious threat to the idea that there is a single set of virtues that is conducive to human flourishing" (Prinz, 2009, p. 136). Consequently, Harman (2000) suggested that we abandon all thought and talk about virtues because thinking in terms of character and virtue "has disastrous effects on people's understanding of each other, on their understandings of what social programs are reasonable to support, and of their understandings of international affairs" (p. 224). As an alternative, Harman suggested that people should be convinced "to look at situational factors and to stop trying to explain things in terms of character traits. We need to abandon all talk of virtue and character, not find a way to save it by reinterpreting it" (p. 224). Similarly, Sumner (1996, p. 79) argues that "the conclusion of Aristotle's argument, the equation of welfare and virtue, has always seemed too good to be true." Finally, even if Aristotle's concept of telos is important, his "so-called orthogenesis view that there is an intrinsic striving ("orthogenesis") toward perfection in living nature is not trustworthy" (Mayr, 2004, p. 24).

Summing up on Aristotle

My review of Aristotelian eudaimonism is brief, simple, and only one of many possible interpretations. It is written by a nonphilosopher, and my selection of sources is somewhat arbitrary (although not completely so). Nevertheless, I hope it will serve as a suitable outline of Aristotle's core ideas about wellbeing (eudaimonia) in the present context. To be brutally short, I suggest that the main idea of Aristotelian eudaimonism may be cut down to the following.

First, Aristotle's theory of the good life is a very broad notion of a life going well and contains only a very thin specification of a telos, or final end (Annas, 1993). Nevertheless, the telos is important because it makes striving for wellbeing the only goal that is truly intrinsic, i.e., worth pursuing for its own sake.

Second, the telos connects with the notion of functioning. The functioning argument juxtaposes goodness with excellent performance, which can be defined as fulfilling an essential capacity. The essential capacity of something is determined by its nature, and for humans, it is to be rational. Proper reasoning will instruct us to act virtuously by cultivating contemplation, or alternatively, practical wisdom that "dispose us to behave in accordance with the doctrine of the mean: we should acquire traits that steer between deficiency and excess" (Prinz, 2009, p. 133). Virtuous behavior also includes the notion of completeness or wholeness. Being eudaimon applies to a person's life *as a whole* and not merely to what he or she thinks or feels about it. Thus, virtues endow us with characteristically human lives (Prinz, 2009, p. 133).

By and large, Aristotelian eudaimonism suggests that our lives can only be good if we fulfill our human nature, i.e., if we perform our humanness well. However, to be useful, these general features must be further specified. Aristotle identified human nature as being actively goal oriented, rational, and social, which he further laid out as acting rationally and in accordance with virtue. But Aristotle's suggestions are 2350 years old and not necessarily the specification we need today. Hence, a review of eudaimonia might well start with Aristotle, but it should not end with him. Building on the principal idea that some elements of our human nature must be fulfilled to call a life well lived, a science of eudaimonic wellbeing must begin by identifying those elements of our nature that, when fulfilled, stimulate a way of living that can reasonably be called good.

Eudaimonic Wellbeing Evolves

The notion of eudaimonia has influenced psychologists for more than a hundred years. For example, William McDougall launched the idea of a "hormic psychology" in the first edition of his voluminous *Introduction to Social Psychology* in 1908. Hormism is a teleological concept, and its basic idea is that activities are not motivated by an urge to maximize pleasure but are rather undertaken "in the pursuit of some goal, for the sake of some result which we foresee and desire to achieve" (McDougall, 1950, p. 446). To a hormist, pleasure is not seen as an end in itself; it is more like a byproduct or "incidental to the pursuit and attainment of some goal toward which some hormic impulse sets" (p. 468).

Somewhat later, Kurt Goldstein articulated a holistic approach to an overarching analysis of humans and other biological organisms. His magnum opus, *The Organism* (Goldstein, 1939), came to play a major role in establishing the "third force" movement of humanistic psychology. Goldstein was educated in neurology and psychiatry, but his theory of self-actualization and organismic living was psychological by content. It was also founded on eudaimonic thinking. Goldstein's key idea was that all organisms have an inborn "tendency to actualize its nature, to actualize 'itself'" (Goldstein, 1939, p. 196). Goldstein advocated the view that organisms are continuously active and self-regulated toward preserving their organic structure and expanding that structure (within limits). The organismic approach contrasts the mechanistic and reductionistic approaches in biology and opposes hedonic and behavioristic ideas in psychology. As discussed below, organismic thinking is consistent with Aristotelian eudaimonism, although Goldstein's theory is not completely Aristotelic. For example, Goldstein's concept of self-actualization does not posit a predefined self (Morley, 1995). Nevertheless, his book inspired scholars such as Maslow, Rogers, de Charms, White, Allport, Jahoda, and many others. Maslow even dedicated his book *Toward a Psychology of Being* to Kurt Goldstein.

Organismic Theories

Although Goldstein disseminated the notion of organismic living to a broad audience, he was not the inventor of the term "organismic." Thinkers such as Leibnitz and Spinoza had prepared the ground for the idea that organisms are holistic, active, and self-regulating systems that consistently strive toward self-preservation and self-affirmation. However, it was the biologists William E. Ritter (1919) who first introduced the word organismic to muster these common characteristics. The term was later adapted and developed by scholars such as Ashby (1946), von Bertalanffy (1952/2014), Hebb (1949), Piaget (1952), Vygotsky (1978), Blasi (1976), and Maslow (1954). The organismic approach is firmly grounded in the term holism, which Smuts (1926) defined as the idea that the whole is more than the sum of its parts (Mayr, 1982, p. 66). Eventually, the concept of holism was expanded to include the notion of emergence, i.e., the way in which new and often unexpected characteristics can arise in a system as a result of interactions among its components (Mayr, 2010; Thagard, 2019). For example, a water molecule, which is a combination of two hydrogen atoms and one oxygen atom, is different from the individual properties the hydrogen and oxygen atoms have on their own. Similarly, a heart can pump blood, whereas none of its components can. A scientifically respectable characterization of emergence has been laid out to occur "when (a) the whole has a property not found in any of its parts, (b) the property of the whole is not simply the sum or aggregate of the properties of the parts, and (c) the property results from the interactions of the parts" (Thagard, 2019, p. 12).

As noted by von Bertalanffy (1952/2014, pp. 18–19), the organismic principles are dynamic, active, and include the interplay between stability and homeostatic maintenance on the one hand and "spontaneous movements" toward growth on the other. Spontaneous activity is the primary modus of operations of an organism, and mechanical (or stimulus response–directed behavior) is "superimposed upon it," von Bertalanffy argued (1952, p. 20). More recently, Ruiz-Mirazo et al. (2000, pp. 211–219) described an organism-centered biology as one that presupposes that "organisms are bounded and informed self-organising systems whose processes cannot be fully explained in mechanical terms." Furthermore, the authors claim that the idea of organismic living expresses "a special emphasis on aspects like autonomy and the capacity of a system to create its own world of meanings" (p. 218).

A final core element in the organismic framework is interaction. Interactions occur not only between parts within the system and between the parts and the system as a whole but also between an organism and its external environment. Mayr therefore argues that the most essential aspect of the organismic approach is relationships. He cites Georges Braque, who declared that "I do not believe in things, I believe in their relationships" (Mayr, 1982, p. 67). These interactions make both the life sciences unique (different from the natural sciences) and each organism unique (different from other members of their species). Every human, as everything else alive, is unique not only in its genetics but also in its genuine life stories of interactions (Mayr, 2010).

Many psychologists of the mid-twentieth century were inspired by the notion of organismic biology (e.g., Deci & Ryan, 1985; Ryan, 1993; Ryan & Deci, 2017). A common core of these perspectives is the belief in an organism's capacity for development toward increased complexity and that increased complexity means better functioning. One approach was formulated by Blasi (1976), who maintained that the organismic model depicted human development as a series of discontinuous upheavals with the capacity to change us in a more functional and thus better direction. The crucial element in the organismic approach, Blasi claims, is the ability to consider certain forms or patterns as privileged or "good." He pointed to Piaget for an example and argued that Piaget's theory is not purely descriptive. The theory specifies what it means for a cognitive structure to develop in optimal ways (Blasi, 1976, p. 38). In contrast, the "tabula rasa" component in behaviorism restricts human development to merely comprise an accumulation of associations between the elements of sensation. For the behaviorist, development is something that happens deterministically, and it cannot be described in terms of improvement or deterioration.

The mechanistic worldview entailed in behaviorism was a major reason why the "Humanistic Revolution," or the "Third Force," emerged in psychology. According to Maslow, one of the movements' leading figures, the promise of an organismic rather than mechanistic understanding of humans was convincing to a long list of psychologists, including (in addition to Maslow himself) writers such as Fromm, Horney, Jung, Buhler, Angyal, Allport, Schachtel, Lynd, and "some Catholic psychologists" (Maslow, 1962, p. 28). More names from the early and mid-twentieth century could easily be added to the list, Kaufman (2016) nominates Erik H. Erikson, and Ryan (1995) mentions Loevinger and Werner. This group of scholars shared two important beliefs about human nature: first, that our goals are not limited to maximizing pleasure and, second, that we, as all living systems, are geared to both preserving our biological structure and extending it. Humans are in other words inherently oriented toward both stability and growth.

Abraham Maslow

Maslow was the archbishop of humanistic psychology, and his great passion was perfection. Maslow sought to understand how psychological health can be refined to "the fullest degree of humanness" (Maslow, 1971, p. 7). He spent much of his career pondering why some people became what he called "superior specimen," while others stagnated at "unhealthy" levels of development. What motivates the best among us? Maslow asked. The answer turned up in his well-known hierarchy of needs (Maslow, 1943). The five basic human needs, or sets of goals, as he also called them, are physiological, safety, love, esteem, and self-actualization. The needs are organized as a five-stage model in which each need builds on the other, and higher needs will therefore not be activated until the previous needs are fulfilled. The hierarchical structure in Maslow's motivational model was not as rigid as typically imagined—the well-known pyramid metaphor did, for instance, not come from Maslow but from a management consultant in the 1960s (Bridgman et al., 2019). Yet, the distinction between lower and higher needs is crucial in Maslow's theory. He was very explicit that lower needs must be properly satisfied before higher needs can be met (e.g., Maslow, 1971, p. 290). But see Rojas et al. (2023) for a recent empirical study that disconfirms Maslow's hierarchical hypothesis.

The notion of lower and higher needs is clearly related to the difference between maintaining stability and facilitating growth. The business of the lower needs, the D-needs, is to overcome deficiencies and secure a feeling of safety. The higher needs are concerned with expansion and the enhancements of being, hence the name B-needs (Maslow, 1962). Needless (sic) to say, Maslow's concept of self-actualization was related to B-needs, and here, Maslow was Aristotelian and organismic in his thinking (Morley, 1995). Actualization is teleologically driven toward a "naturalistic humanness," and Maslow maintained that "Man demonstrates *in his own nature* (italics in original) a pressure toward fuller and fuller Being, more and more perfect actualization of his humanness in exactly the naturalistic, scientific sense that an acorn may be said to be 'pressing toward' being an oak tree, or that a tiger can be observed to 'push toward' being tigerish, or a horse toward being equine" (Maslow, 1962, loc. 2237).

When studying self-actualized people, Maslow noted that their motivation was qualitatively different from that of others. Self-actualizers actively strive toward perfection, constantly seeking opportunities for character growth, character expression, maturation, and development. Maslow's grand idea was that all the desirable traits in a human being are positively correlated (Maslow, 1971, p. 6), and his master plan was to identify a small and selected group of "superior specimen" and start digging into them in depth. By mapping the capabilities of these "best people," Maslow imagined that he would be able to uncover the highest and most universal values of humankind. By means of these "growing tip statistics," he speculated that he could "find ultimate values which are right for mankind by observing the best of mankind" (Maslow, 1961, pp. 5–6). He even argued that he had established an objective method that stood "above cultures," something he could use to analyze the "moral principles common to the entire human spices" (Kendler, 1987, p. 424).

This insight made Maslow enthusiastically exclaim that "There is now emerging over the horizon a new conception of human sickness and of human health, a psychology that I find so thrilling and so full of wonderful possibilities that I yield to the temptation to present it publicly even before it is checked and confirmed, and before it can be called reliable scientific knowledge" (Maslow, 1962, loc. 158). He summarized some of his discoveries in a catalog of capabilities that features the best and healthiest among us. The list is presented in Table 6.1.

Maslow's evidence about self-actualizers' tendency to share the same values and capabilities was tautological, at least in the sense that the individuals he classified as self-actualizers were people who also shared his moral code to begin with. He thus confirmed his ideas about self-actualization by analyzing the character traits of people whose sampling criteria were those very character traits that Maslow wanted to validate (Kendler, 1999).

Table 6.1 Maslow's list of self-actualizing characteristics

1. More efficient perception of reality
2. Acceptance of self, others, and nature
3. Spontaneity
4. Problem centering
5. Detachment
6. Independence of culture and environment
7. Continued freshness of appreciation
8. Limitless horizons
9. Social feeling
10. Deep but selective social relationships
11. Democratic character structure
12. Ethical certainty
13. Unhostile sense of humor
14. Creativeness
15. Resistance to enculturation

Maslow's biases go beyond his selective sampling theory. He was, for instance, embarrassingly elitist—and seriously flawed—in adapting the opinion that "all desirable traits in a human being correlate positively" (Maslow, 1971, p. 6). Consider his method for identifying the best way to lead our lives or determine our ultimate values. Here, Maslow suggested that we could "select the healthiest 2 percent of our population" and use these "good specimen as the chooser for the whole species" (Maslow, 1971, p. 8). Just as the best runners can tell us what the human potential for running is, "the healthiest people (or the most creative, or the strongest, or the wisest, or the saintliest) can be used as biological assays, or perhaps I could say, as advance scouts, or more sensitive perceivers, to tell us less sensitive ones what it is that we value" (pp. 8–9). Maslow even cited Aristotle in claiming that "what the superior man thinks is good, that is what is *really* (italics in original) good" (p. 9).

Maslow's proposal that the self-actualized among us should determine the "healthy values" disagrees with the social epistemology presented in Chap. 1. Feminist thinkers such as Sandra Harding, Helen Longino, and Carol Gilligan argue that it is the open dialog between a multitude of perspectives, what Fleck (1979) referred to as "thought collectives," that secures scientific quality. Maslow's idea that objectivity will be reached by excluding the perspectives of 98% of humankind is not only the opposite of objectivity but also the opposite of humanism.

Carl Rogers

Carl Rogers is remembered as a founding figure in humanistic psychology, but compared with Maslow, he was less of an elitist thinker. Rogers spent much time developing the concept of a fully functioning person, and he shared with many of his peers the idea that individuals are naturally oriented toward realizing their full potential. Rogers referred to this tendency to improve oneself via better organization and personal growth as the *organismic valuing process*. It served as a holistic framework for his thinking and constituted what Rogers believed to be the only true human motive (Maurer & Daukantaitė, 2020; Proctor et al., 2016; Vittersø, 2013). The goal of this never-ending progress is to develop one's full potential and become "the self one truly is" (Rogers, 1961). To realize one's full potential, it is necessary to be embraced by a growth-promoting atmosphere, an environment of trust and transparency. Rogers talked about this phenomenon as unconditional positive regard. When people feel psychologically safe, they will "feel enough trust to gradually dare to open themselves up toward their self, listening to the inner processes and becoming more self-aware, particularly of one's emotional and cognitive movement" (Maurer & Daukantaitė, 2020, p. 2).

Reading Rogers from the vantagepoint of modern psychology can be a disappointment. The theory is conceptually vague, empirically weak, and there is not much integration between Rogers' thinking and modern psychological knowledge. On the surface, his ideas may appear intuitively sound. However, scrutinized in detail, Rogers' message turns out to be either too good to be true or too hard to understand. For example, how should we interpret the scope of the characteristic of being open to experience? Such a person "would have access to all of the available data in the situation, on which to base his behavior; the social demands, his own complex and possibly conflicting needs; his memories of similar situations, his perception of the uniqueness of this situation, etc." (Rogers, 1963, p. 20). But how real is such a person? How can someone "have access to all of the available data in the situation"? It's a little like the virtuous person who "think, feel and act at the right time, about the right things, toward the right people, for the right end, and in the right way" (Badhwar, 2014, p. 143).

And what about living every moment to the fullest without concentrating on either the past or the future? Momentary feelings are important, but so is planning. Gilbert (2006) has even declared that "the human being is the only animal that thinks about the future" (p. 4). There is obviously a trade-off between living in the moment, remembering the past, and planning for the future. This balance is under-communicated by Rogers.

The organismic valuing process is firmly grounded in the individual, and Rogers has been critiqued for being individualistic and Pollyanna theorizing (Joseph & Linley, 2004; O'Dwyer, 2012). Even if the self-realized person is not selfish, Rogers' writing lacks a clear articulation of the person as a cultural being. A full acceptance of the self and one's emotions may constitute a basis for accepting other people, Rogers argues (1961), but it does not account for the sociability and shared intentionality documented in the work of Tomasello or the empathy, compassion, and caring attitude as articulated in feminist morality (Chaps. 1 and 7). This knowledge was not available for Rogers. But it is for us, which illustrates the need to upgrade theories and concepts as new understandings evolve.

A final critique that applies to Rogers' theory can be found in Kagan (1994).[5] Kagan suggests that a carefully developed theory starts with something robust and awaits listing names and concepts until after a reliable functional understanding has been established. "Many psychologists, by contrast, prefer to begin their inquiry by assuming the reality of *a priori*, idealized concepts that they try to find in nature" (p. 75).

Hadley Cantril

Hadley Cantril is not associated with the movement of humanistic psychology, but his theory of wellbeing (Cantril, 1965, 1988) is closer to Aristotelian thinking than is typically acknowledged (e.g., Campbell et al., 1976). Cantril did not use the term eudaimonic, but his concept of "human concerns" is grounded in the idea that humans have the capacity to experience something Cantril referred to as "valued satisfaction." For example, in interpreting the results from his large cross-national study, Cantril noted that "Our data confirm the truth of Aristotle's observation that happiness comes from 'the exercise of vital powers along lines of excellence in a life affording them scope'" (Cantril, 1965, p. 273).

Cantril had a growth perspective on wellbeing, and he thought of humans as having an inborn desire to enrich the values of their lives. The process develops in stages, from the most primitive, which he called "acquiescence to circumstances," to the fifth and highest level of personal development, the stage of "satisfaction and gratification." Individuals who reach this stage will feel that even if they have "arrived" at their final level of development, they still have much to learn. Here is an excerpt of what Cantril thinks about value satisfaction.

> The guiding star for the individual in this process is a capacity unique to the human being as a species; namely the capacity to experience satisfaction that are permeated with value overtones. As human beings, we seem to seek a quality of experience far different from that sought by any other organism we know. Man's capacity to experience value satisfactions propels him to learn and to devise new ways of behaving that will enable him both to extend the range and heighten the quality of value satisfaction and to ensure the repeatability of these value satisfactions already experienced. While the principle of homeostasis and the notion of a drive to reduce "cognitive dissonance" are useful in describing certain limited phases of human behavior, I think both of these accounting models fall short of the mark by overlooking the larger context of this more enduring, overriding characteristics of man. (Cantril, 1965, p. 10)

[5] Kagan's advice is directed toward psychological theories in general and not toward Rogers' theory in particular.

Today, Cantril is not recognized for his Aristotelian thinking and ideas about personal growth and valued satisfaction. He is known for the Cantril ladder, a self-report instrument intended to tap into the evaluative dimension of wellbeing. More concretely, the scale asks about people's idea of "the best possible life" and not particularly about their life satisfaction. The correlations between "the best possible life" version of the Cantril ladder and more classical life satisfaction variables are strong, even if these scales are not identical (Deaton & Stone, 2016; Helliwell et al., 2016; Nilsson et al., 2024;Tsurumi et al., 2021). However, Cantril did not develop his scale to measure life satisfaction; rather, the aim was to map people's values and the extent to which these values were realized in their lives. Cantril explained that the original ladder was developed "as a means of discovering the spectrum of values a person is preoccupied or concerned with and by means of which he evaluates his own life" (Cantril, 1965, p. 22). Hence, Cantril dobbed his scale "the self-anchoring striving scale" and asked survey participants to first define their own "concerns," with reference to their goals, values, and perceptions. Only in the second step came the actual placement on the "ladder of life." But it is only this part of Cantril's ladder that is used today (but see Møller and Roberts (2017) for a recent use of Cantril's original design). Participants in large surveys such as those reported in The World Happiness Report (e.g., Helliwell et al., 2024) are no longer asked *what* their best life consists of, only how close their lives are to the abstract notion of "a best possible life."

Other Pioneers

Norman Bradburn (1969) is associated with studies of affect and a hedonistic perspective on wellbeing (e.g., Campbell et al., 1976). However, Bradburn started his quest for the good life, or the "most fruitful dependent variable in a healthy life," with Aristotle and the *Nicomachean Ethics* (Bradburn, 1969, p. 6). Bradburn examined the development of eudaimonia in the history of ideas and paid attention to its translation into English. In particular, he was interested in how the concept of happiness, which was the traditional translation of eudaimonia, has changed over time. During the Enlightenment, happiness was for instance associated with political rights but came, as we have seen, eventually to change it meaning. Hence, in the USA in the nineteenth century, the meaning of happiness changed toward the ideas of happiness held by thinkers such as Adam Smith and Benjamin Franklin. Then, influenced by the writing of William James, the meaning of a happy life turned more psychological, and the original Aristotelian idea of happiness as a life in accordance with one's nature gradually disappeared (see McMahon, 2006). Bradburn was well aware of the altered meaning given to the term happiness, but he was also inspired by Marie Jahoda's writing on mental health and the idea that happiness comes as a consequence of solving the "problems in living." Interestingly, however, Bradburn concluded his reading of Jahoda with a notion of happiness that, in many respects, was similar "to older pleasure-pain or utility models that view an individual's happiness or well-being in terms of the degree to which pleasure predominates over pain in his life experiences" (Bradburn, 1969, p. 9). Bradburn dobbed his Jahoda-inspired model of happiness "psychological well-being."

A final eudaimonic contribution from the youth of wellbeing research worth mentioning is a paper by the theologian Richard Creel (1983). Drawing on Aristotelian eudaimonism, Creel wanted to establish a science of happiness by the name of eudology: "I am convinced that because of the importance of happiness to most people, because of the methodological advances of social science, and because of the number of social scientists who are conducting eudological studies, that all the historical conditions are present for the formation of a new scientific focus" (Creel, 1983, p. 312). In his call, Creel said little more than "Let us have a science of happiness." This credo was surprisingly similar to what Seligman articulated in his editorial column for the *APA Monitor* 15 years later (Seligman, 1998). But the reception of the two invitations was dramatically different. Whereas Seligman was honored as visionary, Creel was deemed an illusionist. The reason, according to Csikszentmihalyi (1983), was the normative spirit of Creel's proposal and his lack of a falsifiable definition of happiness. As noted in Chap. 1, however, the normative evocation in positive psychology is critically challenged (see also Kristjánsson, 2013; Prinzing, 2021), and Chap. 2 revealed that positive psychologists hardly have agreed upon a falsifiable definition of happiness. Hence, Creel's proposal might have been rejected prematurely.

The Big Three

The popularity of eudaimonic approaches in wellbeing research spurred with Waterman's "Two Concepts of Happiness" article from 1993, with the increased approval for the ideas Ryff (1989) presented in her "Happiness is everything?" paper, and with a much-cited text about eudaimonic wellbeing by Ryan and Deci (2001). Each of the "big three" approaches will be surveyed in turn. However, since the philosopher David Norton's interpretation of eudaimonism has had an imperative impact on Waterman's thinking about eudaimonia and, to some extent, also influenced Ryff's psychological wellbeing theory, I will start with a summary of Norton's philosophy.

David Norton

In his book *Personal Destinies: A Philosophy of Ethical Individualism,* Norton claims that eudaimonia is an individualistic business. According to his reading of Plato and Aristotle, eudaimonism is the ethical doctrine "that each person is obliged to know and live in truth to his *daimon* (italics in original), thereby progressively actualizing an excellence that is his innately and potentiality" (p. ix). To be true to one's daimon means to following one's "personal truths," rather than the truths of others (p. 7). Consequently, "it is every person's primary responsibility first to discover the daimon within him and thereafter to live in accordance with it. (…) Each person is free to adhere to his destiny or deviate from it, but he cannot change it" (Norton, 1976, p. 16). Such an interpretation does not fit commonly accepted understandings of what it means to be eudaimon.

Norton does not really analyze Aristotle in much detail.[6] Rather, he seems to cherry-pick quotes from the Classic Greek philosophers, in addition to more recent ones, to construct his own scheme of ethical reasoning. His theory is essentially grounded in a distinction between three different kinds of truths: "truths of reasons," "truths of facts," and "truths of self" (Norton, 1976, p. 7). Truths of self, or "personal truth," exist within us and are determined by our own daimon. This truth is unique to each and one of us; they belong to our beings; thus, we must avoid living our lives according to "truths that belong to others" (p. 9). In a nutshell, what Norton picks up from Hellenic eudaimonism is that we should be steadfastly obedient to our "inner voices," which is the truth that our personal daimon tells us to follow.

Another controversial element in *Personal Destinies* is the definition of eudaimonia as both a condition and a feeling. According to Norton's ethical individualism, the relation between the two is such that the feeling constitutes the intrinsic reward of the condition "and therefore bears the same name as the condition itself. Provisionally we will describe the feeling of eudaimonia as 'being where one wants to be, doing what one wants to do'" (Norton, 1976, p. 216). This notion of eudaimonia is quite different from Aristotle's definition of the human good as "activity of soul in accordance with virtue" or MacIntyre's slogan that eudaimonia is a state of "being well and doing well in being well" (MacIntyre, 2007, p. 148). Fowers (2016) is also critical to Norton's formulations of eudaimonia. He argues that Aristotle viewed excellence as a matter of cultivating good character and habits, not as an expression of the "truth" of an inner self. The ancient Greeks "did not have a concept of an inner self to which one should or even could be 'true'" (Fowers, 2016, p. 72). The complete lack of sociability or cultural community in Norton's thinking has been criticized, and his philosophy has been called "extremely eccentric" (Keyes & Annas, 2009). Norton's work has even been categorized alongside the ultra-elitist, oligarchic, and anti-humanistic ideology of the writer Ayn Rand (Machan, 1979).

Alan Waterman: Identity and Personal Expressiveness

Waterman's eudaimonic identity theory adopted Norton's individualistic fulfillment ideology in combination with neo-psychoanalytic identity theorists such as Horney, Erikson, and Marcia. Hence, Waterman developed a theory with an individualistic

---

[6] All in all, the discussion of Aristotelian eudaimonism in *Personal Destinies* covers no more than a dozen paragraphs—in a book that runs almost 400 pages.

self-realization perspective and defined eudaimonia as "the feeling accompanying behavior in the direction of, and consistent with, one's true potential" (Waterman, 1984, p. 16). As a synonym for eudaimonia, Waterman used the phrase "feelings of personal expressiveness" (Waterman & Schwartz, 2013, p. 104), which thus reduces his concept of eudaimonia to a feeling. This feeling will "typically accompany efforts at self-realization, including the sense that one is acting in such a way that one is truly being oneself" (Waterman, 2008, p. 236). Predictors of such personal expressiveness are "(a) an unusually intense involvement in an undertaking, (b) a feeling of a special fit or meshing with an activity that is not characteristic of most daily tasks, (c) a feeling of intensely being alive, (d) a feeling of being complete or fulfilled while engaged in an activity, (e) an impression that this is what the person was meant to do, and (f) a feeling that this is who one really is" (Waterman, 1993, p. 679).

Waterman's affective theory categorizes the feelings relevant for wellbeing into two groups: hedonic enjoyment and eudaimonic/expressive feelings.[7] Hedonic enjoyment and eudaimonic feelings can be experienced intensely or not intensely. Thus, Waterman's taxonomy can be schematized in a two-by-two table, in which experiences can be either high or low in hedonic enjoyment or high or low in eudaimonia.

With reference to Elizabeth Telfer, Waterman notes that "from a philosophical perspective, eudaimonia has been deemed a sufficient, but not a necessary, condition for hedonic enjoyment (Telfer 1980)" (Waterman et al., 2008, p. 43). Given that both hedonic and eudaimonic feelings are generated by activities, Waterman argues that "there are three conceivable categories of activities, (a) those for which both hedonic enjoyment and eudaimonia are experienced; (b) those for which hedonic enjoyment, but not eudaimonia, is experienced; and (c) those giving rise to neither hedonic enjoyment nor eudaimonia" (p. 43). However, this is not quite what Telfer argues. She distinguishes between empirical and logical analyses of wellbeing and explains about the former that "eudaimonia is empirically neither necessary nor sufficient for [hedonic] happiness." In contrast, when seen from a logical perspective, "happiness might be part of the definition of eudaimonia and so a logically necessary condition of it" (Telfer, 1980, p. 135).[8] Principally speaking, a person can be happy without being eudaimon. But a person cannot be eudaimon unless he or she is happy.[9] Telfer maintains that eudaimonia and hedonia belong to different categories: "eudaimonia is constituted by a way of life, whereas hedonic happiness is a

[7] Waterman uses the terms eudaimonic feelings and expressive feelings interchangeably.

[8] Since necessity and sufficiency are logically dual to one another, Waterman can turn Telfer's formulation (happiness as necessary for eudaimonia) into his preferred statement of eudaimonia as sufficient for hedonic enjoyment.

[9] In more detail, the reasoning is as follows: to claim that eudaimonia is not necessary for happiness is to say that a person can be happy without being eudaimon. To claim that eudaimonia is not sufficient for happiness is to say that being eudaimonia will not bring happiness. If happiness is part of the definition of eudaimonia, however, it must be necessary for eudaimonia. Consequently, one must be happy to be eudaimon.

reaction to a way of life" (Telfer, 1980, p. 39). She defines hedonic happiness as "being pleased with one's life" and eudaimonia as "a life worth living." These definitions allow Telfer to conclude that eudaimonia is sufficient for hedonia because a person who is leading a life worth living must, by theoretical necessity, be pleased about their life.

However, Waterman defines both hedonic enjoyment and eudaimonia as feeling states, which means that they do not belong to different categories—which is a premise for Telfers' necessary but not sufficient logic about happiness and eudaimonia. Whether eudaimonic feelings are included in hedonic enjoyment is thus an empirical question, not a logical one. Waterman finds some empirical support for his "sufficient but not necessary" proposal. For example, in three studies reported in Waterman et al. (2008), activities low in both hedonic and eudaimonia feelings were more frequently listed than those for any other combination. In total, 2037 of the 2972 reported activities (65.5%) in these studies were rated low–low, whereas 18.2% were rated high–high. Only 2.9% of the activities were reported to be experienced as low in hedonic enjoyment and high in eudaimonia. This is the category that philosophically speaking should be a "theoretical null." However, even if hedonic and eudaimonic feelings are highly correlated and even if eudaimonia is rarely experienced without hedonic enjoyment, one cannot conclude that eudaimonia is sufficient for hedonic enjoyment from empirical data. For example, in a constructed sample of data, three participants may score 5, 4, or 4 on eudaimonic feelings and 4, 0, or 0 on hedonic feelings. In this case, the correlation between eudaimonia and hedonia is 1, but the majority of the participants have very high scores on eudaimonic feelings without having any hedonic feelings at all.

Waterman's conceptualization of eudaimonia is debatable. First, the link to Norton's ethical individualism and the idea that we must identify our own daimon and live according to our personal truths rather than the truths of others is a controversial interpretation of Aristotelian eudaimonism. Second, restricting eudaimonia to a feeling state is also at odds with most understandings of the concept. Finally, the notion that eudaimonic feelings are nested within hedonic feelings, which is what Waterman's "sufficient but not necessary" proposal means, indicates that a eudaimonic feeling is a kind of a hedonic feeling. As illustrated in Fig. 6.1, Waterman's theory suggests that you cannot experience eudaimonic feelings unless you are also in a state of hedonic enjoyment. Such a conceptualization of feelings has little support in the literature on affect and emotions. Chapter 3 examined some of the major affect theories, and none of them defend the view that one feeling

Fig. 6.1 Eudaimonia as sufficient for hedonia

quality is nested within another. Many feelings are seen as basic (i.e., irreducible), resulting from appraisals, or constructed (i.e., as a combination of core affect and emotional concepts). Several examples were given in Chap. 3 to illustrate that you do not have to feel happy (a hedonic feeling) to feel interested (a eudaimonic feeling). According to Waterman, however, it is necessary to be in a state of hedonic enjoyment to feel personal expressiveness, i.e., to be eudaimon.

Carol Ryff: Psychological Wellbeing

Coming from the study of successful aging and lifelong development research, Ryff advanced a theory of psychological wellbeing (PWB) that is often categorized as eudaimonic (e.g., Ryff, 1989, 2018; Ryff & Singer, 2008). The PWB partly emerged as a response to research on subjective wellbeing, which Ryff characterized as a tradition with "little theoretical grounding." She accused most studies of wellbeing of having neglected the fundamental task of "defining the essential features of psychological wellbeing" (Ryff, 1989, p. 1069) and claimed that early, empirical attempts to investigate happiness and life satisfaction had "largely nothing behind it conceptually" (Ryff, 2016, p. 96).

Ryff consulted three theoretical schools when her psychological wellbeing approach was established. She looked at the psychological literature on positive functioning, particularly the writings of Maslow, Rogers, Jung, and Allport. She also analyzed life span theorists such as Erikson, Bühler, and Neugarten. Finally, Ryff was inspired by Jahoda's perspective on mental health.[10] As for balancing these perspectives against each other, Ryff (2018) claims that none of these perspectives stood above the rest. However, there is a similarity between her list of six dimensions of psychological wellbeing (self-acceptance, autonomy, environmental mastery, personal growth, meaning in life, and positive relation) and the six items on Jahoda's (1958) list of mental health indicators (self-acceptance, autonomy, environmental mastery, growth/self-actualization, perception of reality, and integration). A schematic overview of the structure of the PWB and its theoretical heritage is provided in Table 6.2. The setup is based on Ryff (1989, 2016, 2018) and Ryff and Singer (2008).

Psychological wellbeing theory is grounded in a literature with little empirical documentation. To remedy this situation, Ryff developed a self-report instrument, the Ryff scales, which became popular. As of 2018, it has been translated into more than 30 languages, resulting in over 750 publications (Ryff, 2018). An impressive number of health and wellbeing benefits have been found to correlate with the Ryff scales (e.g., Ryff et al., 2021). However, the instrument seems to overlap strongly with mainstream SWB measures, which speaks against the independence Ryff claims for her theory. Early factor analyses of PWB and SWB variables revealed,

[10] Somewhat later (e.g., Ryff & Singer, 2008), Frankl was also added to the list.

Table 6.2 Ryff's six dimensions of psychological wellbeing and some of its theoretical inspirations

Dimension	Description	Theoretical inspiration
Autonomy	Seek a sense of self-determination and personal authority in order to sustain individuality within a larger social context	– Autonomous functioning (Maslow) – Internal locus of evaluation (Rogers) – Deliverance from convention (Jung) – Turning inward in later life (Erikson) – Sense of freedom (Neugarten)
Environmental mastery	Seek to shape one's environment to meet personal needs and desires	– Ability to choose or create suitable environments (Jahoda) – Ability to act on and change one's surroundings (Erikson) – Extend the self into spheres of endeavor that go beyond the self (Allport)
Personal Growth	Making the most of one's talents and capacities. Seeking self-realization and achieving personal potential. Openness toward continued development	– Personal becoming (Maslow) – Being fully functioning (Rogers) – Being fully individuated (Jung) – Confronting new challenges at different periods of life (Erikson, Bühler, Neugarten)
Positive relations	Seek to develop and maintain warm and trusting interpersonal relationships	– Ability to love (Jahoda) – Empathy for all humans and capacity for deep friendship (Maslow) – Warm relating to others (Allport) – Achieving close unions with others and having concern for guiding and directing others (Erikson)
Purpose In life	Find meaning in one's efforts and challenges	– Having beliefs that give one a sense of purpose (Jahoda) – Having a clear comprehension of one's purpose (Allport) – Changing goals and purposes over the life span (Erikson, Jung, Neugarten) – Search for meaning (Frankl)
Self-acceptance	Attempts to feel good about oneself even while aware of own limitations	– Positive self-regard (Maslow) – Maturity (Allport) – Optimal functioning (Rogers) – Acceptance of self (Erikson, Neugarten) – Individuation and acceptance of the dark sides of one's self (Jung)

for instance, a correlation between PWB and SWB of $r = 0.84$ (Keyes et al., 2002), and a more recent study, with slightly different indicators of SWB, reported an $r = 0.96$ between the SWB and the PWB factors (Disabato et al., 2016).

However, the high correlations found between PWB and SWB as second-order factors conceal a variety of correlation sizes for the subcomponents of the scales. For example, in two studies reported by Margolis et al. (2019), environmental mastery correlated approximately 0.70 with life satisfaction. Similarly, self-acceptance correlated with life satisfaction in the range of 0.86 to 0.90. In contrast, personal growth correlated with life satisfaction in the range of 0.21 to 0.31. In other words, not all the dimensions of the Ryff scales are strongly related to SWB.

The Eudaimonic Elements in PWB

Aristotelian eudaimonism was reflected in PWB from the beginning (Ryff, 2018, p. 242), although Aristotle played a minor role in the early versions of the theory. He was, for instance, absent in the 1989 article "Beyond Ponce de Leon and Life Satisfaction," which Ryff takes to be the text in which the details of the theory were first introduced (Ryff, 1989, p. 1071). The more frequently cited "Happiness Is Everything?" paper briefly suggests that personal growth might be the dimension in her theory that comes closest to Aristotle's notion of eudaimonia (Ryff, 1989, p. 1071). However, the article does not offer much in terms of eudaimonic analyses. With reference to a book by Waterman from 1984—with the telling title *The Psychology of Individualism*— eudaimonism is introduced as "the feelings accompanying behavior in the direction of, and consistent with, one's true potential" (Ryff, 1989, p. 1071). Ryff further explains that the daimon part of eudaimonia is "an ideal in the sense of excellence, a perfection toward which one strives, and it gives meaning and direction to one's life." That is all there is about eudaimonia in the "Happiness is Everything?" paper. Even Bradburn, whom Ryff criticizes for being untheoretical and essentially empirical, devotes more space to analyzing Aristotle's concept of happiness than does Ryff. And Bradburn's treatment of Aristotle is short—most of it is covered on pages 6 and 7 in his *Structure of Psychological Well-Being* book (cf. the "Other Pioneers" section above).

Some years after the two 1989 papers, Ryff and her colleagues made the link to Aristotle more explicit. In addition to the personal growth dimension, Keyes et al. (2002) declare that the purpose in life dimension is also eudaimonic. The authors further explain that other dimensions, such as positive relations and self-acceptance, do not reflect "the self-fulfillment meanings of eudaimonic well-being" (p. 1007). The connections between Aristotelian eudaimonism and PWB have also examined elsewhere, for instance, in Ryff and Singer (1998), Ryff and Singer (2008), and Ryff (2014). In these papers, Ryff also draws on Norton (1976), which she considers to be "the most thoroughgoing distillation of Hellenic eudaimonism in contemporary scholarship" (Ryff & Singer, 2013, p. 100). As noted in the "David Norton" section above, however, neo-Aristotelians such as Annas (1993), MacIntyre (2007), and (Fowers, 2016, p. 72) consider Norton's ethical individualism as controversial.

Theoretical Reasoning

Ryff is right in criticizing the weak theoretical foundation of scientific wellbeing. This unfortunate situation was noticed even in the earliest research on wellbeing (Dodge, 1930) and applies to psychology more generally and is sometimes referred to as a "theory crisis" (e.g., Borsboom et al., 2021; Eronen & Bringmann, 2021; Oberauer & Lewandowsky, 2019). But even if Ryff's intention to anchor wellbeing studies on a firm theoretical grounding is highly warranted, one may ask if the PWB stands up to the task. For example, a careful reading of Ryff's texts suggests that her theorizing basically consists of listing up a series of concepts. For example, here is how Ryff theorizes about self-acceptance:

> Self-acceptance reflects the Greek imperative to know ourselves, although positive self-regard was also emphasised as a central feature of mental health (Jahoda), a characteristic of self-actualisation (Maslow), optimal functioning (Rogers), and maturity (Allport) as well as part of self-development (Erikson, Neugarten) and individuation (Jung), which included knowing one's dark side (the shadow). (Ryff, 2014, p. 2)

The following is an explanation of the environmental mastery dimension:

> Environmental mastery is closely aligned with a key characteristic of mental health (Jahoda), namely the capacity to choose or create a living environment suitable to one's needs. Life-span developmental theories (Neugarten) emphasised the ability to control and manipulate complex environments, especially in midlife as well as to act on and change the surrounding context. Maturity (Allport) involved the capacity to extend oneself into significant spheres of endeavor. Thus, active participation in and mastery of one's surrounding environment are key elements of well-being. (Ryff, 2014, p. 3)

With a few exceptions, this is about as detailed Ryff becomes in terms of relating specific content to the concepts of her theory. To most of us, this can hardly be considered enlightening, and a reader must be well versed in the writings of Jahoda, Maslow, Rogers, Allport, Erikson, Neugarten, Jung, Frankl, Aristotle, Mill, Russell, Bühler, and Sartre to understand the theoretical structure of psychological wellbeing.

A final critique of Ryff's work relates to how it downplays the two core elements in almost any theory of wellbeing: what we feel in our lives and how we think evaluatively about it. In Table 6.2, there are no references to affective and judgmental elements in the six dimensions, except for a few associated with the self-acceptance dimension. There are some feelings and evaluative items in the Ryff scales, but I have never seen them presented as core elements in psychological wellbeing. Thus, Ryff falls short of what Sumner (1996) refers to as the criterion of descriptive adequacy. With descriptive adequacy is meant that any theory of wellbeing must fit people's ordinary experience and use of concept. A life without good feelings will hardly stand up against this criterion and neither will the idea that people's own evaluations of the quality of their lives are unimportant for them. As Haybron (2008, p. 8) points out, not even the major schools of ancient ethical thought failed to maintain that the good life was pleasant. Similarly, a talented neo-Aristotelian such as Julia Annas insists that "happiness must involve our enjoying the good things of life. It must be a pleasant life" (Annas, 1993, loc. 7135). Good feelings are simply a part of what Annas calls an intuitive requirement for a theory about wellbeing.

Ed Deci and Richard Ryan: Self-Determination

Self-determination theory (SDT) is a macro theory of human behavior and personality development that concerns motivation, innate psychological needs, and wellbeing (Deci & Ryan, 1985, 2000; Ryan et al., 2013; Ryan & Deci, 2017, 2001).[11] Subscribing to an organismic approach, SDT suggests that people do not have to be pushed or prodded to act. Rather, it is inherent in our nature to act in the direction of increased psychological differentiation. Humans "have an organizational nature, moving developmentally in a direction of greater autonomy—of greater coherence and integration in functioning" (Ryan et al., 2013, p. 61). Integration, therefore, is the ultimate problem of self-determination (Ryan & Deci, 2017, p. 648).

The notion of basic psychological needs is important in SDT. Needs are conceived of in terms of being necessary nutriments for growth and wellbeing (Ryan & Deci, 2017, p. 118), and the theory has identified three universal and innate psychological needs that qualify as such nutriments. They are the need for competence, the need for autonomy, and the need for relatedness (e.g., Deci & Ryan, 2000; Vansteenkiste et al., 2020). Psychological needs are defined as feeling states, which is to say that what humans need is to *feel* autonomous, competent, and related.

> The need for autonomy describes the need of individuals to experience self-endorsement and ownership of their actions (…) Competence refers to feeling effective in one's interactions with the social environment (…) Relatedness refers to both (…) feeling connected and involved with others and having a sense of belonging. (Ryan & Deci, 2017, p. 86)

The self-determination theory has contributed new and genuine knowledge about what we may call the human condition. Deci and Ryan have, like few others, succeeded in developing and promoting insights into how and why environments that foster autonomy, competence, and good social relations are universally important. The SDT has become immensely popular, as illustrated by a recent review that identified no less than 60 meta-analyses on various dimensions of self-determination theory (Ryan et al., 2022). Indeed, in the most updated and comprehensive presentation of the SDT (Ryan & Deci, 2017), its two founders had to surrender to their ambition of gaining a full overview of their theory. Despite their efforts over the last 40 years, Deci and Ryan had to conclude that a full overview of SDT is beyond reach. The field is just too active and too diverse for anyone to cover in completeness. Consequently, a brief resume such as the one I will provide is deemed to be unfinished. Yet, I will try my best to present a reasonable understanding of how Deci and Ryan conceptualize wellbeing.

[11] More specifically, the SDT comprises six "mini theories": cognitive evaluation theory, organismic integration theory, causal orientations theory, basic psychological needs theory, goal content theory, and relationship motivation theory (Ryan & Deci, 2017). The mini theories will not be treated separately in this review.

Wellbeing in SDT

The self-determination theory hypothesizes that the fulfillment of our needs for autonomy, competence, and relations will lead to increased wellbeing. However, these needs are themselves defined as positive feelings, and their fulfillment is defined as satisfaction. This puts the core arguments in SDT in danger of being circular. After all, positive feelings and satisfaction are constituents of wellbeing; thus, one could say that SDT is basically arguing that increased positive feeing and satisfaction lead to increased positive feelings and satisfaction. Alternatively, the theory could be interpreted to say that the kinds of feelings and satisfaction associated with fulfillment of psychological needs lead to the kinds of feelings and satisfaction we associate with wellbeing (e.g., Sheldon et al., 2019).

In a much-cited paper, Ryan and Deci refer to wellbeing as "optimal psychological functioning and experience" (Ryan & Deci, 2001, p. 142). The experiential part and the functioning part are often, but not always, considered to reflect two distinct yet overlapping perspectives on wellbeing, labeled the hedonic approach and the eudaimonic approach, respectively. As briefly mentioned in Chap. 5, the hedonic approach was initially defined as focusing "on subjective well-being, which is frequently equated with happiness and is formally defined as more positive affect, less negative affect, and greater life satisfaction" (Ryan & Deci, 2001, p. 161). The eudaimonic approach "defines well-being in terms of the degree to which a person is fully functioning" (p. 141). This paper refers to the hedonic approach as hedonic wellbeing (HWB) and the eudaimonic approach as eudaimonic wellbeing (EWB). To my knowledge, this is the first use of the term eudaimonic wellbeing in the scientific literature.

Although HWB and EWB are straightforwardly defined as "two distinct yet overlapping perspectives on wellbeing," the role of eudaimonia is not clear. Proponents of self-determination theory frequently switch between defining eudaimonia as a *kind* of wellbeing and a *predictor* of wellbeing. For example, Ryan and Deci announced that they will be "reviewing the two principal approaches to *defining* (italics added) well-being" (Ryan & Deci, 2001, p. 143). They also underscored that the eudaimonic approach "*defines* (italics added) well-being in terms of the degree to which a person is fully functioning" (p. 141). The text further claims that SDT has "embraced the concept of eudaimonia, or self-realization, as a *central definitional aspect* (italics added) of well-being" (p. 146). Ryan and Deci also "wholly concur that well-being *consists in* (italics added) what Rogers (1963) referred to as being fully functioning" (p. 147).

On the other hand, Ryan and Deci claim that "From the perspective of SDT, psychological well-being *results* (italics added) in large part from satisfaction of the basic psychological needs for autonomy, competence, and relatedness" (p. 157). And when SDT is compared with Ryff's psychological wellbeing theory, Ryan and Deci write that the basic psychological needs "are the principal factors that *foster* (italics added) well-being, whereas Ryff and Singer's approach uses them to *define* (italics added) well-being" (Ryan & Deci, 2001, p. 147).

The constituting versus predicting nature of eudaimonic wellbeing is also confusingly mixed up in later writings. In Ryan et al. (2008), the criteria held "for judging a theory of eudaimonia rest in its ability to *predict* (italics added), and when implemented, *bring about* (italics added), outcomes that people value deeply and that can be said to represent wellness" (p. 140). The foci of eudaimonic research, the authors clarify, "are to specify what living well entails and to identify the expected *consequences* (italics added) of such living. These consequences may include hedonic satisfactions, but typically eudaimonic theorists have been especially interested in other outcomes indicative of a good life, such as vitality, intimacy, health, and sense of meaning, among others" (Ryan et al., 2008, p. 140). In Ryan and Deci (2017), it is claimed that the satisfaction of psychological needs "*facilitate* (italics added) growth, integrity, and well-being" (p. 82).

In a chapter on Aristotelian philosophy and self-determination theory, Ryan et al. (2013) argue that "Aristotelian eudaimonism holds that the development of what is best in us is essential to flourishing, and flourishing in turn entails both doing what is objectively good and experiencing subjectively happiness, pleasure, and satisfaction. (…) This central tenet of eudaimonistic ethics is resonant not only with SDT (Deci & Ryan, 2000) but also with humanism more generally" (p. 58). Here, eudaimonia comprises both EWB (doing good) and HWB (feeling good and being satisfied). However, in a subsequent chapter, Ryan and Martela maintain that "eudaimonia should not be understood as referring to any kind of subjective experience or 'richer feeling of happiness' but is rather about a good and valued way of living that can *produce* (italics added) happiness, vitality and wellness as its byproducts" (Ryan & Martela, 2016, abstract). In the main text of the chapter, Ryan and Martela explain that "eudaimonia is rather a depiction of the kinds of pursuits and a manner of living that would most reliably give *rise to* (italics added) a life accompanied by a sense of wellness, vitality and thriving" (p. 111).

The predicting rather than constituting nature that SDT attributes to eudaimonia can also be observed in empirical studies. For instance, Chen et al. (2015) investigated whether satisfaction of the three basic psychological needs "*contributes to* (italics added) participants' well-being," using self-esteem as an indicator of well-being. Similarly, DeHaan et al. (2016) found that "SDT's basic psychological needs are substantially *associated* (italics added) with well-being, and that SDT's basic needs partially *mediate* (italics added) the relation between capabilities and indicators of wellness." This study operationalized wellbeing as life satisfaction, positive affect, absence of negative affect, meaning in life, and vitality. In another study, Reis et al. (2000, p. 429) conclude that "Higher levels of autonomy and competence were *associated* (italics added) with more favorable outcomes on all four measures of well-being." The four measures were positive affect, negative affect, vitality, and a symptom checklist (having a running nose, difficulty in breathing, etc.).

These examples illustrate the unsolved conflict between eudaimonia and wellbeing within the SDT. Over the last 30 years, the approach has alternately described eudaimonia as either an ingredient of wellbeing or as a cause of wellbeing. Throughout their writings, Deci and Ryan have claimed that eudaimonia both includes feelings and excludes feelings; and that eudaimonia both is wellbeing and is not wellbeing. I suspect that the core of this problem stems from the way psychological needs are conceptualized. In the SDT, needs are seen as both consisting in good feelings and being a prerequisite for good feelings, rewards, satisfaction, and full functioning (i.e., wellbeing). I further suspect that the inconsistency about eudaimonia frequently observed in the self-determination literature could be rooted in the vagueness with which important SDT concepts are formulated.

Full Functioning and Eudaimonia

To better understand this vagueness, consider this passage from the 2017 *Self-Determination Theory* book:

> In the SDT view, wellness is better described in terms of thriving or being fully functioning rather than merely by the presence of positive and absence of negative feelings. Thriving is characterized by vitality, awareness, access to, and exercise of one's human capacities and true self-regulation. Fully functioning individuals enjoy a free interplay of their faculties in contacting both their inner needs and states, nondefensively perceiving the circumstances in which they find others and themselves. They can be spontaneous and not constrained or holding back their interests or powers of orientation. They are not compartmentalized in their experience. This type of essential functioning reflects what Perls, Hefferline, and Goodman (1951) described as creative adjustment—an ability to be open, welcoming of novelty, and reflective—able to integrate inner and outer inputs into coherent actions.
>
> In line with Aristotle, we have hypothesized that, on average, when people are functioning in a healthy way, they will also tend to report more happiness or SWB, as well as other signs of wellness, such as lower symptoms of anxiety or depression, greater energy and vitality, more sense of coherence and meaning, less defensiveness, and fewer somatic symptoms. Because they are fully functioning, they will have deeper relationships, greater clarity of purpose, and a sense of, and concern with, meaning (Ryff, 1989). (Ryan & Deci, 2017, p. 241)

The description of thriving and fully functioning (are they synonyms?) certainly includes many fine, human qualities. However, it also reflects a conceptual ambiguity resembling the writings of leading figures in the humanistic psychology movement, such as Carl Rogers. Thus, some of the critique I raised against the humanistic psychology above applies to the SDT as well. For example, what does it mean for someone to "enjoy a free interplay of their faculties," to be "compartmentalized in their experience," or to "nondefensively perceiving" one's circumstances? These phrases bear the mark of the a priori and idealized concepts mentioned in the section about Carl Rogers.

Intrinsic Motivation

Intrinsically motivated behaviors constitute the core organismic element in SDT, and this concept is critical for the theory's alignment with eudaimonia. As far as I understand, Deci and Ryan equalize full functioning with being intrinsically motivated.

An in-depth account of intrinsic motivation is given in Deci (1975). The book states that "Intrinsically motivated behavior is behavior which is motivated by a person's need for feeling competent and self-determining[12] in dealing with his environment. This is a basic motivational propensity which is continually present and will be the primary motivator of behavior unless some other factor interrupts the process" (p. 100).

The propensity that is continually present is an awareness of potential satisfaction. More schematically, Deci's approach starts with a stimulus that makes the person aware of a potential satisfaction. The prospect of being satisfied provides the energy needed to set a goal and pursue it (Deci, 1975, p. 61). There are three kinds of satisfactions one can aim at: (1) homeostatic drive reduction, (2) positive affect, and (3) intrinsic motivation. In other words, intrinsically motivated behavior is conducted in order to reach the goal of a fulfilled psychological need. But the use of an "in order to" language is problematic as an explanation of something intrinsic. To say that we do something in order to obtain something (else than carrying out the activity) is considered a hallmark of extrinsic rather than intrinsic motivation (e.g., Koch, 1956). As Koch explains, by transforming intrinsic motivation into an "in order to" context, the basic characteristic of intrinsic motivation is violated, and the explanation is essentially transformed to a theory of external motivation. "Any anticipation of, or speculation about, the consequences to which the finished work might lead—price, reproof, understanding, misunderstanding, acceptance, rejection—will also vitiate the performance" (Koch, 1956, p. 69).

But Deci objects to this understanding of intrinsic motivation and characterizes it as "not very satisfactory" (Deci, 1975, p. 23). The reason is that "an activity cannot in any meaningful sense be its own reward" (p. 101). Here, Deci simply rejects the idea of intrinsic motivation and rather defends the view that intrinsic behavior is extrinsically motivated. It is the anticipation that an activity will lead to a reward that drives both intrinsic and extrinsic motivation. Deci therefore rejects the established explanation of intrinsic behavior as an activity conducted because it feels good to execute it (e.g., Berlyne, 1960; Deckers, 2015; Gazzaniga & Heatherton, 2003; Mook, 1996; Petri, 1991; Schwartz & Wrzesniewski, 2016; Shah & Kruglanski, 2000).

Deci defines intrinsic activities as behavior motivated by the expectation of reaching a goal, just the way extrinsic activities are motivated. The only difference is that intrinsic behavior is conducted in order to reach an intrinsic goal, whereas extrinsic behavior is conducted in order to reach an extrinsic goal. There is also a third category of goals, called affective, which are motivating because they elicit an expectation of feeling positive affect when the goal is reached.

> When a person is rewarded for achieving a goal, he will feel satisfied. In fact, in the case of intrinsic or affective rewards, it is difficult to separate out the positive affect which is the reward from the feeling of satisfaction. Still we can think of the satisfaction as following the

[12] In 1975, relatedness was not included as a basic need. Relatedness was added later but is regarded as a more distal underpinning of intrinsic motivation (e.g., Deci & Ryan, 2000, p. 235; Ryan, Curren, & Deci, 2013, p. 62).

> feeling which is the reward. The satisfaction is the final step in the sequence and will lead to termination of the sequence. (Deci, 1975, p. 121)

Petri (1991) explains the mechanism of intrinsic rewards in this way: "Intrinsic rewards involve the feelings of competence one obtains *after* (italics added) successfully completing a task. Reaching the goal *leads to* (italics added) the satisfaction of intrinsic motivation because one feels self-confident and able to control one's life" (p. 335).

Other Conceptualizations of Intrinsic Motivation

Deci and Ryan claim that the core elements of STD have remained largely intact since its initiation (Ryan & Deci, 2017, p. 124). Yet, Table 6.3 shows that the conceptualization of intrinsic motivation has changed. Initially, intrinsically motivated behavior was defined as goal-driven activities leading to feelings of self-determination and competence. Later, feelings of interest and joy became more salient features of intrinsic motivation, even though such feelings were considered inconsistent with intrinsic activities in Deci's original theory. In Ryan and Deci's 2017 book, satisfaction became the core intrinsic concept. Hence, whereas satisfaction was initially the state that ended intrinsic motivation, satisfaction has now become the mechanism that drives intrinsic motivation.

Table 6.3 Some definitions of intrinsic motivation in SDT

	Definition	Source
1	Intrinsically motivated behavior is behavior which is motivated by a person's **need for feeling competent and self-determinin**g in dealing with his environment	Deci (1975, p. 100)
2	The **life force** or energy for the activity and for the **development of the internal structure** is what we refer to as intrinsic motivation	Deci and Ryan (1985, p. 8)
3	Intrinsic motivation reflects the **primary propensity of organisms** to engage in activities **that interest them** and, in doing so, to learn, develop, and expand their capacities	Ryan and Deci (2000, p. 16)
4	Intrinsic motivation, or the pursuit of an activity because of its **inherent interest and enjoyability**	Ryan et al. (2008, p. 146)
5	This **natural tendency** to engage in play, exploration, and discovery **for its own sake** is called intrinsic motivation	Ryan et al. (2013, p. 61)
6	Intrinsic motivation refers to activities that are **done for** their inherent satisfactions	Ryan and Deci (2017, p. 117)
7	Intrinsic motivation is defined as spontaneous activity that is **sustained by the satisfactions inherent in the activity itself,** and it is contrasted with activity that is functionally dependent for its occurrence or persistence on separable rewards or reinforcements	Ryan and Deci (2017, p. 99)

The concept of inherent satisfaction is complex. For example, Ryan and Deci hold that feelings of autonomy and competence, and to some degree relatedness, are still a prerequisite for intrinsic motivation—either as experienced directly or interactively as moderating feelings. Deci and Ryan (2000) claim that intrinsically motivated behavior "does not have to be aimed at need satisfaction per se; it may simply be focused on an interesting activity or an important goal if they are in a context that allows need satisfaction" (p. 230). A child does not need to play to feel competent; the authors continue, but the psychological needs must be fulfilled to feel spontaneous pleasure from an activity: "the experiences of autonomy and competence, is necessary for the enjoyment of the activity" (p. 230). Another way of explaining this is given in Ryan and Deci (2017) on p. 117. Here, we learn that an individual will only be "intrinsically motivated for an activity to the degree that he or she finds it inherently interesting and enjoyable, which is in turn a function of proximal basic need satisfactions."

I must admit that I struggle to understand how the elements in SDT relate to eudaimonic wellbeing. If being fully functioning is the eudaimonic element in the SDT (Ryan & Deci, 2001, p. 141) and full functioning is defined as being intrinsically motivated (Deci, 1975, p. 100), then definition 1 in Table 6.3 seems to suggest that being eudaimon means to conduct activities motivated by the hope of feeling competent and self-determined when the behavior stops. In most theories of motivation, such an activity would be categorized as extrinsic, because it is driven by the assumption that it will eventually lead to a reward. When the goal is reached and these feelings kick in, the activity stops, and the needs for autonomy and competence (and relatedness) are fulfilled (Deci, 1975, p. 121). According to definition 7, however, being intrinsically motivated means to be spontaneously involved in an activity that is sustained by the satisfactions inherent in the activity itself. In other words, individuals are eudaimonically well to the degree that they are engaged in activities they find "inherently interesting and enjoyable, which is in turn a function of proximal basic need satisfactions" (Ryan & Deci, 2017, p. 117). Hence, the kind of interest and joy that can make an activity intrinsically motivated is conditioned on the satisfaction of psychological needs, which again are conditioned on reaching the goal of the activity, which is to feel competent and self-determined.

To me, it is unclear whether the SDT argues that all activities motivated by the assumption that they at some point will bring about feelings of autonomy and competence are eudaimonic or whether all activities a person finds interesting and enjoyable in itself are eudaimonic. It is also uncertain whether being eudaimon is a constituting ingredient of wellbeing or if it is a cause of wellbeing.

Other Approaches to EWB

A much-cited review of psychological theories about eudaimonic wellbeing was provided by Huta and Waterman in 2014. After examining 11 approaches to EWB, the authors concluded that four overarching themes describe psychological analyses of eudaimonia: growth, authenticity, excellence, and meaning. In more detail, Huta and Waterman found 12 "definition elements" for eudaimonia, and 2 of these elements were present in all 11 approaches. The two are (1) growth/self-realization/self-actualization/development of potentials/full functioning/maturity and (2) meaning/purpose/long-term perspective/caring about and contributing to the broader context. Elements such as authenticity and excellence were also included in most of the 11 approaches, whereas elements such as self-acceptance, physical health, and subjective wellbeing were included in only a minority of the approaches (cf. their Table 2 for the full list of elements).

In a review published a few years later, Heintzelman (2018) described psychological wellbeing theory and self-determination theory as the two template approaches to the study of eudaimonic wellbeing. Then, she added meaning in life as an extra topic—which appears redundant since meaning in life is already included in Ryff's theory of psychological wellbeing. Heintzelman also mentioned four additional concepts frequently employed in EWB research, namely, "the good life," "flow" experiences, growth (or ego development), and character strengths (quotation marks in original). In another authoritative review, Martela and Sheldon (2019) counted more than 45 different ways of operationalizing EWB and reported that at least 63 distinct constructs have been used empirically to measure the concept. Nevertheless, Martela and Sheldon found that "the most commonly measured single elements include meaning/purpose, competence, autonomy, relatedness, and engagement" (p. 461). Finally, a recent examination by Martela and Ryan (2023) identified two broad understandings of eudaimonia: as meaning and as psychological functioning.

Meaning

As examined at the beginning of this chapter, meaning in life was never central to Aristotle's notion of eudaimonism. But modern approaches to eudaimonic wellbeing need not be Aristotelian through and through, and there might be good reasons why meaning should be included among the ingredients of EWB. However, if we turn from an Aristotelian to a scientific epistemology, a different puzzle about meaning appears. Unlike the Aristotelian worldview, in which everything has a final goal, science has no room for an ultimate purpose in the big scheme of things (e.g., Pross, 2016, p. 33). Life itself has no meaning; it merely occurred by "the accident of history" (Wilson, 2014). Or as Dawkins noted, "evolution has no purpose in mind" (1986, p. 31).

Yet, the principles of natural selection have provided biological organisms with the ability to interpret. Ever since the formation of RNA, "an interpretive arms race has taken place with heritable agents that strove to *make sense* (italics in original) in the previously uninterpretable" (Haig, 2020, p. 306). For humans, making sense is more than a mere capability: it is probably also a need. "The human brain cannot sustain purposeless living. It was not designed for that" (Klinger, 1998, p. 33).

Hence, there is an important distinction between meaning *of* life in the big scheme of things on the one hand and meaning *in* life as an interpretive activity performed by living organisms on the other hand. Only the latter is subjected to psychological analyses (e.g., Martela & Steger, 2016).

An excellent account of this literature is offered by Leontiev (2013). Inspired by his personal encounters with Viktor Frankl in Moscow, Leontiev has long studied purpose and meaning in life. Leontiev suggests that the concept of meaning has three main dimensions: direction of real action, purpose in life, and experience of involvement. These elements can also be recognized in a model proposed by Heintzelman and King (2014), who argues that the concept of meaning entails the three basic dimensions of a sense of purpose, the belief that one's existence has value or significance, and coherence or comprehensibility. Martela and Steger (2016) have adopted a similar taxonomy, defining "meaning in life as emerging from the web of connections, interpretations, aspirations, and evaluations that (1) make our experiences comprehensible, (2) direct our efforts toward desired futures, and (3) provide a sense that our lives matter and are worthwhile" (p. 538). Smith (2017) proposes four partly overlapping dimensions of meaning: (1) belonging, (2) purpose, (3) storytelling, and (4) transcendence.

A somewhat more parsimonious taxonomy was developed by Proulx et al. (2013). These authors suggest that the two important elements of meaning can be summarized as the *what* and the *why* of meaning. Briefly, the *what* of life is about understanding something, whereas the *why* of life relates to the value aspect of life, to find the world "worthy enough to live in" (Shmotkin & Shrira, 2012, p. 146). With the increasing number of elements in the concept of meaning, Emmons proposed what he called the big four taxonomy of personal meaning dimensions: achievement/work, relationships/intimacy, religion/spirituality and self-transcendence/generativity (Emmons, 2003, p. 108).

Another "big four" model of meaning comes from Baumeister, whose pathbreaking book, *Meanings of Life* (Baumeister, 1991), remains a cornerstone in the psychology of meaning. Baumeister suggested that the search for meaning is driven by four individual needs. They are the needs for purpose, values, efficacy, and self-worth. Baumeister considers the four needs to be a checklist for life's meaning and regards a person's meaning of life as "the sum of ways he or she has of satisfying these needs for meaning" (p. 30). Importantly, Baumeister anchors the four needs for meaning in a conceptualization that roughly defines meaning as "shared mental representations of possible relationships among things, events, and relationships. Thus, meaning connects thing" (Baumeister, 1991, p. 15).

What Makes Meaning Eudaimonistic?

Meaning has been gradually introduced as an element of eudaimonia. Waterman was, for instance, never particularly concerned with the notion of meaning, although he paid some lip service to it from time to time. In early texts, he mentioned that people such as Erikson and May showed interest in meaning and purpose in life, but

Waterman's own analyses only commented on meaning in the passing, often in relation to the daimon. One example is Waterman (1993), where he says that "The daimon is an ideal in the sense of being an excellence, a perfection toward which one strives and, hence, it can give meaning and direction to one's life" (p. 678). Variants of this sentence can be found throughout his writings, as in Waterman (1981, p. 767), Waterman (1984, p. 16), Waterman et al. (2008, p. 42), and Waterman (2013, p. 6).

In her "Is Happiness Everything?" paper, Ryff (1989) briefly affirms that meaning is an indicator of eudaimonia, but she did not connect the purpose in life dimension to the concept of eudaimonia directly in that paper. It was not until 2002 that purpose in life became an explicit eudaimonic dimension in the PWB (Keyes et al., 2002). Ryff (2014) argues that eudaimonia is related to meaning-making because meaningful living captures the essence of the two great Greek imperatives: to know thyself and to become what you are (p. 2). Ryff further explains that the purpose in life dimension draws heavily on the existential perspectives of Victor Frankl, which is related to eudaimonia because it has to do with fulfillment (see the "Fulfillment" section below). Allport's concept of maturity is also a part of the purpose dimension in PWB, and maturity can be associated with eudaimonia as a growth component.

Ryan and Deci (2001) describe eudaimonic wellbeing as an approach that focuses on meaning and self-realization (p. 141). However, the authors did not spend much effort explaining the meaning part of eudaimonia in that paper, but they briefly referred to King and Napa (1998) and McGregor and Little (1998) for support. The King and Napa reference reports that both happiness and meaning are important elements in folk theories about the good life but do not examine how meaning is related to eudaimonia. McGregor and Little refer to "doing well" (i.e., goal efficacy) as an indicator of happiness and "being yourself" (i.e., goal integrity) as an indicator of meaning. The notion of being yourself can be associated with eudaimonia, and integrity is an integrated part of being fully functioning.

From its marginal role in the early literature, meaning in life has gradually become a more dominant part of eudaimonic wellbeing (e.g., Delle Fave et al., 2011; Dolan, 2015; Graham et al., 2018; Heintzelman, 2018; Huta & Ryan, 2010; Kashdan et al., 2008; OECD, 2013; Ryff, 2014; Steptoe et al., 2015; Stone & Krueger, 2018; Stone & Mackie, 2013; Tov, 2018). The developmental psychologist Jack Bauer even declares that "If I had to choose a single word to represent the many facets of eudaimonia as it is typically studied, I would choose meaning" (Bauer, 2016, p. 149). Although Bauer admits that it is unsatisfactory to use one word to account for the entire bandwidth of a complicated concept such as eudaimonia, he still defends the move by referring to Baumeister's thorough examination of meaning. To Bauer, Baumeister's theory can explain why the notion of meaning is able to carry such a heavy conceptual load and how it connects with eudaimonia. Hence, a closer look at Baumeister's work is in its place.

Meaning Versus Happiness

Although not discussed explicitly in the 1991 book, Baumeister's conceptualization of meaning has clear associations with the notion of eudaimonia. In his later writings, Baumeister also makes the connection explicit (e.g., Baumeister et al., 2013). Here, and in follow-up studies (summarizes in Baumeister, 2018), he identifies important differences between happiness and meaning, and his analysis has obvious parallels to the distinction between hedonic wellbeing and eudaimonic wellbeing. The empirical results of Baumeister's studies revealed, for instance, that happiness was associated with living in the present, whereas meaning was associated with living in the past and the future. Happiness correlated positively with pleasure and ease, whereas meaning did not. Happiness was associated with an identity as a taker, whereas meaning was associated with an identity as a giver. Being argumentative in a social relation was associated with less happiness but greater meaning. Similarly, having had many bad events in one's life was linked to lower happiness but was positively correlated with meaning. Finally, time spent caring for children had a negligible effect on happiness but a significant impact on meaning.

Thus, Baumeister (2018) concludes that "our work suggests two different versions of the good life, with different pathways. A happy life is one of ease and enjoyment, focused on taking pleasure in the present. The meaningful life is oriented toward the future, concerned with constructing and expressing the self, and heavily involved in complex sociocultural activities" (p. 33).

Some caveats of these studies should be mentioned. First, the happiness and meaning variables in Baumiester's studies were highly correlated, in the range of 0.60 to 0.70. This strong correlation between meaning and happiness has frequently been reported in other studies as well (e.g., Heintzelman, 2018; Tov & Lee, 2016).[13] Hence, the distinctions between happiness and meaning reported above only appeared after the shared variance between the two concepts was partialed out, which means that the distinctiveness between happiness and meaning only applies to a relatively small proportion of the variance in the two concepts.

Some parts of Baumeister's "happiness-meaning paradigm" have been conceptually replicated. For example, Tov and Lee (2016) used an experience sampling methodology to compare life satisfaction and meaning against a set of affective variables. Overall, the authors found that the affective profiles of satisfaction and meaning were very similar but also that some differences could be recognized. For example, interpersonal conflicts and impactful negative events were initially associated with both less satisfaction and less meaning. However, after controlling for affect and satisfaction, these negative experiences were associated with greater meaning. Satisfaction was found to covary more strongly with affective discrepancy than with meaning. Tov and Lee also observed an effect they referred to as affective discrepancy, which means a prevalence of positive affect over negative affect. This

[13] In the Tov and Lee's (2016) study, the correlation between meaning and satisfaction as latent factors was $\psi = 0.85$.

effect was stronger for satisfaction than for meaning, and after partialing out the covariance between the two variables, the effect was uniquely related to satisfaction but not meaning. Tov and Lee suggested that this result indicates that life satisfaction is more "hedonic" than is meaning in life. Another distinction between satisfaction and meaning was that for some participants in some situations, negative affect was positively correlated with meaning but negatively correlated with satisfaction.

Meaning and Information Processing

Related to the debate on how meaning and happiness differ, the role of meaning as a eudaimonic concept can also be examined from a cognitive point of view. For example, Greenfield (2009) claims that a pleasant mind tends to wipe out the neurological pathways needed to form a coherent understanding of life, i.e., the *what* aspect of meaning. For new concepts to become understandable, cognitive frameworks must be built gradually. To create such structures, a process of slowly exercising the use of symbols over and over is often necessary, and according to Greenfield, such a slow exercise is not particularly pleasant. Rather, building a complex understanding involves a series of perceptual sequences that connect symbols and logic in a way that often stretches beyond the immediate here-and-now. Anatomically, the prefrontal cortex must therefore be active and integrated with other brain structures to make this happen. However, episodes of intense pleasure, Greenfield argues, tend to prevent the incorporation of such moments into a meaningful life story.

In addition to the neuropsychological evidence, Greenfield (2009) found support for her position in the literature on religious rituals. Referring to the anthropologist Harvey Whitehouse (2004), she points out that religious commitment is partly established by the execution of a low-arousal and high-frequency kind of behavior that is based upon repetition. This kind of commitment seems to be elicited by long-term rumination on questions on meaning. The dominant experience during such activities is not pleasure but a sense of meaning.

Greenfield's analyses of the relations between meaning and pleasure fit amazingly well with Jill Bolte Taylor's description of her feelings during the stroke (Taylor, 2008). As mentioned in previous chapters, Taylor's left hemisphere grew increasingly silent as she became detached from her memories of the past and her ability to make plans for the future. "Every moment seemed to exist in perfect isolation," as she puts it, and she found it almost impossible to concentrate or keep her mind on the task at hand. The feeling accompanying this state, however, gave her a comfortable sense of grace. "I'm no authority, but I think the Buddhists would say that I entered the mode of existence they call Nirvana." The pleasantness of a state of mind is, according to Taylor, unable to cope or understand. In her own words, "Even the simplest of calculations, by definition, requires recognition of the relationship between different entities, and my mind was no longer capable of creating combinations" (Taylor, 2008, p. 50). At the same time, her experiences were delightful, so wonderful that she seriously wondered if she, given that she could have the choice, would prefer to stay in this state of "nirvana" rather than being a successful neuroscientist.

Fulfillment

Fulfillment is a core element of meaning in both philosophical and psychological literature on meaning (Klinger, 1998). To Viktor Frankl, searching for meaning was a way of fulfilling one's values. Although his profound *Man's Search for Meaning* (Frankl, 1945) had a unique spiritual, existential, and scientific impact, the idea of meaning as fulfillment was more fully elaborated in later work, particularly in *The Will to Meaning* (Frankl, 1970). Here, Frankl sees meaning from the perspective of self-transcendence, and he believes that to find meaning in life, people must go beyond themselves and become committed to purposes beyond their personal benefit. Because of its self-transcendent nature, Frankl considered meaning to stand in contrast to being happy (Magen, 1998, p. 8). According to Magen, it is this self-transcendence that gives life its worth and a feeling of fulfillment (p. 37).

Fulfillment was also important to Aristotle and other ancient eudaimonist thinkers. In a thorough treatment of the topic, Gewirth (1998) claims that self-fulfillment is often considered the inclusive content of a good, happy human life and the ultimate goal of human striving. According to some conceptualizations, Gewirth explains, "self-fulfillment consists in carrying to fruition one's deepest desires or one's worthiest capacities. It is a bringing of oneself to flourishing completion, an unfolding of what is strongest or best in oneself, so that it represents the successful culmination of one's aspirations or potentials. In this way self-fulfillment betokens a life well lived, a life that is deeply satisfying, fruitful, and worthwhile" (Gewirth, 1998, p. 3).

Baumeister describes fulfillment as a "positive, desirable state, based on a concept of a substantial improvement over present circumstances" (Baumeister, 1991, p. 70), and in his theory, the need for purpose is presented as a kind of fulfillment that reflects a state of feeling good after reaching goals (p. 33). However, Baumeister warned against the glorified and idealized prose with which fulfillment often is described. Fulfillment often involves an "utopic air" and can appear "too good to be true." However, the aspiration to reach such rare states or goals is not uncommon. Baumeister refers to a study by Levinson et al. (1978) showing that people (only males took part in this study) tend to believe that if they reach a certain level of success, all their problems and worries will disappear. Similarly, Freedman (1978) observed that young people in his study often dreamt of a quiet and peaceful life in the countryside, believing that the harmonic but hardworking life on a farm would make them happy. However, Freedman's data revealed that people who live on farms or in small villages are not happier than others. Baumeister refers to such unrealistic ideas about how good a life will be once one's dreams and striving are realized as the myth of fulfillment. Three archetypical fulfillment myths are common: the story of the lotus eaters from Homer's "Odyssey," the idea of the Holy Grail, and the story of Faust (Baumeister, 1991, pp. 70–73).[14]

Paradoxically, another link between eudaimonia and meaning might be extracted from existentialism. The links between goals, feelings, and purpose are, for instance, a central theme in Camus' philosophical essay "The Myth of Sisyphus" (Camus, 1942/1955). According to Greek mythology, Sisyphus, who is condemned for all eternity to roll a rock up a hill only to have it roll back down, was used by Camus as a metaphor for the absurdity of our human condition. The French philosopher, novelist, and Nobel laureate considers our existence to be inherently meaningless; thus, we are forced to create our own meaning in life. It is only through an individual's own actions and choices that the fundamental indifference in the universe can be dealt with, Camus tells us, before he concludes that the struggle of life "is enough to fill a man's heart. One must imagine Sisyphus happy" (p. 89). Although Camus briefly mentions Aristotle in the book, he is not making the connection between a good life and a rational life explicit, even if that link is important to both philosophers. For Aristotle, as we have seen, being rational means to live in accordance with universal virtues. For Camus, rationality means finding meaning in one's personal struggle against the innate absurdity of life. But according to Sagi and Sagi (2002), both Aristotle and Camus championed the full realization of human capacity (cited in Aronson, 2022, p. 19). Other ways of connecting Aristotelian eudaimonism and Camus' existentialism can be found in Fendt (2019, 2020), Eubanks and Petrakis (1999), and Fabian (2020).

Personal Growth

Growth is frequently mentioned as an element of eudaimonia, and the notion of personal growth can be traced back to the axial age (800–200 BCE). In the "Odyssey," for example, something called a "growth cycle" was supposed to be completed after adventurous voyages had been embarked on. The idea was that a journey changed the traveler's understanding of themselves (Jourard & Landsman, 1980). In old Chinese ethics, the striving toward personal betterment was elaborated by Confucius and others (Wong, 2013; Yu, 1998), and the ancient pan-African belief system, Ubuntu, articulated an ethic about how individuals can only develop as humans through other persons (Ramose, 2002). The classical Greek era also concerned itself with striving toward personal growth. The Socratic "know thyself" and Aristotle's theory of virtues can be seen as advice about sound developments. For

[14] Lotus from Greek "lotos" can refer to several plants but is described in the "Odyssey" as a flower that gives anyone who eats them an overwhelming feeling of happiness that includes a loss of interest in doing anything else. The Holy Grail comes from the King Arthur legends and is the name of the cup that Jesus used at the Last Supper. Faust is the protagonist in Goethe's play. Faust is famous for his pact with the devil, which gave Faust unlimited knowledge and earthly pleasures until he wants the present moment to last. Then, the devil may come to claim Faust's soul.

the ancient Greeks, personal growth was a moral concern. It was based on the conviction that an individual (given that he was a male and part of the elite of a society) should develop into the "man-he-could-be-if-he-realized-his-essential-nature" (MacIntyre, 2007).

The earliest appearance of the term personal growth in psychology seems to be in a book from 1898 entitled *Social and Ethical Interpretations in Mental Development* (Baldwin, 1906). As suggested by the title and in a review of the book (Dewey, 1898), personal growth was considered by Baldwin to be an ethical concept, and the change process was only possible through certain social experiences. The normative element of personal growth was also noticeable in the work of Allport (1961), who depicted the goal of personal growth to be about "propriate striving."

Thus, the concept of personal growth was originally very broad and dynamic and included intellectual, personality, and moral elements. In more recent conceptualizations, personal growth is still broad and dynamic, but throughout the twentieth century, the moral element has been downplayed. The value element in personal growth is at least less explicitly articulated. For example, Jourard and Landsman (1980) define personal growth as a change in the way one experiences the world and one's own being. However, not all kinds of change are growth. Any increase in a person's cardiovascular status, intellectual performance, or artistic achievement would typically not count as personal growth. To provide some perspective, Kagan (2014) asks whether an adolescent's ability to vandalize a school compared with the gentle innocuous play of a 2-year-old should count as personal growth.

The concept of personal growth is, in other words, not merely about becoming bigger, which is what growing literally means (Jackson, 2009, p. 269). For example, Jourard argues that "one can speak of growth only when the changes enhance the person's ability to cope with challenges in existence" (Jourard & Landsman, 1980, p. 229). The need to restrict the meaning of personal growth brings back the issue of normativity because the criteria for inclusion and exclusion are unavoidably value based. Personal growth is therefore a dual-character concept (Chap. 1), as it always refers to something normative. It comprises a value-laden kind of improvement and is direction toward capabilities that are essential to our humanness, to a touch of "the better angels of our nature." It is not easy to pinpoint what these improvements are exactly, and for this reason, I suspect that the idea of personal growth will remain imprecise and idealized for a long time.

Maslow, Rogers, and other humanistic psychologists associated personal growth with fulfillment, self-actualization, or full functioning. Waterman (e.g., Waterman & Schwartz, 2013) relates it to people's struggle toward the type of being they wish to become, although he does not discuss the concept much. For Carol Ryff, personal growth is a dimension of psychological wellbeing, even the most eudaimonic dimension among the six dimensions. Deci and Ryan often include growth as a core element in their descriptions of the organismic perspective on life. For example, in Ryan (1995, p. 397), we can read that "many psychological theorists have assumed that the psyche contains its own natural or inherent principles that promote growth, integration, and the resolution of psychological inconsistencies and conflicts."

Elsewhere, they say that "within each individual, we observe a natural tendency toward growth and development, which represents an ongoing tendency toward organismic integration" (Ryan & Deci, 2017, p. 8). However, when the SDT becomes more specific, it treats personal growth as an outcome (e.g., Martela & Ryan, 2023, p. 6) and typically narrows the term down to represent an intrinsic goal, i.e., a goal or aspiration that is rewarding in its own right. Personal growth is also described as an individualistic goal and almost always contrasts with community-oriented goals.[15]

Life Span Development Approaches

Life span development studies examine the concept of personal growth in much detail, as exemplified in the personality and life stories paradigm (e.g., Bauer, 2016; Bauer et al., 2020; McAdams, 2006; McAdams & McLean, 2013). According to Bauer et al. (2008), the process of creating growth can be observed in a narrative that differentiates, elaborates, integrates, or otherwise strives to make greater sense of various experiences, as well as in narratives with a temporal structure that suggests progress. Interestingly, the correlation between personal growth, as operationalized by Bauer, and typical indicators of hedonic wellbeing, such as life satisfaction and overall happiness, is not very strong. According to Bauer, "People who can think complexly and deeply about their lives (suggesting wisdom) are just as likely to be happy as not" (Bauer et al., 2019, p. 84).

Another tradition within life span studies, summarized in Law and Staudinger (2016), suggests that personal growth comprises three facets:

1. It involves cognitive insight into oneself, others, and the world.
2. It requires complex emotion regulation as indexed by a tolerance of ambiguity.
3. A motivation that transcends self-interest and is focused on the well-being of others.

Following these criteria, Law and Staudinger argue that several theories of psychosocial maturation are not really about personal growth. For instance, Erik H. Erikson's theory of psychosocial development is about adjustment and adaptation rather than growth. The process of adaptation is by nature oriented toward assimilation and stability rather than toward accommodation and change. In contrast, personal growth refers to a continuous striving for new experiences, i.e., toward learning. It concerns successful accommodation in Piagetian terms and correlates with openness to experience and eudaimonic wellbeing. In Erikson's final developmental state, however, the ability to adapt is the central mechanism. It is described as a conflict between integrity and despair in which the positive outcome of the conflict, integration, will provide satisfaction.

[15] In all but one of the 20 times personal growth is mentioned in the book *Self-Determination Theory* (Ryan & Deci, 2017), it is supplemented with a community goal or an other-oriented goal.

Importantly, such integration often results in reduced growth. Abandoning aspirations and difficult life goals might well lead to satisfaction, but it will not lead to continued growth and goal attainment. Erikson's theory can therefore be characterized as a hedonic theory of wellbeing (Staudinger & Kunzmann, 2005). For that reason, it is not surprising that Staudinger and her colleagues find that measures of adjustment are associated with life satisfaction and personality traits such as conscientiousness, agreeableness, and emotional stability, whereas measures of personal growth are only weakly correlated with life satisfaction. Under some circumstances, the association is even negative (e.g., Law & Staudinger, 2016).

Wisdom

Wisdom is a complex concept but an important element of personal growth. Staudinger and Kunzmann (2005) consider it even as the prototype of human growth, the endpoint of human development. Staudinger and her colleagues also argue that wisdom has a moral element because a person cannot be truly wise unless they consider both seeking the good for themselves and seeking the good for others. Based on the Berlin wisdom paradigm, the concept is separated into two subdimensions: personal wisdom (referring to judgments and insight about a person's own life) and general wisdom (focusing on the life of others and on life in general). Personal wisdom and general wisdom comprise values. Wisdom refers to changes that can be classified according to increases in certain virtues, such as insight, integrity, and self-transcendence. Wisdom is, in other words, defined by the orientation toward balancing one's own good with that of others.

Schwartz (2011) emphasizes practical wisdom as the most important character humans must develop to exercise moral will and moral skill and to flourish as human beings. Being practical wise means knowing how to read the social context, to properly interpret guiding principles in different contexts, to take the perspective of another, to improvise and balance conflicting aims, and to have well-educated emotions and intuition. It takes exercise to develop wisdom, with trial, error, and feedback as important ingredients in the process. Schwartz argues that managers who replace opportunities for such practices with rules and incentives create a downward spiral in organizations that constrains employees' potential for knowing and doing the right thing in any particular situation.

References

Allport, G. W. (1961). *Pattern and growth in personality*. Holt, Rinehart and Winston.
Annas, J. (1993). *The morality of happiness [Kindle]*. Oxford University Press.
Annas, J. (1998). Virtue and eudaimonism. *Social Philosophy and Policy, 15*(1), 37–55. https://doi.org/10.1017/S0265052500003058
Annas, J. (2003). Virtue ethics and egoism. *A Priori, 2*, 20–31.

Annas, J. (2008). The phenomenology of virtue. *Phenomenology and the Cognitive Sciences, 7*, 21–34.
Annas, J. (2011). *Intelligent virtue [Kindle]*. Oxford University Press.
Aristotle. (trans. 1908). *The Nicomachean ethics [Kindle]* (W. D. Ross, Trans.). Enhanced Media, 2017.
Aronson, R. (2022). Albert Camus. In E. N. Zalta (Ed.), *The Stanford encyclopedia of philosophy* (Spring 2022 ed.). Retrieved from https://plato.stanford.edu/archives/win2022/entries/camus/
Ashby, W. R. (1946). Dynamics of the cerebral cortex: The behavioural properties of systems in equilibrium. *The American Journal of Psychology, 59*(4), 682–686.
Badhwar, N. K. (2014). *Well-being: Happiness in a worthwhile life [Kindle]*. Oxford University Press.
Baldwin, J. M. (1906). *Social and ethical interpretations in mental development* (4th ed.). Macmillan.
Bauer, J. J. (2016). Eudaimonic growth: The development of the goods in personhood (or: Cultivating a good life story). In J. Vittersø (Ed.), *Handbook of Eudaimonic well-being* (pp. 147–174). Springer International Publishing. https://doi.org/10.1007/978-3-319-42445-3_10
Bauer, J. J., McAdams, D. P., & Pals, J. L. (2008). Narrative identity and eudaimonic well-being. *Journal of Happiness Studies, 9*(1), 81–104.
Bauer, J. J., King, L. A., & Steger, M. F. (2019). Meaning making, self-determination theory, and the question of wisdom in personality. *Journal of Personality, 87*(1), 82–101. https://doi.org/10.1111/jopy.12381
Bauer, J. J., Park, S. W., Kamide, H., Pesola, N. V., Kamble, S. V., Graham, L. E., DeBrosse, J., & Waddar, M. S. (2020). Growth motivation and well-being in the U.S., Japan, Guatemala, and India. *Journal of Happiness Studies, 21*(3), 899–919. https://doi.org/10.1007/s10902-019-00099-6
Baumeister, R. F. (1991). *Meanings of life*. Guilford Press.
Baumeister, R. F. (2018). Happiness and meaningfulness as two different and not entirely compatible versions of the good life. In J. P. Forgas & R. E. Baumeister (Eds.), *The social psychology of living well* (pp. 21–33). Routledge.
Baumeister, R. F., Vohs, K. D., Aaker, J. L., & Garbinsky, E. N. (2013). Some key differences between a happy life and a meaningful life. *The Journal of Positive Psychology, 8*(6), 505–516. https://doi.org/10.1080/17439760.2013.830764
Berlyne, D. E. (1960). *Conflict, arousal, and curiosity*. McGraw-Hill.
Besser-Jones, L. (2015). Eudaimonism. In G. Fletcher (Ed.), *The Routledge handbook of philosophy of well-being [Kindle]*. Routledge.
Blasi, A. (1976). Concept of development in personality theory. In J. Loevinger (Ed.), *Ego development* (pp. 29–53). Jossey–Bass.
Bok, S. (2010). *Exploring happiness. From Aristotle to brain science [Kindle]*. Yale University Press.
Borsboom, D., van der Maas, H. L., Dalege, J., Kievit, R. A., & Haig, B. D. (2021). Theory construction methodology: A practical framework for building theories in psychology. *Perspectives on Psychological Science, 16*(4), 756–766.
Bradburn, N. M. (1969). *The structure of psychological well-being*. Aldine.
Bradford, G. (2015). Perfectionism. In G. Fletcher (Ed.), *The Routledge handbook of philosophy of well-being [Kindle]* (pp. 124–134). Routledge.
Bridgman, T., Cummings, S., & Ballard, J. (2019). Who built Maslow's pyramid? A history of the creation of management studies' most famous symbol and its implications for management education. *Academy of Management Learning & Education, 18*(1), 81–98. https://doi.org/10.5465/amle.2017.0351
Campbell, A., Converse, P. E., & Rodgers, W. L. (1976). *The quality of American life*. Sage.
Camus, A. (1942/1955). *The myth of Sisyphus [Kindle]* (J. O'Brian, Trans.). Pinguin.
Cantril, H. (1965). *The pattern of human concerns*. Rutgers University Press.
Cantril, H. (1988). *Psychology, humanism, and scientific inquiry: The selected essays of Hadley Cantril*. Transaction Books.

Chen, B., Vansteenkiste, M., Beyers, W., Boone, L., Deci, E. L., Van der Kaap-Deeder, J., Duriez, B., Lens, W., Matos, L., Mouratidis, A., Ryan, R. M., Sheldon, K. M., Soenens, B., Van Petegem, S., & Verstuyf, J. (2015). Basic psychological need satisfaction, need frustration, and need strength across four cultures. *Motivation and Emotion, 39*(2), 216–236. https://doi.org/10.1007/s11031-014-9450-1
Creel, R. (1983). Eudology: The science of happiness. *New Ideas in Psychology, 1*, 303–312.
Crisp, R. (2017). Well-being. In E. N. Zalta (Ed.), *The Stanford encyclopedia of philosophy*. Retrieved from http://plato.stanford.edu/archives/fall2011/entries/well-being/
Csikszentmihalyi, M. (1983). A "Columbus fallacy". *New Ideas in Psychology, 1*(3), 313–314.
Darley, J. M., & Batson, C. D. (1973). "From Jerusalem to Jericho": A study of situational and dispositional variables in helping behavior. *Journal of Personality and Social Psychology, 27*(1), 100–108. https://doi.org/10.1037/h0034449
Dawkins, R. (1986). *The blind watchmaker [Kindle]*. Norton.
Deaton, A., & Stone, A. A. (2016). Understanding context effects for a measure of life evaluation: How responses matter. *Oxford Economic Papers, 68*(4), 861–870. https://doi.org/10.1093/oep/gpw022
Deci, E. L. (1975). *Intrinsic motivation*. Plenum Press.
Deci, E. L., & Ryan, R. M. (1985). *Intrinsic motivation and self-determination in human behavior*. Plenum Press.
Deci, E. L., & Ryan, R. M. (2000). The "what" and "why" of goal pursuits: Human needs and the self-determination of behavior. *Psychological Inquiry, 11*(4), 227–268. https://doi.org/10.1207/S15327965PLI1104_01
Deckers, L. (2015). *Motivation: Biological, psychological, and environmental*. Psychology Press.
DeHaan, C. R., Hirai, T., & Ryan, R. M. (2016). Nussbaum's capabilities and self-determination theory's basic psychological needs: Relating some fundamentals of human wellness. *Journal of Happiness Studies, 17*(5), 2037–2049. https://doi.org/10.1007/s10902-015-9684-y
Delle Fave, A., Brdar, I., Freire, T., Vella-Brodrick, D., & Wissing, M. (2011). The eudaimonic and hedonic components of happiness: Qualitative and quantitative findings. *Social Indicators Research, 100*(2), 185–207. https://doi.org/10.1007/s11205-010-9632-5
Dewey, J. (1898). A book review on social and ethical interpretations in mental development by James Mark Baldwin [Social and ethical interpretations in mental development, James Mark Baldwin]. *The Philosophical Review, 7*(4), 398–409. https://doi.org/10.2307/2177135
Disabato, D. J., Goodman, F. R., Kashdan, T. B., Short, J. L., & Jarden, A. (2016). Different types of well-being? A cross-cultural examination of hedonic and eudaimonic well-being. *Psychological Assessment, 28*(5), 471–482. https://doi.org/10.1037/pas0000209
Dodge, R. (1930). *"Autobiography". i C. Murchison: A history of psychology in autobiography, Vol 1* (pp. 99–121). Clarc University Press.
Dolan, P. (2015). *Happiness by design: Finding pleasure and purpose in everyday life [Kindle]*. Penguin.
Doris, J. M. (1998). Persons, situations, and virtue ethics. *Noûs, 32*(4), 504–530. http://www.jstor.org/stable/2671873
Emmons, R. A. (2003). Personal goals, life meaning, and virtue: Wellsprings of a positive life. In C. L. M. Keyes & J. Haidt (Eds.), *Flourishing. Positive psychology and the life well-lived* (pp. 105–128). American Psychological Association.
Eronen, M. I., & Bringmann, L. F. (2021). The theory crisis in psychology: How to move forward. *Perspectives on Psychological Science, 16*(4), 779–788.
Eubanks, C. L., & Petrakis, P. A. (1999). Reconstructing the world: Albert Camus and the symbolization of experience. *The Journal of Politics, 61*(2), 293–312.
Fabian, M. (2020). The coalescence of being: A model of the self-actualisation process. *Journal of Happiness Studies, 21*(4), 1487–1508. https://doi.org/10.1007/s10902-019-00141-7
Fendt, G. (2019). Reason, feeling, and happiness: Bridging an ancient/modern divide in the plague. *Philosophy and Literature, 43*(2), 350–368.
Fendt, G. (2020). Camus and Aristotle on the art community and its errors. *Labyrinthe, 22*, 40–59.

Fleck, L. (1979). *Genesis and development of a scientific fact*. The University of Chicago Press.
Fowers, B. J. (2016). Aristotle on eudaimonia: On the virtue of returning to the source. In J. Vittersø (Ed.), *Handbook of eudaimonic well-being* (pp. 67–83). Springer International Publishing. https://doi.org/10.1007/978-3-319-42445-3_4
Frankl, V. (1945). *Man's search for meaning. An introduction to logotheraphy*. Washington Square Press.
Frankl, V. (1970). *The will to meaning*. Plume.
Frede, D. (2006). Pleasure and pain in Aristotle's ethics. In R. Kraut (Ed.), *The Blackwell guide to Aristotle's Nicomachean ethics* (pp. 255–275). Blackwell.
Freedman, J. (1978). *Happy people: What happiness is, who has it, and why*. Harcourt Brace Jovanovich.
Gazzaniga, M. S., & Heatherton, T. F. (2003). *Psychological science. Mind, brain, and behavior*. Norton.
Gelman, S. A., & Rhodes, M. (2012). Two-thousand years of stasis. In K. S. Rosengren, S. Brem, E. M. Evans, & G. Sinatra (Eds.), *Evolution challenges: Integrating research and practice in teaching and learning about evolution* (pp. 3–21). Oxford University Press.
Gewirth, A. (1998). *Self-fulfillment*. Princeton University Press.
Gilbert, D. (2006). *Stumbling on happiness*. Harper Press.
Goldstein, K. (1939). *The organism: A holistic approach to biology derived from pathological data in man*. American Book Publishing. https://doi.org/10.1037/10021-000.
Gotthelf, A. (1976). Aristotle's conception of final causality. *The Review of Metaphysics, 30*(2), 226–254. https://doi.org/10.2307/20126919
Graham, C., Laffan, K., & Pinto, S. (2018). Well-being in metrics and policy. *Science, 362*(6412), 287–288. https://doi.org/10.1126/science.aau5234
Greenfield, S. (2009). *ID. The quest for meaning in the 21st century*. Sceptre.
Grene, M. (1972). Aristotle and modern biology. *Journal of the History of Ideas, 33*(3), 395–424. https://doi.org/10.2307/2709043
Haig, D. (2020). *From Darwin to Derrida: Selfish genes, social selves, and the meanings of life [Kindle]*. Mit Press.
Haney, C., Banks, W. C., & Zimbardo, P. G. (1973). A study of prisoners and guards in a simulated prison. *Naval Research Reviews, 9*(1–17), 14–65.
Harman, G. (2000). The nonexistence of character traits. *Proceedings of the Aristotelian Society (Hardback), 100*(1), 223–226. https://doi.org/10.1111/j.0066-7372.2003.00013.x
Haybron, D. M. (2008). *The pursuit of unhappiness. The elusive psychology of well-being*. Oxford University Press.
Haybron, D. M. (2016). The philosophical basis of eudaimonic psychology. In J. Vittersø (Ed.), *Handbook of Eudaimonic well-being* (pp. 27–53). Springer International Publishing. https://doi.org/10.1007/978-3-319-42445-3_2
Hebb, D. O. (1949). *The organization of behavior: A neuropsychological theory*. Wiley.
Heintzelman, S. J. (2018). Eudaimonia in the contemporary science of subjective well-being: Psychological well-being, self- determination, and meaning in life. In E. Diener, S. Oishi, & L. Tay (Eds.), *Handbook of subjective well-being*. DEF publishers. https://doi.org/nobascholar.com
Heintzelman, S. J., & King, L. A. (2014). Life is pretty meaningful. *American Psychologist, 69*(6), 561–574. https://doi.org/10.1037/a0035049
Held, V. (2006). *The ethics of care: Personal, political, and global*. Oxford university press.
Helliwell, J., Huang, H., & Wang, S. (2016). The distribution of world happiness. In J. Helliwell, R. Layard, & J. Sachs (Eds.), *World happiness report 2016* (pp. 8–48). http://worldhappiness.report/
Helliwell, J. F., Layard, R., Sachs, J. D., De Neve, J.-E., Aknin, L. B., & Wang, S. (Eds.). (2024). *World happiness report 2024* (21th ed.). Sustainable development solutions network. https://worldhappiness.report/

Huta, V., & Ryan, R. M. (2010). Pursuing pleasure or virtue: The differential and overlapping well-being benefits of hedonic and eudaimonic motives. *Journal of Happiness Studies, 11*, 735–762. https://doi.org/10.1007/s10902-009-9171-4

Huta, V., & Waterman, A. S. (2014). Eudaimonia and its distinction from hedonia: Developing a classification and terminology for understanding conceptual and operational definitions. *Journal of Happiness Studies, 1425–1456.* https://doi.org/10.1007/s10902-013-9485-0

Jackson, T. (2009). *Prosperity without growth*. Earthscan.

Jahoda, M. (1958). *Current concepts of positive mental health*. Basic Books.

Joseph, S., & Linley, P. A. (2004). Positive therapy: A positive psychological theory of therapeutic practice. In P. A. Linley & S. Joseph (Eds.), *Positive psychology in practice* (pp. 354–368). Wiley.

Jost, L. J. (2002). Introduction. In L. J. Jost & R. A. Shiner (Eds.), *Eudaimonia and well-being* (pp. ix–xxxiii). Academic Printing & Publishing.

Jost, L. J., & Shiner, R. A. (Eds.). (2002). *Eudaimonia and well-being*. Academic Printing & Publishing.

Jourard, S. M., & Landsman, T. (1980). *Healthy personality: An approach from the viewpoint of humanistic psychology*. Macmillan.

Kagan, J. (1994). Distinctions among emotions, moods, and temperamental qualities. In P. Ekman & R. J. Davidson (Eds.), *The nature of emotion. Fundamental questions* (pp. 74–78). Oxford University Press.

Kagan, J. (2014). Presuppositions in developmental inquiry. In L. Cirillo & S. Wapner (Eds.), *Value presuppositions in theories of human development [Kindle]* (pp. 63–78). Psychology Press (Original work published in 1986).

Kashdan, T. B., Biswas-Diener, R., & King, L. A. (2008). Reconsidering happiness: The costs of distinguishing between hedonics and eudaimonia. *The Journal of Positive Psychology, 3*(4), 219–233. https://doi.org/10.1080/17439760802303044

Katz, L. D. (2016). Pleasure. In E. N. Zalta (Ed.), *The Stanford encyclopedia of philosophy* (Winter 2016 ed.). Retrieved from https://plato.stanford.edu/archives/win2016/entries/pleasure/

Kaufman, S. B. (2016). *How to be an optimal human*. https://blogs.scientificamerican.com/beautiful-minds/how-to-be-an-optimal-human/

Kendler, H. H. (1987). *Historical foundations of modern psychology*. Brooks/Cole Publishing Company.

Kendler, H. H. (1999). The role of value in the world of psychology. *American Psychologist, 54*(10), 828.835.

Keyes, C. L. M., & Annas, J. (2009). Feeling good and functioning well: Distinctive concepts in ancient philosophy and contemporary science. *Journal of Positive Psychology, 4*(3), 197–201. https://doi.org/10.1080/17439760902844228

Keyes, C. L. M., Shmotkin, D., & Ryff, C. D. (2002). Optimizing well-being: The empirical encounter of two traditions. *Journal of Personality and Social Psychology, 82*(6), 1007–1022. https://doi.org/10.1037/0022-3514.82.6.1007

King, L., & Napa, C. K. (1998). What makes a life good? *Journal of Personality and Social Psychology, 75*(1), 156–165.

Klinger, E. (1998). The search for meaning in evolutionary perspective and its clinical implications. In P. T. P. Wong & P. S. Fry (Eds.), *The human quest for meaning. A handbook of psychological research and clinical applications* (pp. 27–50). Lawrence Erlbaum.

Koch, S. (1956). Behavior as "intrinsically" regulated: Work notes towards a pre-theory of phenomena called "motivational". In M. R. Jones (Ed.), *Nebraska symposium on motivation* (pp. 42–86). University of Nebraska Press.

Korsgaard, C. M. (2008). *The constitution of agency: Essays on practical reason and moral psychology*. Oxford University Press.

Kraut, R. (2015). Aristotle on well-being. In G. Fletcher (Ed.), *The Routledge handbook of philosophy of well-being [Kindle]* (pp. 20–28). Routledge.

Kraut, R. (2022). Aristotle's ethics. In E. N. Zalta (Ed.), *The Stanford encyclopedia of philosophy* (Spring 2022 ed.). Retrieved from https://plato.stanford.edu/archives/fall2022/entries/aristotle-ethics/

Kristjánsson, K. (2013). *Virtues and vices in positive psychology* [Kindle]. Cambridge University Press. https://doi.org/10.1017/cbo9781139177818

Law, A., & Staudinger, U. M. (2016). Eudaimonia and wisdom. In J. Vittersø (Ed.), *Handbook of eudaimonic well-being* (pp. 135–146). Springer International Publishing. https://doi.org/10.1007/978-3-319-42445-3_9

Leontiev, D. A. (2013). Personal meaning: A challenge for psychology. *The Journal of Positive Psychology, 8*(6), 459–470. https://doi.org/10.1080/17439760.2013.830767

Levinson, D. J., Darrow, C., Klein, E., Levinson, M., & McKee, B. (1978). *The seasons of a man's life*. Ballentine Books.

Lewin, K. (1931). The conflict between Aristotelian and Galileian modes of thought in contemporary psychology. *The Journal of General Psychology, 5*(2), 141–177. https://doi.org/10.1080/00221309.1931.9918387

Lewin, K. (1936). *Principles of topological psychology*. McGraw-Hill.

Liberman, V., Samuels, S. M., & Ross, L. (2004). The name of the game: Predictive power of reputations versus situational labels in determining prisoner's dilemma game moves. *Personality and Social Psychology Bulletin, 30*(9), 1175–1185.

Machan, T. R. (1979). Recent work in ethical egoism. *American Philosophical Quarterly, 16*(1), 1–15.

MacIntyre, A. (2007). *After virtue [Kindle]* (3rd ed.). University of Notre Dame Press.

Magen, Z. (1998). *Exploring adolescent happiness. Commitment, purpose, and fulfillment*. Sage.

Margolis, S., Schwitzgebel, E., Ozer, D. J., & Lyubomirsky, S. (2019). A new measure of life satisfaction: The Riverside life satisfaction scale. *Journal of Personality Assessment, 101*(6), 621–630. https://doi.org/10.1080/00223891.2018.1464457

Martela, F., & Ryan, R. M. (2023). Clarifying eudaimonia and psychological functioning to complement evaluative and experiential well-being: Why basic psychological needs should be measured in national accounts of well-being. *Perspectives on Psychological Science, 18*(5), 1121–1135. https://doi.org/10.1177/17456916221141099

Martela, F., & Sheldon, K. M. (2019). Clarifying the concept of well-being: Psychological need satisfaction as the common core connecting eudaimonic and subjective well-being. *Review of General Psychology, 23*(4), 458–474. https://doi.org/10.1177/1089268019880886

Martela, F., & Steger, M. F. (2016). The three meanings of meaning in life: Distinguishing coherence, purpose, and significance. *The Journal of Positive Psychology, 11*(5), 531–545. https://doi.org/10.1080/17439760.2015.1137623

Maslow, A. H. (1943). A theory of human motivation. *Psychological Review, 50*(4), 370–396.

Maslow, A. (1954). *Motivation and personality*. Harper and Row.

Maslow, A. H. (1961). Eupsychia—The good society. *Journal of Humanistic Psychology, 1*(2), 1–11.

Maslow, A. (1962). *Toward a psychology of being [Kindle]*. Van Nostrand.

Maslow, A. (1971). *The farther reaches of human nature*. Penguin Compass.

Maurer, M. M., & Daukantaitė, D. (2020). Revisiting the organismic valuing process theory of personal growth: A theoretical review of rogers and its connection to positive psychology [Review]. *Frontiers in Psychology, 11*. https://doi.org/10.3389/fpsyg.2020.01706

Mayr, E. (1982). *The growth of biological thought. Diversity, evolution, and inheritance*. Harvard University Press.

Mayr, E. (2004). *What makes biology unique?: Considerations on the autonomy of a scientific discipline*. Cambridge University Press.

Mayr, E. (2010). What is the meaning of "life"? In C. E. Cleland & M. A. Bedau (Eds.), *The nature of life: Classical and contemporary perspectives from philosophy and science* (pp. 88–101). Cambridge University Press. https://doi.org/10.1017/CBO9780511730191.009

McAdams, D. P. (2006). *The redemptive self.* Oxford University PRess.

McAdams, D. P., & McLean, K. C. (2013). Narrative identity. *Current Directions in Psychological Science, 22*(3), 233–238. https://doi.org/10.1177/0963721413475622
McDougall, W. (1950). The hormic psychology. Supplementary chapter 7. In *An introduction to social psychology* (pp. 444–494). https://brocku.ca/MeadProject/McDougall/1926/1950_s07.html
McGregor, I., & Little, B. (1998). Personal projects, happiness, and meaning: On doing well and being yourself. *Journal of Personality and Social Psychology, 74*(2), 494–512.
McMahon, D. (2006). *The pursuit of happiness. A history from the Greeks to the present.* Allen Lane.
Megone, C. (1994). Quality of life: Starting from Aristotle. In S. Baldwin, C. Godfrey, & C. Propper (Eds.), *Quality of life: Perspectives and policies* (pp. 28–41). Routledge.
Merritt, M. (2000). Virtue ethics and situationist personality psychology. *Ethical Theory and Moral Practice, 3*(4), 365–383. https://doi.org/10.1023/A:1009926720584
Michalos, A. C., & Robinson, S. R. (2012). The good life: Eighth century to third century BCE. In K. C. Land, A. C. Michalos, & M. J. Sirgy (Eds.), *Handbook of social indicators and quality of life research* (pp. 23–61). Springer. https://doi.org/10.1007/978-94-007-2421-1_2
Milgram, S. (1963). Behavioral study of obedience. *The Journal of Abnormal and Social Psychology, 67*, 371–378. https://doi.org/10.1037/h0040525
Mischel, W. (1973). Toward a cognitive social learning reconceptualization of personality. *Psychological Review, 80*, 252–283.
Moen, O. M. (2015). Hedonism before Bentham. *Journal of Bentham Studies, 17*(1), 1–18. https://doi.org/10.14324/111.2045-757X.007
Møller, V., & Roberts, B. J. (2017). South African hopes and fears twenty years into democracy: A replication of Hadley Cantril's pattern of human concerns. *Social Indicators Research, 130*(1), 39–69. https://doi.org/10.1007/s11205-015-1131-2
Mook, D. G. (1996). *Motivation: The organization of action* (2nd ed.). Norton.
Morley, J. (1995). Holistic biology and the organismic foundations of humanistic psychology. *The Humanistic Psychologist, 23*(3), 358–364. https://doi.org/10.1080/08873267.1995.9986836
Nakamura, J., & Csikszentmihalyi, M. (2014). The concept of flow. In M. Csikszentmihalyi (Ed.), *Flow and the foundations of positive psychology: The collected works of Mihaly Csikszentmihalyi* (pp. 239–263). Springer. https://doi.org/10.1007/978-94-017-9088-8_16
Nilsson, A. H., Eichstaedt, J. C., Lomas, T., Schwartz, A., & Kjell, O. (2024). The Cantril Ladder elicits thoughts about power and wealth. *Scientific Reports, 14*(1), 2642. https://doi.org/10.1038/s41598-024-52939-y
Norton, D. L. (1976). *Personal destinies: A philosophy of ethical individualism.* Princeton University Press.
Nussbaum, M. C. (2001). *Upheavals of thought. The intelligence of emotions.* Cambridge University Press.
Nussbaum, M. C. (2004). Mill between Aristotle & Bentham. *Daedalus, 133*(2), 60–68. https://doi.org/10.1162/001152604323049406
Nussbaum, M. C. (2008). Who is the happy warrior? Philosophy poses questions to psychology. *The Journal of Legal Studies, 37*(S2), s81–s113. https://doi.org/10.1086/587438
Oberauer, K., & Lewandowsky, S. (2019). Addressing the theory crisis in psychology. *Psychonomic Bulletin & Review, 26*(5), 1596–1618. https://doi.org/10.3758/s13423-019-01645-2
O'Dwyer, K. (2012). "The quiet revolutionary": A timely revisiting of Carl Rogers' visionary contribution to human understanding. *International Journal of Existential Psychology and Psychotherapy, 4*(1), 67–78.
OECD. (2013). *OECD Guidelines on measuring subjective well-being.* https://doi.org/10.1787/9789264191655-en
Oishi, S. (2018). Culture and subjective well-being: Conceptual and measurement issues. In E. Diener, S. Oishi, & L. Tay (Eds.), *Handbook of subjective well-being. Noba Scholar Handbook series: Subjective well-being.* DEF Publishers. nobascholar.com. https://doi.org/nobascholar.com

Oishi, S., & Westgate, E. C. (2022). A psychologically rich life: Beyond happiness and meaning. *Psychological Review, 129*(4), 790–811. https://doi.org/10.1037/rev0000317

Oishi, S., Graham, J., Kesebir, S., & Galinha, I. C. (2013). Concepts of happiness across time and cultures. *Personality and Social Psychology Bulletin, 39*(5), 559–577. https://doi.org/10.1177/0146167213480042

Petri, H. (1991). *Motivation: Theory, research, and applications* (3rd ed.). Wadsworth Publ.

Piaget, J. (1952). *The origins of intelligence in children*. International Universities Press.

Prinz, J. (2009). The normativity challenge: Cultural psychology provides the real threat to virtue ethics [journal article]. *The Journal of Ethics, 13*(2), 117–144. https://doi.org/10.1007/s10892-009-9053-3

Prinzing, M. (2021). How to study well-being: A proposal for the integration of philosophy with science. *Review of General Psychology, 25*(2), 152–162. https://doi.org/10.1177/10892680211002443

Proctor, C., Tweed, R., & Morris, D. (2016). The Rogerian fully functioning person: A positive psychology perspective. *Journal of Humanistic Psychology, 56*(5), 503–529. https://doi.org/10.1177/0022167815605936

Pross, A. (2016). *What is life?: How chemistry becomes biology*. Oxford University Press.

Proulx, T., Markman, K. D., & Lindberg, M. J. (2013). Introduction: The new science of meaning. In K. D. Markman, T. Proulx, & M. J. Lindberg (Eds.), *The psychology of meaning* (pp. 3–14). American Psychological Association.

Ramose, M. B. (2002). Globalization and Ubuntu. In P. Coetzee & A. Roux (Eds.), *The African philosophy reader* (pp. 626–650). Routledge.

Reis, H. T., Sheldon, K. M., Gable, S. L., Roscoe, J., & Ryan, R. M. (2000). Daily well-being: The role of autonomy, competence, and relatedness. *Personality and Social Psychology Bulletin, 26*(4), 419–435.

Ritter, W. E. (1919). *The unity of the organism, or, the organismical conception of life*. Gorham Press.

Rogers, C. R. (1961). *On becoming a person. A therapist's view of psychotherapy*. Houghton Mifflin Co.

Rogers, C. R. (1963). The concept of the fully functioning person. *Psychotherapy: Theory, Research & Practice, 1*(1), 17–26. https://doi.org/10.1037/h0088567

Rojas, M., Méndez, A., & Watkins-Fassler, K. (2023). The hierarchy of needs empirical examination of Maslow's theory and lessons for development. *World Development, 165*, 106185. https://doi.org/10.1016/j.worlddev.2023.106185

Romero, A. (2012). When whales became mammals: The scientific journey of cetaceans from fish to mammals in the history of science. *New Approaches to the Study of Marine Mammals*, 3–30.

Roosevelt, E. (1983). *You learn by living. Eleven keys for a more fulfilling life [Kindle]*. Harper Perennial.

Ross, W. D. (2009). *Aristotle: The Nicomachean ethics*. Oxford University Press.

Ross, L., & Nisbett, R. E. (2011). *The person and the situation. Perspectives of social psychology*. McGraw Hill.

Ruiz-Mirazo, K., Etxeberria, A., Moreno, A., & Ibáñez, J. (2000). Organisms and their place in biology [journal article]. *Theory in Biosciences, 119*(3), 209. https://doi.org/10.1007/s12064-000-0017-1

Russell, D. C. (2013). Virtue ethics, happiness, and the good life. In D. C. Russell (Ed.), *The Cambridge companion to virtue ethics [Kindle]* (pp. 7–28). Cambridge University Press.

Ryan, R. (1993). Agency and organization: Intrinsic motivation, autonomy and the self in psychological development. In J. Jacobs (Ed.), *Nebraska symposium on motivation: Development and psychopathology* (Vol. 40, pp. 1–56). University of Nebraska Press.

Ryan, R. M. (1995). Psychological needs and the facilitation of integrative processes. *Journal of Personality, 63*, 397–428.

Ryan, R. M. M., & Deci, E. L. (2000). When rewards compete with nature: The undermining of intrinsic motivation and self-regulation. In C. Sansone & J. M. Harackiewics (Eds.), *Intrinsic and extrinsic motivation. The search for optimal motivation and performance* (pp. 13–54). Academic Press.

Ryan, R. M. M., & Deci, E. L. D. (2001). On happiness and human potentials: A review of research on hedonic and eudaimonic well-being. *Annual Review of Psychology, 52*, 141–166. http://psych.AnnualReviews.org/cgi/reprint/52/1/141.pdf

Ryan, R. M., & Deci, E. L. (2017). Self-determination theory: Basic psychological needs in motivation, development, and wellness [Kindle]. *Guilford.* Publications.

Ryan, R. M., & Martela, F. (2016). Eudaimonia as a way of living: Connecting Aristotle with self-determination theory. In J. Vittersø (Ed.), *Handbook of Eudaimonic well-being* (pp. 109–122). Springer International Publishing. https://doi.org/10.1007/978-3-319-42445-3_7

Ryan, R. M. M., Huta, V., & Deci, E. L. (2008). Living well: A self-determination theory perspective in eudaimonia. *Journal of Happiness Studies, 9*(1), 139–170. https://doi.org/10.1007/s10902-006-9023-4

Ryan, R. M., Curren, R. R., & Deci, E. L. (2013). What humans need: Flourishing in Aristotelian philosophy and self-determination theory. In *The best within us: Positive psychology perspectives on eudaimonia* (pp. 57–75). American Psychological Association. https://doi.org/10.1037/14092-004

Ryan, R. M., Duineveld, J. J., Di Domenico, S. I., Ryan, W. S., Steward, B. A., & Bradshaw, E. L. (2022). We know this much is (meta-analytically) true: A meta-review of meta-analytic findings evaluating self-determination theory. *Psychological Bulletin, 148*, 813–842. https://doi.org/10.1037/bul0000385

Ryff, C. D. (1989). Happiness is everything, or is it? Explorations on the meaning of psychological well-being. *Journal of Personality and Social Psychology, 57*, 1069–1081. https://doi.org/10.1037/0022-3514.57.6.1069

Ryff, C. D. (2014). Self-realisation and meaning making in the face of adversity: A eudaimonic approach to human resilience. *Journal of Psychology in Africa, 24*(1), 1–12. https://doi.org/10.1080/14330237.2014.904098

Ryff, C. D. (2016). Beautiful ideas and the scientific enterprise: Sources of intellectual vitality in research on eudaimonic well-being. In J. Vittersø (Ed.), *Handbook of Eudaimonic well-being* (pp. 95–107). Springer International Publishing. https://doi.org/10.1007/978-3-319-42445-3_6

Ryff, C. D. (2018). Well-being with soul: Science in pursuit of human potential. *Perspectives on Psychological Science, 13*(2), 242–248.

Ryff, C. D., & Singer, B. (1998). The role of purpose in life and personal growth in positive human health. In P. T. P. Wong & P. S. Fry (Eds.), *The human quest for meaning. A handbook of psychological research and clinical applications* (pp. 213–235). Lawrence Erlbaum.

Ryff, C. D., & Singer, B. H. (2008). Know thyself and become what you are: A eudaimonic approach to psychological well-being. *Journal of Happiness Studies, 9*(1), 13–39. https://doi.org/10.1007/s10902-006-9019-0

Ryff, C. D., & Singer, B. (2013). Know thyself and become what you are: A eudaimonic approach to psychological well-being. In A. Delle Fave (Ed.), *The exploration of happiness* (pp. 97–116). Springer.

Ryff, C. D., Boylan, J. M., & Kirsch, J. A. (2021). Eudaimonic and hedonic well-being. An integrative perspective with linkages to sociodemographic factors and health. In M. T. Lee, L. D. Kubzansky, & T. J. VanderWeele (Eds.), *Measuring well-being: Interdisciplinary perspectives from the social sciences and the humanities*. Oxford University Press.

Sagi, A., & Sagi, A. (2002). *Albert Camus and the philosophy of the absurd* (Vol. 125). Rodopi.

Schwartz, B. (2011). Practical wisdom and organizations. *Research in Organizational Behavior, 31*, 3–23. https://doi.org/10.1016/j.riob.2011.09.001

Schwartz, B., & Wrzesniewski, A. (2016). Internal motivation, instrumental motivation, and eudaimonia. In J. Vittersø (Ed.), *Handbook of Eudaimonic well-being* (pp. 123–134). Springer International Publishing. https://doi.org/10.1007/978-3-319-42445-3_8

Seligman, M. E. P. (1998). *What is the 'good life'?* Edotorial. APA Monitor.

Shah, J. Y., & Kruglanski, A. W. (2000). The structure and substance of intrinsic motivation. In C. Sansone & J. M. Harackiewics (Eds.), *Intrinsic and extrinsic motivation. The search for optimal motivation and performance* (pp. 105–127). Academic Press.
Sheldon, K. M., Corcoran, M., & Prentice, M. (2019). Pursuing eudaimonic functioning versus pursuing hedonic well-being: The first goal succeeds in its aim, whereas the second does not. *Journal of Happiness Studies, 20*(3), 919–933. https://doi.org/10.1007/s10902-018-9980-4
Shields, C. (2022). Aristotle. In E. N. Zalta (Ed.), *The Stanford encyclopedia of philosophy* (Spring 2022 ed.). Retrieved from https://plato.stanford.edu/archives/spr2022/entries/aristotle/
Shmotkin, D., & Shrira, A. (2012). On the distinction between subjective well-being and meaning in life: Regulatory versus reconstructive functions in the face of a hostile world. In *The human quest for meaning: Theories, research, and applications* (2nd ed., pp. 143–163). Routledge/ Taylor & Francis Group.
Smith, E. E. (2017). *The power of meaning: Crafting a life that matters*. Random House.
Staudinger, U. M., & Kunzmann, U. (2005). Positive adult personality development. Adjustment and/or growth? *European Psychologist, 10*(4), 320–329.
Steptoe, A., Deaton, A., & Stone, A. A. (2015). Subjective wellbeing, health, and ageing. *The Lancet, 385*(9968), 640–648. https://doi.org/10.1016/S0140-6736(13)61489-0
Stone, A. A., & Krueger, A. B. (2018). Understanding subjective well-being. In J. E. Stiglitz, J.-P. Fitoussi, & M. Durand (Eds.), *For good measure: Advancing research on well-being metrics beyond GDP* (pp. 163–202). OECD Publishing.
Stone, A. A., & Mackie, C. (2013). *Subjective well-being: Measuring happiness, suffering, and other dimensions of experience*. National Academies Press.
Sumner, L. W. (1996). *Welfare, happiness, and ethics*. Clarendon Press.
Sumner, L. W. (2002). Happiness then and now. In L. J. Jost & R. A. Shiner (Eds.), *Eudaimonia and well-being* (pp. 21–39). Academic Printing & Publishing.
Taylor, J. B. (2008). *My stroke of insight [Kindle]*. Hodder & Stoughton.
Telfer, E. (1980). *Happiness*. St. Martin's Press.
Thagard, P. (2010). *The brain and the meaning of life [Kindle]*. Princeton University Press.
Thagard, P. (2019). *Mind-society: From brains to social sciences and professions (treatise on mind and society)*. Oxford University Press.
Tov, W. (2018). Well-being concepts and components. In E. Diener, S. Oishi, & L. Tay (Eds.), *Handbook of subjective well-being. Noba Scholar Handbook series: Subjective well-being*. DEF publishers. DOI: nobascholar.com. https://doi.org/nobascholar.com
Tov, W., & Lee, H. W. (2016). A closer look at the hedonics of everyday meaning and satisfaction. *Journal of Personality and Social Psychology, 111*(4), 585–609. https://doi.org/10.1037/pspp0000081
Tsurumi, T., Yamaguchi, R., Kagohashi, K., & Managi, S. (2021). Are cognitive, affective, and eudaimonic dimensions of subjective well-being differently related to consumption? Evidence from Japan. *Journal of Happiness Studies, 22*(6), 2499–2522. https://doi.org/10.1007/s10902-020-00327-4
Van Zyl, L. (2018). *Virtue ethics: A contemporary introduction [Kindle]*. Routledge.
Vansteenkiste, M., Ryan, R. M., & Soenens, B. (2020). Basic psychological need theory: Advancements, critical themes, and future directions. *Motivation and Emotion, 44*(1), 1–31. https://doi.org/10.1007/s11031-019-09818-1
Vittersø, J. (2013). Functional well-being: Happiness as feelings, evaluations and functioning. In S. David, I. Boniwell, & A. C. Ayers (Eds.), *The Oxford handbook of happiness* (pp. 227–244). Oxford University Press.
von Bertalanffy, L. (1952/2014). *Problems of life. An evaluation of modern biological and scientific thought*. Martino Publishing. (Original work published in 1952).
Vygotsky, L. S. (1978). *Mind in society: The development of higher psychological processes*. Harvard University Press.
Walsh, D. M. (2015). *Organisms, agency, and evolution*. Cambridge University Press. https://doi.org/10.1017/CBO9781316402719

Waterman, A. S. (1981). Individualism and interdependence. *American Psychologist, 36*, 762–773.
Waterman, A. S. (1984). *The psychology of individualism*. Praeger.
Waterman, A. S. (1993). Two conceptions of happiness: Contrasts of personal expressiveness (Eudaimonia) and hedonic enjoyment. *Journal of Personality and Social Psychology, 64*(4), 678–691. https://doi.org/10.1037/0022-3514.64.4.678
Waterman, A. S. (2008). Reconsidering happiness: A eudaimonist's perspective. *Journal of Positive Psychology, 3*(4), 234–252.
Waterman, A. S. (2013). Introduction: Considering the nature of a life well-lived—Intersections of positive psychology and eudaimonist philosophy. In *The best within us: Positive psychology perspectives on eudaimonia* (pp. 3–17). American Psychological Association. https://doi.org/10.1037/14092-001
Waterman, A. S., & Schwartz, S. J. (2013). Eudaimonic identity theory. In A. S. Waterman (Ed.), *The best within us: Positive psychology perspectives on eudaimonia* (pp. 99–118). American Psychological Association. https://doi.org/10.1037/14092-006
Waterman, A. S., Schwartz, S. J., & Conti, R. (2008). The implications of two concepts of happiness (Hedonic enjoyment and eudaimonia) for the understanding of intrinsic motivation. *Journal of Happiness Studies, 9*(1), 41–79. https://doi.org/10.1007/s10902-006-9020-7
Weiss, R. (1979). Aristotle's criticism of eudoxan hedonism. *Classical Philology, 74*(3), 214–221. https://doi.org/10.1086/366501
Whitehouse, H. (2004). *Modes of religiosity. A cognitive theory of religious transformation*. Altamira Press.
Wilson, E. O. (2014). *The meaning of human existence [Kindle]*. WW Norton & Company.
Wong, D. (2013). Chinese ethics. In E. N. Zalta (Ed.), *The Stanford encyclopedia of philosophy*. http://plato.stanford.edu/archives/spr2013/entries/ethics-chinese/
Yu, J. (1998). Virtue: Confucius and Aristotle. *Philosophy East and West, 48*(2), 323–347. https://doi.org/10.2307/1399830

Chapter 7
Steps Toward a Humanistic Theory of Wellbeing

Introduction

No one will get cake until everyone has had bread. Einar Gerhardsen.[1]

The science of wellbeing asks *how* and *why* a live is well lived. Thus, a good theory must "tell us what it is for someone's life to go well or badly" (Sumner, 1996, p. 1). The answers proposed by the humanistic theory of wellbeing are grounded in basic knowledge about human nature, such as what life is and what makes life possible (e.g., Pross, 2016). Biologists acknowledge that to survive, the chemical structures we call life must have a built-in valuation mechanism that provides the organism with "value hints," i.e., signals about what it should care about and what it must avoid. In primitive life forms, this information is regulated by a chemical process called chemotaxis. In sentient beings, equipped with a central nervous system and the ability to experience subjectivity, value hints can appear as feelings. In humans, equipped with concepts such as care, morality, and objectivity, value hints are transformed into intricate and multidimensional information processes and include both feelings and thinking as these are developed in social interactions (e.g., Damasio, 2021).

The varieties of human valuations can be organized in accordance with three, universal human needs: the need for stability, the need for change, and the need to and for care. This theoretical structure efficiently categorizes the major kinds of wellbeing into a hierarchical taxonomy and avoids the ad hoc list making often seen in the wellbeing literature (cf. Chap. 6). The humanistic theory of wellbeing further suggests that the fulfillment of these universal needs enables us to lead good lives, in the sense of allowing us to*perform our humanness well.*

[1] Norwegian Prime Minister (1945–1951 and 1955–1965).

J. Vittersø, *Humanistic Wellbeing*, https://doi.org/10.1007/978-3-031-69292-5_7

Needs for Stability and Change

A sign in a southwestern bar in the USA got the interplay between stability and change about right. It says:

> I ain't what I've been.
> I ain't what I'm going to be.
> I am what I am.

The verse is mentioned in Bruner et al. (1986/1957) to illustrate how a classification—of one's identity in this example—can remain stable even if what it represents change. More generally, the sign captures fundamental insight into how life must be both stable and changeable.

As spelled out in Chap. 1, this principle can be observed in everything biological, from the DNA molecule to central evolutionary mechanisms. Life involves chemical reactions, and chemical reactions are regulated by a balance between stability and instability. Fundamentally speaking, living organisms therefore operate by dynamically steering between their need for stability and their need for change (e.g., Pross, 2016). One powerful illustration comes from the way in which organic structures are regulated by the laws of nature, particularly by the second law of thermodynamics. Very roughly, we might say that things in the natural world move toward chaos and disorder and that the second law explains why. To survive in the world of thermodynamics entropy (i.e., disorganization), animated organisms must be able to hold back the constant push toward disorganization. Erwin Schrödinger, who in 1946 published a breakthrough in biological chemistry, realized how life became possible when an organisms evolved the ability to maintain order and coherence in the face of the constant exchange of matter and energy with their environments. Schrödinger reasoned that the capacity to hold back the second law of thermodynamics is what makes biological organisms different from nonliving entities. The capacity to maintain stability is therefore nothing less than the essence of life. By eating, drinking, and breathing, a biological organism can counteract the principle of entropy and maintain "itself stationary at a fairly high level of orderliness" (Schrödinger, 2010/1946, p. 64).

Stability and Homeostasis

Homeostasis has been introduced throughout this book as an intricate set of regulatory procedures structured around the need to preserve stability by maintaining essential physiological and psychological elements within a narrow range of values (e.g., Billman, 2020; Cummins, 2020; Damasio, 2018; Lercher, 2018; Lewis, 2018; Rodolfo, 2000). As illustrated in the principles by which a thermostat regulates the temperature in a room,[2] homeostasis enables a body to initiate responses that move it toward a target value. A well-known example is the maintenance of a core body temperature at 37 °C, but numerous other processes are controlled by homeostatic principles, such as breathing, heart rate, blood pressure, energy balance, pH, visceral operations, and a variety of endocrine processes (e.g., Damasio, 2018; Lewis, 2018). Homeostasis is not only a stabilizing regulator of minds and bodies. The atmosphere is, for instance, involved in the homeostatic regulation of life on our planet. Lercher (2018) explains that "higher temperatures cause increased phytoplankton growth in the oceans, which produces airborne gases and organic matter that seeds cloud droplets; more and denser clouds, in turn, lead to an increased reflection of sunlight back into space and thus contribute to temperature homeostasis" (p. 121).

But the regulation of stability is not limited to homeostasis. A bird constantly flapping its wings is an example of how an airborne state is kept stable. At a yet grander scale, the existence of species such as the cyanobacteria—which have lived on Earth for several billion years (Pross, 2016, p. 75)—is a stunning example of what Dawkins (2016) refers to as the principle of "the survival of the most stable."

Change

Stability is not enough to keep biological structures alive; it is the dynamic interaction between stability and change that ensures survival. For example, Pross (2016, p. 75) likened the stability–change duality of life to a water fountain: it remains the same even if its water is constantly turning over. By analogy, the cells in our bodies are regularly replaced with new cells, even if our bodies remain the same. Some changes are nevertheless more fundamental than others. Larvae turns into insects, eggs become chickens, and human babies grow into adults. People may also change more spectacularly, as when the civil rights movement activist Rosa Parks went from a victim to a catalyst or when Nelson Mandela went from prisoner to statesman (Sapolsky, 2017, p. 175).

More principally, organisms are dependent on their environments and must also be open to them. Biological structures therefore need to adjust their responses and accommodate the changing demands of their surroundings. As mentioned in Chap. 1, Blasi once claimed that "the organism must die or change its structural laws to meet environmental demands" (Blasi, 1976, p. 35). Although not always as dramatically expressed as in the Blasi quote, the notion that both stability and change are universal needs is well acknowledged. Block has, for instance, pointed out that "under the widest range of conditions, organisms undergo transformations from the

[2] The homeostatic, or cybernetic, process in a thermostat has four components: (1) a system variable (the phenomenon to be regulated), (2) a monitor, (3) a set point (or more correctly, a set zone), and (4) a correcting mechanism (see Carver and Scheier (2001) for a useful introduction and Clark (1996) for a technical account).

status of relatively undifferentiated entities to relatively differentiated and integrated adult forms" (Block, 1982, p. 287). Similarly, Nurse (2020, p. 129) explains that "living entities are chemical, physical and informational machines. They construct their own metabolism and use it to maintain themselves, grow and reproduce." McGilchrist (2012, loc. 192) maintains that "All systems in nature, from particles to the greater universe, from the world of cellular processes to that of all living things, depend on a necessary balance of the forces for stasis with the forces for flow." Jasanoff (2019, p. 1) points out that life depends on "both the variety and the relative stability of biological organisms."

Psychologists have also had a long-standing interest in the dynamics between stability and change. Half a century ago, Charlotte Bühler concluded that "the individual tries to maintain its equilibrium at the same time that it expands" (1951, pp. 320–321). Maslow's hierarchy of needs (reviewed in Chap. 6) comprises the two main categories of d-needs and b-needs. The former deals with stability, while the latter deals with change. In the same spirit, Gordon Allport argued that stability and change are steering principles that we both want and need in our lives (Allport, 1955, p. 66). He considered hedonism to be a stability motivator and the term "propriate stiving" to be a change motivator (Allport, 1961, p. 199). He also thought of stability and change as core dimensions in the study of individual differences, a perspective that has reappeared in concurrent personality psychology. For instance, DeYoung and colleagues (DeYoung, 2006; DeYoung & Weisberg, 2018) proposed that a major source of human personality variation can ultimately be tied to a motivation for either stability (protection of goals, interpretations, and strategies from disruption of impulses) or plasticity (exploration and creation of new goals, interpretations, and strategies). Other personality psychologists have argued in a similar vein (e.g., Bleidorn et al., 2021; Kiley & Vaisey, 2020). Indeed, individuals differ in their preferences for stability and change to the extent that the philosopher John Stuart Mill considered it "commonplace" to have one political party for order or stability and one for progress or change (Mill, 1859, loc. 771). Recent research has convincingly confirmed that conservative people prefer stability, whereas liberals prefer change (e.g., Churchland, 2018b; Johnson, 2014; Wojcik et al., 2015).

We also find a strong argument for the stability/change dynamics in the work of Piaget, particularly in his ideas about equilibration, which was briefly introduced in Chap. 3. Piaget's concept of equilibration is abstract and hard to grasp (e.g., Chapman, 1992) but essentially implies an adjustment between a person's cognitive structures and his or her environment (Ginsburg & Opper, 1969, p. 14). Among developmental psychologists, this balance is known as the interaction between two factors: assimilation and accommodation. Briefly, Piaget defines assimilation as the integration of external elements into evolving or completed structures (Block, 1982, p. 282). Thus, it contributes to stability by maintaining a sense of continuity in our understanding of the world. Change is avoided by fitting new experiences into existing frameworks. In contrast, accommodation is defined as any modification of an assimilatory scheme or structure by the elements it assimilates. Accommodation facilitates change because it requires individuals to modify their cognitive structures in response to novel information. To Piaget, the foremost tendency of all organisms is to survive and remain the same. However, there are limits to how much an organism can oppose radical change, and structural transformations must sometimes occur. According to Piaget, optimal human functioning thus works by the following imperative: "Assimilate if you can; accommodate if you must!" (Block, 1982, p. 286).

John Bowlby is another developmental psychologist with a keen interest for the interplay between stability and change (Bowlby, 1973; van der Horst et al., 2008). He recognized that children have an innate drive to explore their environments and that this exploration is crucial for cognitive and social change. However, these phases of growth and development can become overwhelming and stressful, which is why children also seek back to their caregivers for a "secure base" or a "haven of safety" (Bowlby, 1973, p. 146). The interaction between the comfort and protection experienced in their secure base, and the growth and development occurring in the phases of exploration, nicely illustrates the dynamic interaction between stability and change. A similar pattern of stability-and-change dynamics has also been reported by Bühler et al. (1928), whose views were briefly mentioned above. Some of the observations Bühler used as evidence for her conclusions came from a study of 6-month-old children exposed to a strange stimulus. The first response Bühler noted was fearful behavior often involving crying and movement, which is indicative of displeasure. The next time the stimulus appears, the response is still dominated by movements and vocalizations indicative of displeasure. However, at the third exposure, the 6-month-old children started paying closer attention to the stimulus and no longer showed signs of displeasure. Finally, at the fourth exposure, the baby looks attentively at the stimulus with interest for approximately 15 s (cited in Berlyne, 1960, p. 204).

The interplay between safety and exploration has also been observed in other species, such as birds. Izard and Ackerman (2000) refer to a report by Lorenz (1950), who recorded the behavior of a raven in this way: "From a high limb of a tall tree, the bird studies an object on the ground. The raven flies closer for a better look, then returns to a limb a bit closer than it first perch. It flies down again and this time back up to a limb yet closer to the object. This process continues until the raven lands by the object and begins actively exploring it" (Izard & Ackerman, 2000, p. 257).

Need to and for Care

Chapter 1 noted that all organisms care about what happens to them. Although this principle applies to everything alive, the caring capacity of mammals has evolved to be particularly powerful, and this is due to a strong selection pressure on sociability. In no mammals have the need to care for others been developed to higher levels of sophistication than it has for *Homo sapiens* (e.g., Bloom, 2013; Gopnik, 2009; Keltner, 2009; Tomasello, 2019). Hence, an important premise for the humanistic theory of wellbeing is that this joint need for maintaining both one's own wellbeing and that of others is essential to understanding the notion of a good life.

The neurological basis for the expansion of self-care into other care is described in a nontechnical way by the philosopher Patricia Churchland (e.g., Churchland, 2018a, 2018b). She argues that organisms are structured to care about their most basic values, which are the values of being alive and being well. Such caring is thus "a ground-floor function of nervous systems" (Churchland, 2018a, p. 30). Churchland maintains that there has been a selection pressure on mammals for the expansion of self-caring into other-caring. Many processes participate in making mammalian brains able to care, but three factors stand out: (1) urges to care about the welfare of self, offspring, mates, and affiliates; (2) the capacity to evaluate and predict what oneself and others will feel and do, in particular circumstances; and (3) a neural reward-and-punishment system linked to internalizing social practices and applying them suitably—more generally, linked to learning the expectations and ways of parents, siblings, and other groups (Churchland, 2018a, p. 61).

This sociability originated almost certainly in maternal behavior, and much is now known about the mechanisms that gradually converted self-care into care for offspring. A mother rat, for instance, "behaves as though the newborn pups are included in her basic homeostatic ambit—they must be fed, cleaned, and kept warm, as well as protected from the assorted dangers of the world, just as she must keep herself fed, warm, clean, and safe from the dangers of the world" (Churchland, 2018a, p. 30).

Churchland refers to the selection pressure toward caring as the "snuggle for survival" (Churchland, 2018b, p. 19). Humans are masters of such snuggle, equipped as we are with brains that ensure that we become attached to our families and closed ones and are powerfully motivated to cooperate with them, even when doing so entails going against our own interests. These processes have been creatively described by Paul Bloom:

> A young woman meets a much younger man and takes him into her home. He suffers from serious limitations. He cannot walk or talk or even sit up; he cannot be left alone and must be fed and bathed. He often screams and cries at night, and she spends the first years with him in a sleep-deprived fog. Still, this is the most important relationship of her life. She would die for him. She dedicates many years to nursing him as he gradually becomes able to walk, to toilet himself, and to speak. After they have been together for a bit over a decade, he becomes interested in other women and begins to date, and eventually he leaves her home and marries someone else. The woman continues to love and support him, helping to raise the children that he has with his new wife. If this younger man were a grown stranger, the woman's actions would be seen as saintly or insane. But this description summarizes a typical relationship between mother and son. (Bloom, 2013, p. 159)

Care Ethics

The young woman in Bloom's story is not primarily seeking to further her own individual interests. Her interests are obviously intertwined with those of the "much younger man" that she fosters. People who look after a particular other often do so because their interests are inseparable from the interests of the persons they care for: "Persons in caring relations are acting for self-and-other together" as Held puts it (2006, p. 12). Held, who was introduced in Chap. 1, argues that care is our most fundamental value, more essential than justice, for example. There can be care without justice, she maintains, but there can be no justice without care.

An ethics of care has according to Held (2006, pp. 9–13) five essential features. First, the moral salience of care ethics involves attending to and meeting the needs of the particular others, for whom responsibility is taken. Second, the ethics of care values emotion. To understand what would be morally best for us to do and to be, emotions should be emphasized rather than rejected. Third, the view that more abstract reasoning about a moral problem is better than less abstract reasoning is abandoned. The abstract and impartial perspective on which a universal set of moral principles is grounded is potentially in conflict with an ethics anchored in the obligation to apply a specific kind of care to a small group of particular others. But the relational interests embedded in care ethics make the tension between the particular and the universal less critical. The relational view is also a view of persons engaged in developing human morality, and this perspective might enable us to respect both a universal and a particular ethics. Fourth, the traditional notions about the distinction between the public and the private are reconceptualized. Given the asymmetry of this privacy notion, such as how "the law has not hesitated to intervene into women's private decisions concerning reproduction but has been highly reluctant to intrude on men's exercise of coercive power within the 'castles' of their homes" (p. 12), the ethics of care address family matters such as unequal power relations, economic dependencies, sexual abuse, and domestic violence as moral rather than private issues. Fifth, humans are conceived of as relational rather than rational.

The relational approach to human nature is important but overlooked in dominant moral theories. Held criticizes liberal theories of justice and Kantian thinking for having adopted a liberal idea of individuals as rational, autonomous, and self-interested agents, for whom cooperation only takes place if it benefits the individual interests of those involved. She refers to the philosopher Michael Sandel, who explains how liberal theories essentially hold humans to be distinct individuals first and only secondly form relationships (Held, 2006, p. 13).

Sandel has pointed out that economists often promote a worldview in which the selfish individual is the solution to our moral considerations. The economic perspective "saves society from squandering its scarce supply of virtue," by, for example, economizing the rare resource of love (Sandel, 2011, p. 127). Sandel refers to Lawrence Summers, a renowned economist within this tradition, who makes altruism look like a zero-sum game. We only dispose a scarce amount of altruism, Summers argues, and we should therefore not waste it. He suggests that "Reckless expenditure of altruism in social and economic life not only deplete the supply available for other public purposes. They even reduce the amount we have left for our families and friends" (Sandel, 2011, p. 129).

Rather than seeing care and altruism as a scarce recourse that we individualistically must conserve and handle with caution, the ethics of care "sees persons as relational and interdependent, morally and epistemologically. Every person starts out as a child dependent on those providing us care, and we remain interdependent with others in thoroughly fundamental ways throughout our lives. That we can think and act as if we were independent depends on a network of social relations making it possible for us to do so" (Held, 2006, pp. 13–14). These mechanisms of cooperation and relational understanding are elaboratively presented in Tomasello's moral theory and will be examined next.

Becoming a Moral and Caring Human Being

The caring needs comprise the need *to* care, as well as the need *for* care. The need to care is accounted for in Tomasello's theory of human development (Tomasello, 2019), particularly in its moral elements (Tomasello, 2016). Tomasello is a developmental psychologist and primatologist who briefly was introduced in Chap. 1. His contribution to the literature on human phylogeny and ontogeny is extensive and recently summarized in the impressive tome *Becoming Human* (2019). In it, Tomasello describes how changes in the environmental circumstances in our evolutionary past drew early humans—perhaps they were *Homo heidelbergensis*—toward new and more sophisticated forms of cooperation. One radical transformation took place approximately 400,000 years ago and altered the way we shape our goals and values, what Tomasello refers to as intentionality, i.e., the ability to share attention, intentions, and goals with others. These new skills enabled our ancestors to understand not only that my wellbeing is vitally dependent on your wellbeing but also that *our* wellbeing depends on *us* taking care of *one another*. A "second-person" morality was thus established as the "me" was favorably subordinated to an "us." This second-personal agency created a normative sense of "ought," a cooperative pressure and a rational understanding of responsibility vis-à-vis a collaborative partner. This was the shift from an individual to a joint intentionality.

A more essential game changer was needed, however, to enable the ethical thinking possessed by modern human beings: a "third-person" or "objective" morality. It started to emerge about 200,000 years ago, when small bands of hunters and gatherers grew into larger tribes. Competition between the groups as they expanded prepared a tighter organization among in-group populations, as collaborators refined a practice of labor division. This mutual collaboration led to an institutionalization of the rights and duties associated with the diversity of tasks required by the new lifestyle. Consequently, the idea of objectivity matured—i.e., the understanding that some tasks and perspectives are not mine or yours but rather are universal.

Such a group-minded mentality with the capacity to think in terms of objectivity was a great comparative advantage for the newly evolved modern human. By committing themselves to a collective rather than to particular persons, social institutions and more abstract affiliations with in-group members evolved. The novel common ground laid the foundation for cultural conventions and a cultural identity that grew from a conformity to social norms and cultural practices, such as how to talk, how to dress, and how to solve day-to-day problems. Sympathetic concern for a partner's wellbeing was transformed into loyalty for the group and an objectification of values.

The universal goodness gradient referred to as a valuation mechanism throughout this book was now scaled up to operate beyond a single organism or a dyadic interaction. It became applicable at the level of groups: *our* way of talking, dressing, and solving problems is good—and better than the practices of other groups. Moreover, common in-group rules were established about how to treat one another on a general basis, universal ideas about rightness and wrongness evolved, and the concept of morality was born. A moral value is not mine or yours; it is ours. With moral objectivity came individual responsibility: if the conventions were broken, the uncooperativeness had to be explained. "In this way, modern humans internalized not only moral actions but moral justifications and created a reason-based moral identity within the community" (Tomasello, 2018, p. 75). This innovative understanding implies that a major concern became not only what "they" think of me but importantly what "we," including "I," think of me. "The essence of this account is thus a kind of 'we is greater than me' psychological orientation, which gives moral notions their special powers of legitimacy in personal decision making" (p. 75). The third-person perspective, i.e., the objectivity generated by culture, ensured that notions of right and wrong were established as universal truths, at least within the group. This was the shift from a joint intentionality to a collective intentionality.

The relatively recent insights into cooperative, caring, and solidaric human phylogeny are not a discovery of a happy Shangri-La of peace and harmony. Social interactions have always faced many challenges, and cooperative and culturally shaped intentionality tendencies can be thwarted or misused for purposes other than those of a common good and the creation of sustainable societies inhabited by happy people. For example, we are mentally equipped for a collaborative life in small groups, geared for solving moral problems within tribal societies. Humans are more poorly equipped to solving conflicts and moral disagreements in large societies or across groups (Greene, 2013). But again Tomasello: "if we are to solve our largest challenges as a species, which threaten all human societies alike, we had best be prepared to think of all of humanity as a 'we'" (2018, p. 75).

From this perspective, Tomasello's theory contrasts with previous (mis)understandings about human nature. The tradition after Hobbes, for instance, in which selfish individuals are believed to be forced into collaboration for strategic and self-centered reasons, is inconsistent with updated insights about human nature. As cultural beings, contemporary humans are born into and identify themselves with a society. Social norms are not always enforced upon us from the outside but can be internalized as a collective commitment. In most instances, but certainly not all, cultural values of right and wrong operate as a cooperative rationality that makes us consider them as "ours" and not something "they" force upon "me." We don't obey them to act strategically; we stick to them because we are convinced that is the right thing to do.

Individuals are therefore not determined to become selfish because of their genetic constitution, as Dawkins legendarily suggested in *The Selfish Gene*. He writes, "I shall argue that a predominant quality to be expected in a successful gene is ruthless selfishness. This gene selfishness will usually give rise to selfishness in individual behavior. (...) Much as we might wish to believe otherwise, universal love and the welfare of the species as a whole are concepts that simply do not make evolutionary sense" (Dawkins, 2016, p. 3). True enough, Dawkins goes on to tell us that facts about evolution should not be taken as arguments about human morality, and he warns readers against making such an interpretation of his message. However, his cautions have not been strong enough to prevent rich and influential people from using Dawkins' self-centric views to justify their own ruthless egoism (see, for instance, Taplin (2017)). Dawkins has also argued that "if you wish, as I do, to build a society in which individuals cooperate generously and unselfishly toward a common good, you can expect little help from biological nature" (Dawkins, 2016, p. 3). Tomasello's theory suggests that the last part of Dawkins' postulate is misleading. Human's cultural environment has provided a selection pressure toward a genetic constitution that favors cooperation and a social orientation. Besides, "modern evolutionary theory emphasizes hat organisms inherit their environments as much as they inherit their genes: a fish inherits not only fins, but also water" (Tomasello, 2019, p. 7).

The idea of selfishness also has a strong standing in economics and in the promotion of a *Homo economicus* (Annett, 2022; Kahneman, 2003; Kwak, 2017; Offer & Söderberg, 2016). As briefly exemplified above, many economists believe that humans are born to act as selfish agents whose decisions are solely guided by the aim of maximizing their individual utility and are unaffected by emotions and morality. The predictions made on this basis, however, are not always very convincing:

> Many of the economists who have received the Alfred Nobel Memorial Prize for Economic Science work within the paradigms of rational choice theory and statistical modeling. Yet is a noteworthy fact that *not a single one of them has been awarded the prize for confirmed empirical predictions* (italics in original). By an ironic contrast, on the one occasion it was awarded on that basis it went to Daniel Kahneman for his work in behavioral economics, notably for the discovery of loss aversion. (Elster, 2009, p. 20)

Paradoxically, it seems that the concept of the economic man describes apes better than humans. For example, Jensen et al. (2007) trained chimpanzees to play an adopted version of the Ultimatum game, and when playing it, the apes behaved like a *Homo economicus*. In contrast, when humans play, they behave more like *Homo sociabilies*. An ordinary ultimatum game proceeds like this. Two anonymous individuals are invited to share a sum of money. One of them, the proposer, suggests a way to split the money, and the other player, the responder, accepts or rejects the proposal. If the responder accepts, the money is split per the proposal; if the responder rejects, both receive nothing. If the players were economically rational, the proposer should offer the responder the smallest possible unit of money, and the responder should accept it. But that is not how humans behave. The proposer typically offers the responder somewhere between 30% and 40% of the total. Offers smaller than that are typically rejected (e.g., Camerer & Thaler, 1995; Henrich et al., 2006). Contrary to human players, apes in the study reported by Jensen, Call, and Tomasello did not make fair offers in a systematic manner nor did they systematically refuse to accept unfair offers during the play. The authors therefore concluded that "one of humans' closest living relatives behaves according to traditional economic models of self-interest, unlike humans, and this species does not share the human sensitivity to fairness" (Jensen et al., 2007, p. 109).

A Taxonomy of Wellbeing

Taxonomies can be defined as "the theory and practice of delimiting kinds or organisms and of classifying them" (Mayr, 1982, p. 146). The idea began with Aristotle. Starting with the Greek word *taxis*, meaning order, Aristotle proposed a hierarchical classification system based on binomial definitions. In his landmark work entitled *History of Animals*, Aristotle (1991) started at the highest possible level, living organisms, which he then divided into two groups: plants and animals. At the next level, he divided plants into those with a soft stem and those with a wooden stem and so on. The logic developed by Aristotle resembles the familiar game Twenty Questions. Here, the use of binary questions effectively divides a phenomenon into two parts, and each step dramatically narrows down the possible answers. By this strategy, a well-arranged conceptual structure quickly appears because so many irrelevant possibilities are eliminated.

Modern science makes good use of the taxonomic structure developed by Aristotle. Thagard argues for instance that kind hierarchies and part hierarchies "structure most of our conceptual systems, providing backbones of which other conceptual relations can hang" (Thagard, 1992, p. 28), and when Kuhn proposed that science makes progress by means of scientific revolutions, changes in taxonomic categories were an important part of his empirical examples (Kuhn, 1970, Postscript). More concretely, cognitive psychologists will typically use such hierarchical structures in the form of an IS-A KIND OF taxonomy, or an IS-A taxonomy for short (e.g., Holyoak & Morrison, 2005; Murphy, 2002). A simple example is provided in Fig. 7.1.

Categories that are represented high-up in the taxonomy are superordinate, and lower-level categories are subordinate. Murphy (2002) explains that a taxonomic hierarchy is a special kind of network in the sense that the IS-A structure allows only so-called set inclusion relations. For instance, a dog is subordinate to mammals, which again is subordinate to animals. The structure is also asymmetric, which means that even if all dogs are mammals, all mammals are not dogs. The

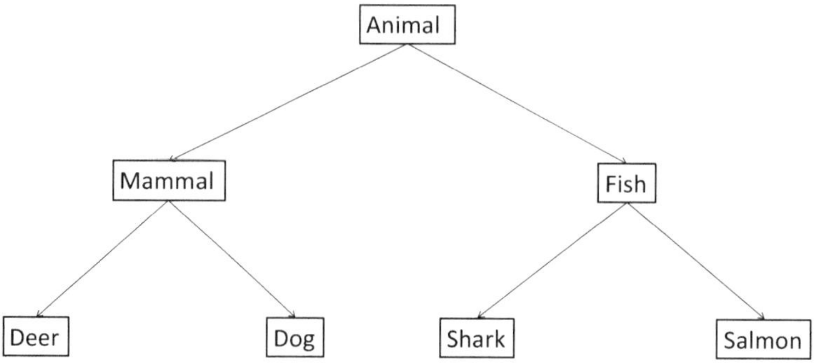

Fig. 7.1 The principles of an IS-A taxonomy

taxonomy handles individual differences within a category, as well as distinctions between sub-types. For example, in my family, we have a dog named *Kipp*, and he is a Griffon Bruxellois, a dog bred along with German Shepard, Labrador Retriever, and hundreds of other breeds.

A good taxonomy is useful for other purposes as well, and using whales as an example, Thagard (1992) provides a good illustration of some of them. As a start, it should be recognized that a natural classification of whales is difficult (Romero, 2012). It was, for instance, not until the tenth edition of Linnaeus's *Systema Naturae,* which appeared in 1758, that they were classified as sea mammals. Until then, whales had been thought of as a fish, located in accordance with the Aristotelian principle of categorizing animals based on the teleological doctrine of purposiveness and on where they lived. Hence, Aristotle operated with the three overarching categories of animals, which were "air dwellers," "land dwellers," and "sea dwellers."[3] Despite this misclassification, many of Aristotle's observations about whales remain accurate.

However, the reclassification of whales generated an important improvement in biological knowledge. As Thagard (1992, p. 22) points out, the new taxonomic localization enabled us to *explain* whale behavior (for example, why they breastfeed their babies); it enabled us to make *deductive inferences* (if "Grace" is a whale, then she has fins), *analogical inferences* (whales are somewhat akin to dolphins, so they may also be intelligent), and *generalizations* (whales will probably have blubber under their skin).

A similar function is aimed at in the taxonomy that organizes the core concepts in the humanistic theory of wellbeing. A happy feeling is, for example, a kind of harmony feelings which is a kind of spontaneous good–bad evaluation (SGBE), which is a kind of hedonic wellbeing. In contrast, being engaged in an activity is an opportunity feeling, which means that it facilitates change and growth rather than stability and is thus a kind of eudaimonic wellbeing. Engagement has different functions and phenomenology than does emotional happiness. To illustrate,

[3] The typology is from https://microbiosuu.weebly.com/aristotle.html#

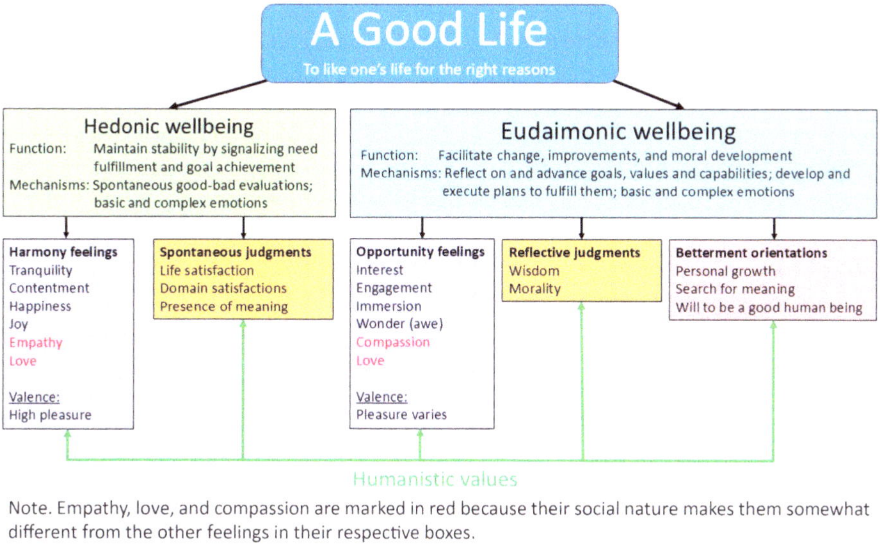

Fig. 7.2 A taxonomy of core concepts in the theory of humanistic wellbeing

consider a challenging task that only can be accomplished in a state of homeostatic imbalance. A hunger strike, for example, is basically inconsistent with the need for stability and a physiological equilibrium and will hardly if ever be motivated by or accompanied by harmony feelings. However, a hunger strike can be motivated and accompanied by opportunity feelings. Hence, the feelings of hunger, thirst, and fatigue that normally urge us to redirect our activities to regain homeostatic balance can be suppressed by feelings such as engagement, interest, or immersion. Opportunity feelings can therefore motivate us to suppress the impulse to a quick return to equilibrium and inspire us instead to continue an ongoing activity until its goal has been reached. Opportunity feelings are therefore different from harmony feelings, even if both can be highly valued. Figure 7.2 illustrates how the IS-A principle applies to the other elements in the taxonomy of humanistic wellbeing.

Hedonic Wellbeing

To some, like me, it is convenient to use the Aristotelian taxonomic principle and divide the overarching concept of wellbeing into two broad, subordinate kinds and then use the Greek terms hedonic and eudaimonic to name them. This procedure was also proposed by Ryan and Deci (2001), the authors who first introduced the term eudaimonic wellbeing (see Chap. 5). Ryan and Deci simply renamed subjective wellbeing (SWB) into hedonic wellbeing (HWB) and then invented the phrase eudaimonic wellbeing to name indictors of a good life that did not fit the mainstream definition of wellbeing as consisting of high life satisfaction and a surplus of positive over negative affect. For example, Ryan and Deci argued that thriving or being fully functioning is not well captured by the concept of SWB/HWB, so they rather classified thriving and full functioning as a kind of eudaimonic wellbeing (EWB; Ryan & Deci, 2001, p. 141). As pointed out in Chap. 5, however, the inclusion of life satisfaction as an indicator of HWB is problematic. Hedonia means pleasure, and life satisfaction is not the same as pleasure; consequently, the two should not be merged under the same taxonomic heading. Hence, Ryan and Deci later abandoned their initial conceptualization of HWB and redefined it as "just positive affect and negative affect" (Deci & Ryan, 2008, p. 2).[4]

Nevertheless, the use of HWB as a synonym for SWB remains popular (e.g., Chen et al., 2013; Oishi & Westgate, 2022; Tov & Lee, 2016), and the humanistic theory of wellbeing also uses the term HWB with at least a slight resembles to the traditional definition of SWB. But there are significant differences between HWB[5] and default SWB as well. For example, replacing the term "subjective" with the term "hedonic" has some benefits. If a dimension of wellbeing is named subjective, it is indicated that other dimensions in the taxonomy are not subjective. Hence, unless the notion of SWB includes all the possible indicators of wellbeing that are not objective, the term is misleading. For example, Ryff's psychological wellbeing scales are not included in the default setup of SWB measures but are used as alternatives or supplements to SWB. However, that does not mean that Ryff's approach to wellbeing is not subjective. Essentially, PWB is just as subjective as SWB is, and that puts the vocabulary in wellbeing research in an awkward situation. This problem can be avoided by referring to what appears as only a subset of subjective indicators of wellbeing as hedonic rather than subjective. Other kinds of subjective indicators could be called something else, such as psychological wellbeing or eudaimonic wellbeing.

Another distinction between HWB and default SWB is that the former comprises an indicator named harmony feelings, whereas SWB comprises an indicator named positive affect. The difference is not trivial.

---

[4] A quick remark on names. Applying a historical term with slightly new meanings is not uncommon. For example, the word diaspora holds a different meaning today than it had originally. The term derived from the ancient Greek verb *diaspeirō*, which means "to scatter about." According to the Merriam-Webster online dictionary, it can be used both to denote "Jews living outside Israel" and "people settled far from their ancestral homeland." Similarly, eudaimonia literally means "a good guardian spirit" (Chap. 6) but has been given a more flexible meaning in the wellbeing literature.

[5] In the remaining part of this chapter, the term hedonic wellbeing (HWB) refers to the conceptualization offered by the humanistic theory of wellbeing.

Harmony Feelings

Recall from Chap. 3 that feelings are not the same as affect and that in the humanistic theory of wellbeing affect is conceived of as an umbrella term under which subcategories such as temperament, mood, emotion, feelings, and evaluation are located. Among these, feeling is proposed to be the critical indicator of wellbeing. It is what we *feel* that most directly constitutes the affective essence of what it means to be well. By contrast, the default SWB approach does not offer a principal specification of which affective elements or mechanisms it considers relevant for wellbeing—besides that they should be positive.

Previous chapters have pointed out that the concept of feelings comprises four subdimensions: pleasure/valence, quality, intensity, and duration. These dimensions have different functions and operate with some independence from each other. The SWB literature has shown some concern for the distinction between intensity and duration, and most wellbeing researchers argue that frequency is more central to a person's wellbeing than is intensity (e.g., Diener et al., 1991; Helliwell et al., 2019; Kushlev et al., 2020; Parducci, 1968). Yet, Chap. 2 noted that Kahneman's peak–end rule emphasizes how intensity also can be important (Fredrickson & Kahneman, 1993; Kahneman et al., 1997).

The the main concern about wellbeing and feelings should be directed towards the dimensions of valence and quality. That is at least what the HTW argues. But the default SWB model does not even separate the two dimensions (e.g., Schimmack, 2008; Schimmack et al., 2000) it rather uses the term pleasure as a synonym for either emotional happiness or, more broadly, for the overarching concept of positive affect (e.g., Diener et al., 2009). The humanistic theory of wellbeing claims, however, that it is more useful to let pleasure refer to the valence dimension of a feeling state and to let quality denote what such states feel like phenomenologically. The variety of what it feels like to experience a "positive affect" is large, and in terms of quality it often makes little sense to collapse all these feelings into a single grab-bag category and think of them as either "positive affect" or "pleasure."

Chapter 5 summarized how pleasure developed prehistorically in tandem with displeasure to advance the regulation of homeostasis as organisms evolved to become more complex. The primordial function of pleasure is thus to provide a signal about the return to homeostatic equilibrium, whereas displeasure is a signal about an increasing distance from such a balanced state (Panksepp, 1998, p. 182). Overall, pleasure therefore works as an update about how we are doing in terms of fulfilling needs and achieving goals. In contrast, feeling qualities inform us about the nature of a situation and contribute to separating stimuli and events into qualitatively distinct entities. Cabanac (2009) has, for example, argued that feeling qualities critically assist us in the process of categorizing, or giving meaning to, our inner and outer environments. Pleasure, on the other hand, informs us about the goodness and badness of a situation.

The notion of harmony feelings emphasizes both the valence dimension and the quality dimension, and feelings such as tranquility, contentment, happiness, and joy are prototypical quality exemplars of this concept. The valence dimension often pairs with the qualities of harmony feelings, yet pleasure is not a constituent of these feelings. Harmony feelings have their distinct qualities generated as so-called psychological primitives, which means that they are irreducible and cannot be further decomposed into lower-level states. With reference to the communicative theory of emotions (e.g., Oatley, 1992, and Chap. 3), a feeling such as happiness is not supposed to be composed of pleasure, arousal, and an emotional concept, which is what Barrett's theory of constructive emotions proposes (e.g., Barrett, 2017, and Chap. 3).

The distinction between the valence dimension and the quality dimension of a feeling state has not been subjected to much empirical examination in the wellbeing literature. One reason is that survey participants hardly are asked to distinguish between the valence dimension and the quality dimension of a feeling, at least not when responding to ordinary affect items. However, more tailormade study designs are available and can bypass this problem. One such approach was illustrated by Wilson-Mendenhall et al. (2013) and discussed in Chap. 3. The study introduced a procedure that allowed participants to keep the quality of a feeling constant while varying the amount of pleasure (and arousal) to be reported. The "chocolate study" by Small et al. (2001), which was mentioned in Chap. 3, is another example of such a design. The study showed that eating chocolate in a hungry state typically produces feelings of both sweetness and pleasure. However, eating chocolate after you are full no longer feels pleasant, although the taste is still sweet.

Empathy and love are social emotions and therefore marked in red in Fig. 7.2. Their social nature makes them different from the other harmony feelings. For example, when we empathize with the feelings of another person, the experience is not necessarily harmonic—it can for instance be painful. As noted by Bloom (2017), empathy may have negative consequences, such as making the person experiencing them emotionally overwhelmed or biased in unfortunate ways. Excessive empathy can also lead to a wrongful desire for self-denial or cross over to controlling domination (Held, 2006, p. 95). Even Darwin was aware of the possible negative consequences of empathic feelings: "If we put ourselves in other's places, we will share their suffering, and this will not give us pleasure. Hence, the feeling of sympathy cannot easily be explained as deriving from the quest for pleasure" (cited in Gruber, 1974, p. 321). Whether empathy is a harmony feeling or not can therefore be discussed, but I believe it is permissible to regard it as harmonious, at least for now.

Love is another social feeling with fussy taxonomic borders. It comes in different shapes and can for instance be directed toward a romantic partner, toward one's children, or toward others we care deeply about. Love can also be felt toward our caregivers. Love is basically harmonic, particularly in an early phase, as when we fall in love. But love can also develop and become profoundly mature. In those cases, I have categorized love as an opportunity feeling (see below).

Spontaneous Judgments

The term spontaneous judgments is preferred over cognitive wellbeing, which is the term typically used in the SWB tradition. The core indicator in both vocabularies is life satisfaction, a concept with clear affective characteristics (Chap. 4). This is one reason why the name cognitive can appear misleading as a descriptor of life satisfaction. Its affective nature is also an argument for categorizing life satisfaction as a spontaneous good–bad evaluations (SGBE; see Chap. 1).

Life satisfaction and other spontaneous judgments are strongly correlated with harmony feelings. That is an argument for considering it as an indicator of hedonic wellbeing. The Greek word hêdonê means pleasure, but as pointed out throughout the book, pleasure is a concept that can be classified as subordinate to a more general evaluative capacity. The HTW argues that life satisfaction also is a member of the same SGBE concept. That opens for the possibility that both pleasure and life satisfaction are related but separable kinds of hedonic wellbeing. This is admittedly a speculative idea, but it is not without merit. For example, if the function of pleasure and harmony feelings is to maintain the universal need for stability, and if life satisfaction and other spontaneous judgments operate in a similar fashion, then the hypothesis that hedonia refers to a latent SGBE mechanism makes sense. If harmony feelings and spontaneous judgments also are highly correlated, the hypothesis is strengthened. Variables correlate for a reason, and one possibility is that they share the same underlying, or latent, concept. This is what Borsboom et al. (2021) refer to as the positive manifold argument of theory building, which again is the foundation for reflective factor models (e.g., Bollen & Lennox, 1991). The taxonomy presented in Fig. 7.2 is not a latent variable model, so strictly speaking, the correlational argument is not needed to justify it or, more correctly, make it empirically falsifiable. However, since studies typically show that indicators of harmony feelings and spontaneous judgments are highly correlated, often in the area of 0.70 or even higher (e.g., Glatz & Eder, 2020; Glatzer, 1984; Schimmack & Oishi, 2005; Sirgy, 2012), the positive manifold argument makes the taxonomic structure more robust. Nevertheless, the hypothesis that harmony feelings and spontaneous judgments are functionally connected to the universal need for stability remains the main argument for classifying them as hedonic.

HWB also differs from default SWB in its definition of life satisfaction (Chap. 4). The humanistic theory of wellbeing considers life satisfaction to be a quick and automatized System 1 kind of judgment, generated by a SGBE that functionally serves to maintain the universal need for stability. In contrast, the SWB model defines life satisfaction as a reflective System2 kind of concept. For instance, Diener (2006, p. 401) referred to life satisfaction as "a report of how a respondent evaluates or appraises his or her life taken as a whole. It is intended to represent a broad, reflective appraisal that a person makes of his or her life." As debated throughout this book, however, much evidence speaks against the notion that measures of life satisfaction signify this definition.

The humanistic theory of wellbeing categorizes the presence of meaning in life as a spontaneous judgment and thus an indicator of HWB. This constitutes another controversy between the concept of hedonic wellbeing and the concept of subjective wellbeing. It was Steger et al. (2006) who introduced the distinction between presence of meaning and search for meaning (see Chap. 6), and the humanistic theory of wellbeing considers the former to be an indicator of hedonic wellbeing and the latter to be an indicator of eudaimonic wellbeing. Mainstream opinion in the science of wellbeing seems less concerned about the presence of/search for distinction in the study of meaning but rather speaks more generally about meaning in life and classifies it as an indicator of eudaimonic wellbeing (e.g., Heintzelman, 2018; OECD, 2013) or as a separate dimension of wellbeing that is neither hedonic nor eudaimonic (e.g., Oishi & Westgate, 2022).[6]

There are two major reasons why the presence of meaning in life can be considered an indicator of HWB. The first is functional and maintains that the presence of meaning is a stabilizing factor in a person's life. For example, Baumeister argues that stability is a key feature of meaning (e.g., Baumeister, 1991, p. 360) and emphasizes that humans use meaning as part of "their never-ending quest to achieve stability" (Baumeister, 2013). One might even speculate that the meaninglessness in the myth of Sisyphus (Chap. 6) is the instability of the result of his work. If the rock had remained on the mountaintop, at least for a while, Sisyphus efforts would not have been in vain. To better see why this may be, consider a study by Ariely et al. (2008). The authors experimentally demonstrated that participants who were paid for assembling Bionicle Lego models that were immediately disassembled by the experimenter rated their efforts as less meaningful than did participants who, after assembling the same models and receiving the same payment, did not have the result of their work destroyed until somewhat later.

Moreover, studies by Oishi and colleagues show that people who lead either a happy life or a meaningful life prefer to maintain social order and the status quo. In contrast, people who lead psychologically rich lives seem to embrace social change (Oishi & Westgate, 2022, p. 799). Oishi and Westgate define a happy life as "one characterized by high life satisfaction and a high positive-to-negative affect ratio" (p. 791), and they consider it to have core features such as comfort, joy, and security. The key features of a meaningful life are significance, purpose, and coherence. The last wellbeing category in this tripartite model is the rich life, which is recognized by features such as variety, interest, and perspective change. The Oishi and Westgate study also suggests that both a happy life and a meaningful life rely on an exploitation strategy in which people take advantage of familiar environments that are available to them. A psychologically rich life, on the other hand, relies on an exploration strategy, in which resources are pursued by expanding horizons and broadening social ties (Oishi & Westgate, 2022, p. 803). However, there are also arguments that speak against the idea that meaning in life is related to stability. For example, the

[6] It should be noted that some proponents of SWB have clustered meaning in life and life satisfaction together in a common category, referred to as "global life judgments" (see Chap. 2 and Diener (2009, p. 71)). However, there is no consensus about this taxonomic proposal.

study by Oishi and Westgate revealed that people who prefer to lead a happy life value security, stability, and comfort, whereas those leading a meaningful life aspire to make a difference in the world (Oishi & Westgate, 2022, p. 803).

The second reason why meaning in life can be a hedonic concept is empirical and points to the strong correlations typically found between meaning and the other indicators of HWB. The experience of meaning in one's life can, for instance, be very pleasant. The correlation argument again appeals to the reflectivity of a latent model. Such attributes are not assumed in the humanistic wellbeing taxonomy, but they make the classification more robust.

Eudaimonic Wellbeing

The HTW suggests that eudaimonic wellbeing (EWB) has a three-dimensional structure, comprising the components of opportunity feelings, reflective judgments, and betterment orientations. All three reflect the idea that a good life must be dynamic in the sense of moving toward something better. The main function of these subdimensions is therefore associated with the universal need for change. Basically, EWB concerns the capability and motivation to formulate and reflect on complex plans and goals we have reason to value, as well as the experiences connected with the execution of such plans. EWB is also about judging what is right and wrong in life. This conceptualization is inspired by Aristotelian eudaimonism in several ways, most radically by including normative, i.e., objective, elements. However, the values themselves and the reasons to consider them eudaimonic are not Aristotelian.

The humanistic theory of wellbeing is grounded in an organismic perspective on life, with its inherent notion of organisms as autonomous, yet interactionist, entities that strive toward some kind of fulfillment (Chap. 6). The organismic approach also makes the HTW somewhat reminiscent of Aristotle's thinking. Moreover, the theory is vaguely Aristotelian in a "perfectionist" way, expressed as a will to improve and become "a better version" of oneself. Finally, the concepts of wisdom and morality, which are considered by the HTW as kinds of reflective judgments, are not very far apart from the Aristotelian notions of rationality and virtues.

Opportunity Feelings

An important characteristic of opportunity feelings, or eudaimonic feelings, is their active, exploratory nature and ability to provide a fundamental basis for learning (Smith et al., 2014, p. 20). Some researchers even refer to opportunity feelings as "knowledge emotions" (e.g., Silvia, 2006) or as emotions of attraction (Oatley, 1992). These feelings are also related to the experiential part of what Oishi and colleagues refer to as psychological richness (e.g., Oishi et al., 2019, 2020; Oishi &

Westgate, 2022). Chapter 3 examined the properties of opportunity feelings in detail and noted that pleasure often is absent from the experience of an opportunity feeling (e.g., Silvia, 2006; Vittersø, 2016). This attribute not only separates opportunity feelings from harmony feelings but also makes their phenomenological qualities more salient than their valence dimension. Typical opportunity feelings are engagement, interest, immersion, wonder, and awe. Motivationally, these feelings stimulate the urge to overcome a challenge, to be deeply interested in figuring things out, or to expand ones understanding of the world. Love and compassion are social feelings included in the category of opportunity feelings.

Some emotion theories conceptualize happiness in ways that makes it resemble an opportunity feeling. For example, Oatley and Johnson-Laird's communicative theory of emotion suggests that happiness often occurs during activities that lead to final achievements, rather than as the result of reaching goals (Chap. 3). According to this theory, happiness is typically prompted by the incorporation of new elements into an activity, i.e., when the plan that leads to a goal is progressing well (Oatley, 1992, p. 48). This account resembles the way in which feeling engaged is explained in the HTW. Oatley and Johnson-Laird's theory even uses the terms happiness and engagement interchangeably from time to time.

But the humanistic theory of wellbeing is concerned with the distinction between the smooth running of familiar and easy activities on the one hand and the effortful and explorative pursuit of a challenging goal on the other. Only the former is referred to as emotional happiness in the HTW, and it is categorized as a harmony feeling. In contrast, effortful engagement in overcoming a challenge and the enthusiastic exploration of new understandings are associated with feelings such as interest, immersion, and wonder. These experiences are classified as opportunity feelings.

The distinction between happiness as a harmony feeling and happiness as an opportunity feeling is nicely formulated by Sapolsky (2017), who accounts for the difference with reference to the neurotransmitter dopamine. Sapolsky explains that dopamine mediates the rewarding experience of reaching a goal through a motivation to work hard to reach it. Dopamine binds the reward to a hardworking process, Sapolsky says. "It fuels the goal-directed behavior needed to gain that reward" (p. 88). Dopamine is "not about the happiness of reward. It's about the happiness of pursuit of reward that has a decent chance of occurring" (Sapolsky, 2017, p. 88). In the HTW, therefore, harmony feelings are about the "happiness of reward," while opportunity feelings are about the "happiness of pursuit." To avoid terminological confusion, only the "happiness of reward" is called happiness.

Compassion and love are classified as pro-social opportunity feelings, although they are not prototypical exemplars of opportunity feelings. Both compassion and love have the capacity to develop over time and to become complex emotions of care (e.g., Goetz et al., 2010; Oatley, 2018). In Chap. 3, a profound kind of love was described in the words of Proust as something that fills us with "a precious essence" (Proust, 1981, p. 48). Compassion, but not love, can extend beyond those emotionally dare to us and include people we do not know and who are very different from us (Singer, 2015).

Reflective Judgments

Wellbeing is grounded in feelings and thinking about goodness and badness. The thinking part of such evaluations, referred to by the HTW as judgments, assigns value to states and situations. Judgments are not perceptions of these states and situations; they are not thoughtful matter-of-facts statements in the sense of determining *what* something is. Evaluation is something else, and the idea of spontaneous judgments assumes that the perception of a state or situation will be valued automatically, as an unconscious System 1 process. In contrast, the concept of reflective judgment is combining a more careful process of understanding what something is with the evaluative process of assigning a value to it. As argued in Chap. 3, such reflective perceptions and background beliefs may *influence* on the good–bad judgment in important ways.

A good illustration of the interaction between background beliefs and good–bad evaluations is provided by Hsee (1996). In a small set of studies, he asked participants to imagine that they were in the marked for a secondhand music dictionary. Dictionary A had 10,000 entries and was described to be "like new." Dictionary B had 20,000 entries and had "cover torn, otherwise like new." When presented separately, Dictionary A was more highly valued than Dictionary B. However, when presented together, Dictionary B became the most valuable. After all, the number of entries is more important for a good dictionary than its cover. Hsee therefore argues that the value of an attribute cannot be evaluated on its own. It can only be evaluated in comparison to something else.

The humanistic theory of wellbeing asserts that evaluations of wellbeing also are made in comparison to something but that many comparisons are made unconsciously and automatically in the biological valuation mechanism referred to as SGBE. However, some evaluative processes can be transformed from a System 1–regulated SGBE to a System 2–regulated judgment process in which updated knowledge feeds into the evaluative process somewhat analogically to the dynamics illustrated in Hsee's dictionary example. The proposal is that evaluative comparisons can be made reflective by deliberatively adding thoughtful elements to the judgmental process. Two such thoughtful elements are wisdom and morality. The inclusion of these two as ingredients of wellbeing makes the concept interactionist and multidimensional in the sense that feelings and spontaneous good–bad evaluations are not its only constituents. For humans, the HTW recommends, reflections about who we are and why we feel and think as we do should be included in the decision of how good life is.

Reflections are not limited to the thinking part of wellbeing. They may apply to feelings as well, even if feelings typically have a spontaneous nature and even if Frijda has argued that reflection tends to destroy the true nature of an emotional experience (Frijda, 1986, p. 243). Our feelings can to some extent be regulated and controlled by will and reflexivity (e.g., Clore, 2011; Marcel, 2003; Oatley, 2004), and what we may call "raw feelings" are not necessarily the best indicators of wellbeing. As noted by Held (2006, p. 10), feelings ought to "be reflected on and educated."

Psychotherapy is one example of how changes in the way we feel about ourselves and our environments can be brought about by reflecting upon them and thus improving the quality of our lives (e.g., Beck, 1987; Southward et al., 2021). Other ways of regulating our emotions by thinking thoroughly about them also exist (e.g., Davidson, 2018; Gross, 2015; Pennebaker, 2012). A striking example of how a reflexive development of self-knowledge can affect the most fundamental feelings in a life comes from the memoirs of Joanna Field, who was briefly introduced in Chap. 3 as the pen name of Marion Milner. In December 1926, Milner started to keep a diary, in the hope of finding out what it was that she "really wanted" in life (Field, 1981/1934, p. 173). Optimistically, she estimated that a few weeks, or months at most, would suffice to give her "the facts of her life" and that these insights would be what was needed to make the changes she was longing for.

Milner wanted to discover her inner purpose by understanding her own mind. But the diary project surprised her. First, it did not take weeks or months but 7 years to complete the endeavor. Seven years of critical introspection, diary writing, and careful analyses of perceptions and experiences were necessary to articulate a satisfactory purpose for her life and to work out plans and practices that could help her achieve it.

Milner's most astonishing discovery was that the best part of her life had been hidden for her. The culprit that prevented the discovery of her true values was something Milner named "blind thoughts." A blind thought is a kind of "chatter," a childish concern with worries, anger, and doubts that was not at all important for her essential goals in life. For example, one diary entry expressed a concern about whether she would manage to get her hair cut before going to work (p. 7). It was not that this particular worry was a major problem in itself; the problem was that the blind thought fed her with trivial worries and kept on bothering her by being disproportionally preoccupying and alarming. Like a little child who mistakenly believes that when her mother leaves her, it is forever, Milner observed that she too was unable to limit the range and imagined consequences of her chattering mind. Moreover, the blind thoughts were often vague and lacked a clear meaning in the moments she was experiencing them. Only upon reflection could Milner see that the blind thoughts were "thieves of happiness." Her reflections generated an even greater reward, since the things she gradually learned to appreciate were not necessarily those that maximized emotional happiness. Little by little, Milner discovered that happiness in itself might be quite irrelevant. She gradually learned to care less about the unpleasant element of a valuable activity. Emotional happiness, Milner realized, was only half the story of a good life and then, and only then, could she comprehend the meaning of William Blake's poem "Auguries of Innocence":

> It is right it should be so;
>   Man was made for joy and woe;
>   And when this we rightly know,
>   Thro' the world we safely go.

Betterment Orientations

Betterment orientations have to do with the will to improve, a motivation to perform important life tasks with some kind of perfection or elegance. A concrete specification of the standards against which perfection should be evaluated is hard to work out, but it might involve features such as intrinsic values, effort, and purposiveness (e.g., Bradford, 2015). Perfectionism might also be conditioned on having complex plans and bringing them to fruition (e.g., Hurka, 1993). But these standards need not be oriented toward the best possible performance for a certain activity in an absolute sense. An amateur painter can be successful in their betterment orientations without producing art that compare with the best paintings in the world.

MacIntyre's (2007) notion of a practice is an example of a betterment process. Grounded in the Aristotelian notion of telos, a practice can roughly be seen as a goal-directed activity that is contingent on the use of appropriate means to reach the goal. The core idea is therefore that the proper value of an activity is only available through the achievements and satisfactions inherent to the practice itself (e.g., Schwartz & Wrzesniewski, 2016). For example, the value of a Nobel prize is not defined by the physical token of a medal; it's worth is rooted in the practice that leads to the achievement, and no external reward can replace the value inherent in that activity.

A practice is more precisely defined as "any coherent and complex form of socially established cooperative human activity through which goods internal to that form of activity are realized in the course of trying to achieve those standards of excellence which are appropriate to, and partially definitive of, that form of activity, with the result that human powers to achieve excellence, and human conceptions of the ends and goods involved, are systematically extended" (MacIntyre, 2007, p. 175). Boyle (1987) uses the example of a democracy to make MacIntyre's concept of a practice more concrete. Boyle explains that in liberal democracies, politics cannot be good unless it is motivated by a genuine wish for societal improvement. Without the democratic values embedded in democratic activities, politics declines to empty rhetoric and cynical fights for power, Boyle argues (1987, loc. 157).

Schwartz and Wrzesniewski (2016) use education to illustrate the principles of a practice. The authors maintain that the goal of teaching is to train students and that the goodness of teaching can only be judged against what students learn. Measuring the quality of teaching by other indicators, such as salary or popularity, is misplaced. The value of a practice is attainable through certain ways of performing the activity, and, importantly, success must be evaluated by standards that change as the skills of the practitioner improve. According to the humanistic theory of wellbeing therefore, betterments are dynamic, they can occur at different levels of performance, and they are judged according to continuously changing standards.

Betterments typically require time and effort (e.g., Annas, 2008; Ericsson & Pool, 2016), which is one reason why they are eudaimonic rather than hedonic. Marion Milner's journey to a better life is a good example of the striving that might be needed to change, and so is the story Paul Bloom (2021) tells about his gradual understanding of why pleasure is not the only good thing in life. The initial idea behind his book *The Sweet Spot* was hedonic: to show how suffering—contra-intuitively enough—can give rise to pleasure. The right kind of pain will, in the end, lead to more pleasure or better pleasure. Hence, the enhancement of pleasure remains the ultimate goal of human behavior, even for painful and strenuous activities. Bloom therefore planned to call his book *The Pleasures of Suffering*. But then things changed. In the process of writing the book, Bloom gradually realized that challenges and suffering can be valuable in themselves. They are not merely means toward pleasantness. In the preface, he writes: "A lot of people think that humans are natural hedonists, caring only about pleasure. I want to convince you that a close look at our appetite for pain and suffering shows that this view of humanity is mistaken. It turns out that we are inclined toward something deeper and more transcendent" (Bloom, 2021, p. xiii).

The economist and Catholic Anthony Annett (2022) ponders on how his professional and moral understandings gradually changed as new insights evolved with careful observation and varied personal experience. From his job at the International Monetary Fund (IMF), where he served as a speech writer for people such as Dominique Strauss-Kahn and Christine Lagarde, Annett came to see that the theories he was brought up with as a student of economics did not fit the empirical landscape of the real world. For instance, faith in the notion of a free marked got a serious crack with the global financial crisis of 2008. The crisis was an eye-opener, but the evidence had been around for a while. Annett realized that the moral foundation of standard economic theory, i.e., that the pursuit of short-term self-interest is good for everyone, was simply not true. The steady rise in economic and social inequality, financial instability, and environmental devastation can no longer be ignored but calls for a new worldview (Annett, 2022, p. 15). For Annett, the decisive moment came with the inauguration of Pope Francis in March 2013. The teaching of the new Pope touched something deep in Annett, "a feeling that our global economy is on the wrong path, driven by the wrong values, headed in the wrong direction" (Annett, 2022, p. 14). In 2014, Annett left the IMF to work with Jeffery Sachs on the intersection of ethics, economics, and sustainable development.

The educational psychologist William Perry characterized changes like those described above as "an intellectual Pilgrim's Progress" (cited in Hofer & Pintrich, 2012). Perry's seminal work on intellectual and ethical growth among college students in the USA in the 1950s and 1960s showed how the complexity of their moral understanding grew during their undergraduate years (e.g., Perry, 1999). In the stage model Perry developed, he depicted an early phase of ethical development in which students tend to view knowledge and authority in simplistic, black-and-white terms. Gradually, complexity is added to their ethical comprehension, and at the highest of Perry's stages, students are able to critically evaluate various moral perspectives, make informed judgments, and take principled stands on issues.

In the humanistic theory of wellbeing, betterments are organized around the concept of betterment orientations, which has three major subdimension. The first is personal growth, a concept that was examined in Chap. 6. The other is a search for meaning, which was also discussed in Chap. 6. Frankl's original writings (Frankl,

1945, 1970) and more recent interpretations of if (e.g., Von Devivere, 2018) were suggested to be useful sources for further refinement of this concept and subsequent measurements. The third dimension of betterment orientations is referred to as a will to be a good human being. Nothing much is formulated about this indicator of eudaimonia in the current version of the HTW. Potentially, a vast literature can be identified as relevant, depending on how this very broad and vague notion is to be specified. One appropriate philosophical tradition is nicely summarized by Neiman (2015), whereas Jasanoff (2019) presents an interesting perspective on the crossroad between biology, social sciences, and philosophy. However, it will take much work to develop this concept further.

Humanistic Wellbeing and Normativity

Common ground has it that philosophical approaches to wellbeing are normative, whereas scientific approaches are descriptive (Chap. 1). By implication, if a scientist reports that a survey participant is pleased or satisfied, this is not a value judgment about that person but merely a description of a psychological state. In contrast, when a philosopher calls a person pleased or satisfied, it is typically taken to be a value judgment and to indicate that life is going well for this person (Chap. 2).

The humanistic theory of wellbeing objects to this demarcation, and throughout this book, I have instead argued that scientists are, and should be, normative about wellbeing. For example, Chap. 1 noted that it is impossible to communicate about human doings and whereabouts outside a normative framework and that concepts such as happiness and wellbeing even have a dual character in the sense that they jointly entail both descriptive and normative qualities. It makes little sense to say that a person is happy or well without also indicating that it is good for them to be happy and well. Hence, one reason for the value argument embedded in the HTW relates to the lack of credibility of the alternative. Is it really trustworthy for a scientist to state that a person's wellbeing is unrelated to whether that person's life goes well or badly? I don't think so, and here, I lean on Naomi Oreskes. Her excellent book *Why Trust Science?* (2019) explains that scientists cannot hang up their values and biases outside the laboratory as an overcoat (p. 52). Hence, if scientists claim that they are value-free, Oreskes argues, "it comes across as false, for they are claiming the impossible" (Oreskes, 2019, p. 152). If it is impossible to live without values, scientists should admit their subjective position and stop acting as if their work is value-free.

Another reason for making theories of wellbeing value-based is that without a normative stand, any self-declared happy or satisfied person must be accepted as being well off, regardless of the causes of these states. Chapter 1 pointed out the problem with this position. For example, it is nothing logically wrong with stating that Frank was emotionally happy after a day spent killing his parents (Gilbert, 2006, pp. 36–37). Chapter 1 also referred to studies showing that both harming and hurting people can produce pleasure and positive affect (Chester, 2017; Sapolsky,

2017). Yet, if wellbeing researchers continue to insist that a life is well lived regardless of whether it is spent hurting others or helping them, they will end up making their work scientifically impotent. A central argument for including normativity in a theory of wellbeing is therefore the consequence of not doing so. In the philosophical literature, this problem has been discussed under labels such as "the happy immoralists" (Cahn, 2004) or "the happy villain" (Badhwar, 2014).

The Happy Villain

Genghis Kahn is supposed to have said that "the greatest happiness is to scatter your enemy, to drive him before you, to see his cities reduced to ashes, to see those who love him shrouded in tears, and to gather into your bosom his wives and daughters."[7] Although the story about Genghis is hard to verify and may appear extreme, it is not too far out to be relevant for the happy villain argument. Instances of "evil pleasures," i.e., getting pleasure from inflicting harm on others, abound in the past and in the present. The brutal slaughters that ancients Romans found amusing when visiting the Colosseum, the schadenfreude reported from torturing criminals in the Middle Ages, and the joy some seem to take, even today, from bullfighting and other hurtful "entertainments" are but a few examples. Hence, the problem of evil pleasures is a challenge for any theory of wellbeing that leaves definitional ownership exclusively to the realm of subjectivity.

To further illustrate this dilemma, consider what happened with the self-reported wellbeing in South Africa after apartheid was abolished. According to a longitudinal survey presented by Møller (2001), the total level of life satisfaction and happiness decreased with the introduction of democracy in South Africa in 1994. In other words, the end of a cruel government resulted in a less satisfied population. What political guidance should SWB researchers advocate based on these observations? It is illogical to advise people not to lead good lives, but if wellbeing is unconditionally defined as a good life, that is what one must end up with in this example. In contrast, if the indicators of wellbeing are conditioned on a set of humanistic values to count as evidence for a good life, this dilemma is avoided.

Comparable examples have more recently been provided by Flanagan et al. (2023). These authors noted that during the pandemic, when an alarmingly high number of US citizens suffered and died from COVID-19, alongside news about the increasing number of teenagers struggling with mental health problems, "Gallup reported that Americans had reached the highest level ever of the percentage of the population who consider themselves 'thriving'" (Flanagan et al., 2023, p. 29). Similarly, Oishi and Westgate (2022) have observed that "happiness is sometimes associated with system justification, resistance to change, and insensitivity to

[7] https://history.stackexchange.com/questions/23975/what-was-the-context-of-this-famous-genghis-khan-quote

inequality and social injustice" (p. 792). Phillips et al. (2017, p. 179) report that "happiness is positively related to traits such as selfishness (Tan & Forgas, 2010), a lack of empathy (Devlin et al., 2014), and risky behavior such as alcohol consumption, binge eating, and drug use (Cyders & Smith, 2008; Bergman & Scott, 2001)." These and comparable examples speak against the argument that wellbeing should be given top priority in a "first things first" policy regime (Flanagan et al., 2023, p. 191). Hence, wellbeing should either be ranked below values such as universal human rights, justice, equality, eradication of poverty, and sustainable development, as Flanagan and coauthors suggest, or be conditioned on not violating these values, as the HTW suggests. The conditioned position offered by the humanistic theory of wellbeing is justified by the argument that scientists can include values as a background assumption.

Values as a Background Assumption

The values as background assumption argument follows the logic of scientists' moral obligations in general. Douglas (2009) has reminded us that scientists have the same moral duties as the general population, and these responsibilities include respecting human rights and the "do-no-harm" commitment (e.g., Arnold, 2001). Scientists are further committed to a set of more specific ethical obligations (e.g., National Academy of Sciences, 2009). For example, any scientist who conducts research with human participants needs to protect the interests of the research subjects. Scientists are also obliged to act in ways that serve the public. These liabilities can be seen as a mandatory part of the background assumptions upon which a scientist is required to act. Hence, consensus already exists that some ethical values must be incorporated in the background assumption that scientists are committed to obey.

The HTW suggests that for the science of wellbeing, these ethical principles can be taken one step further. This is the idea: if scientists accept that moral values are a legitimate part of their background assumptions, they must believe that, overall, a commitment to an adequate morality makes our lives better. Given that the study object of wellbeing research is the good life, it can therefore be argued that the inclusion of moral values in a theory of wellbeing makes the theory better.

One way to decide if a scientific theory is good, is by applying the logic of abduction. Abduction means to make an inference to the best explanation (e.g., Thagard, 2012), and this idea was comprehensively elaborated by Charles Peirce. Drawing on Peirce's thinking, Borsboom et al. (2021) suggest that the concept of abduction can be briefly laid out as follows: "theory T putatively explains phenomenon P" means "if the world were as T says it is, P would follow as a matter of course" (p. 759).

To be more concrete, the phenomenon to be explained by a theory of wellbeing is how and why a life is well lived. The hypothesis proposed by the HTW is that being well follows from performing our humanness well, which in turn depends on fulfilling the three universal needs for stability, change, and care. Among these three, the need to and for care is most relevant for the normative argument. Humans are caring, collaborative, and cultural beings. Our humanness can therefore not be carried out well unless we are committed to some rules of cooperation that are grounded in a set of shared values. This is the essence of the normative argument on offer in the HTW.

The justification of the normative claim springs out of feminist epistemology and its reasoning about background assumptions. Recall from Chap. 1 that scientific theories cannot be derived directly from empirical facts. It is not the relation between a fact and a theoretical statement that determines whether the theory is correct; it is the background assumption we hold about that relation (Longino, 1979). For example, observing that the sun traverses the sky can only be taken as evidence that the earth is circling the sun in the context of a certain set of background assumptions, such as a heliocentric cosmology. Longino further explains that the function of background beliefs is analogous to the function of background conditions in causal interaction. For example, striking a match will cause a flame. However, with no oxygen in the atmosphere, a flame will not result from striking the match. "But we do not regard the presence of oxygen as a cause of the match's igniting. The presence of the oxygen is rather an enabling condition of the causal interaction" (Longino, 1979, p. 40).

A similar reasoning is adopted to justify the normative element of the HTW. Even if a moral principle cannot be logically derived from empirical facts, a relationship between values and a scientific knowledge structure can be established with reference to background assumptions. To bring the humanistic theory of wellbeing to bear on a set of basic humanistic values means to accept these values as a background assumption. The relationship between humanistic values and wellbeing is therefore a bit like the relationship between an oxygenic atmosphere and striking a match. The values do not affect wellbeing causally but prevent it from lighting up if violated.

In science, background assumptions are grounded in institutions that organize communities of academics and these institutions justify the practice of science. According to Longino, scientific communities permit background assumptions to acquire stability and legitimacy through surviving criticism. "Justificatory practices must therefore include not only the testing of hypotheses against data but also the subjection of background assumptions (and reasoning and data) to criticism from a variety of perspectives" (Longino, 2008, p. 80). Similarly, Amartya Sen (2009) suggests that norms can be justified as reasonable from discussions among open-minded individuals. Common ground about values can be established in a process of "welcoming information and through reflecting in arguments coming from diverse quarters, along with undertaking interactive deliberations and debates on how the underlying issues should be seen" (Sen, 2009, p. 43).

To make the concept of wellbeing contingent upon humanistic values is not to say that indicators such as pleasure or life satisfaction bu neccesity will increase as a consequence of adhering to these values. Neither is it to say that activities must be aimed at humanistic values to be good. We can perform our humanness well while engaging in activities not directly related to humanistic values. Getting lost in a book, listening to music, or being absorbed in a challenging puzzle have little direct bearing on human rights or caring for, rather than harming, others. Nevertheless, such activities are important sources of wellbeing for many people. Thus, the right reason argument suggests that subjective liking is disqualified as an indicator of wellbeing if it comes from activities that violate the humanistic values. But the right reason argument does not suggest that activities motivated for nonnormative reasons cannot contribute to good lives.

References

Allport, G. W. (1955). *Becoming: Basic considerations for a psychology of personality*. Yale University Press.

Allport, G. W. (1961). *Pattern and growth in personality*. Holt, Rinehart and Winston.

Annas, J. (2008). The phenomenology of virtue. *Phenomenology and the Cognitive Sciences, 7*, 21–34.

Annett, A. M. (2022). *Cathonomics: How catholic tradition can create a more just economy [Kindle]*. Georgetown University Press.

Ariely, D., Kamenica, E., & Prelec, D. (2008). Man's search for meaning: The case of Legos. *Journal of Economic Behavior & Organization, 67*(3–4), 671–677. https://doi.org/10.1016/j.jebo.2008.01.004

Aristotle. (1991). *History of animals* (Vol. 3). Harvard University Press.

Arnold, D. G. (2001). Coercion and moral responsibility. *American Philosophical Quarterly, 38*(1), 53–67. www.jstor.org/stable/20010022

Badhwar, N. K. (2014). *Well-being: Happiness in a worthwhile life [Kindle]*. Oxford University Press.

Barrett, L. F. (2017). *How emotions are made: The secret life of the brain [Kindle]*. Houghton Mifflin Harcourt.

Baumeister, R. F. (1991). *Meanings of life*. Guilford Press.

Baumeister, R. F. (2013, 16 September). The meanings of life. *Aeon Magazine*. https://aeon.co/essays/what-is-better-a-happy-life-or-a-meaningful-one

Beck, A. T. (1987). Cognitive models of depression. *Journal of Cognitive Psychotherapy, an International Quarterly, 1*, 5–37.

Bergman, M. M., & Scott, J. (2001). Young adolescents' wellbeing and health-risk behaviours: gender and socio-economic differences. *Journal of Adolescence, 24*(2), 183–197. https://doi.org/10.1006/jado.2001.0378

Berlyne, D. E. (1960). *Conflict, arousal, and curiosity*. McGraw-Hill.

Billman, G. E. (2020). Homeostasis: The underappreciated and far too often ignored central organizing principle of physiology. *Frontiers in Physiology, 11*, 200. https://doi.org/10.3389/fphys.2020.00200

Blasi, A. (1976). Concept of development in personality theory. In J. Loevinger (Ed.), *Ego development* (pp. 29–53). Jossey–Bass.

Bleidorn, W., Hopwood, C. J., Back, M. D., Denissen, J. J., Hennecke, M., Hill, P. L., Jokela, M., Kandler, C., Lucas, R. E., & Luhmann, M. (2021). Personality trait stability and change. *Personality Science, 2*, 1–20.

Block, J. (1982). Assimilation, accommodation, and the dynamics of personality development. *Child Development, 53*, 281–295.

Bloom, P. (2013). *Just babies: The origins of good and evil [Kindle]*. Crown Publishers.

Bloom, P. (2017). *Against empathy: The case for rational compassion [Kindle]*. Random House.

Bloom, P. (2021). *The sweet spot. The pleasures of suffering and the search for meaning [Kindle]*. Random House.
Bollen, K. A., & Lennox, R. (1991). Conventional wisdom on measurement: A structural equation perspective. *Psychological Bulletin, 110*(2), 305–314.
Borsboom, D., van der Maas, H. L., Dalege, J., Kievit, R. A., & Haig, B. D. (2021). Theory construction methodology: A practical framework for building theories in psychology. *Perspectives on Psychological Science, 16*(4), 756–766.
Bowlby, E. J. M. (1973). *Separation: Anxiety and anger: Attachment and loss Volume 2* (Vol. 2). Random House.
Boyle, J. (1987). *On MacIntyre's 'after virtue' [Kindle]*. The World & I Online.
Bradford, G. (2015). Perfectionism. In G. Fletcher (Ed.), *The Routledge handbook of philosophy of well-being [Kindle]* (pp. 124–134). Routledge.
Bruner, J. S., Goodnow, J. J., & Austin, G. A. (1986/1957). *A study of thinking*. Routledge. (Original work published 1957)
Bühler, C. (1951). Maturation and motivation. *Dialectica, 5*(3–4), 312–361.
Bühler, C., Hetzer, H., & Mabel, F. (1928). Die Affectwirksamkeit von Fremheitsindrücken im ersten Lebensjahr. *Z. Psychol. Abt, 1*(107), 30–49.
Cabanac, M. (2009). *The fifth influence. The dialectics of pleasure*. iUniverse.
Cahn, S. M. (2004). The happy immoralist. *Journal of Social Philosophy, 35*(1), 1.
Camerer, C., & Thaler, R. H. (1995). Anomalies: Ultimatums, dictators and manners. *Journal of Economic Perspectives, 9*(2), 209–219.
Carver, C. S., & Scheier, M. F. (2001). *On the self-regulation of behavior*. Cambridge University Press.
Chapman, M. (1992). Equilibration and the dialectics of organization. In H. Beilin & P. Pufall (Eds.), *Piaget's theory. Prospects and possibilities* (pp. 39–59). Lawrence Erlbaum.
Chen, F. F., Jing, Y., Hayes, A., & Lee, J. (2013). Two concepts or two approaches? A bifactor analysis of psychological and subjective well-being. *Journal of Happiness Studies, 14*(3), 1033–1068. https://doi.org/10.1007/s10902-012-9367-x
Chester, D. S. (2017). The role of positive affect in aggression. *Current Directions in Psychological Science, 26*(4), 366–370. https://doi.org/10.1177/0963721417700457
Churchland, P. S. (2018a). *Braintrust: What neuroscience tells us about morality [Kindle]*. Princeton Science Library.
Churchland, P. S. (2018b). *Conscience. The origins of moral intuition [Kindle]*. Norton.
Clark, R. N. (1996). *Control system dynamics*. Cambridge University Press.
Clore, G. L. (2011). Thrilling thoughts: How changing your mind intensifies your emotions. In R. M. Arkin (Ed.), *Most underappreciated: 50 prominent social psychologists talk about hidden gem* (Vol. 50, pp. 67–71). Oxford University Press.
Cummins, R. A. (2020). Homeostasis. In F. Maggino (Ed.), *Encyclopedia of quality of life and Well-being research* (pp. 1–4). Springer International Publishing. https://doi.org/10.1007/978-3-319-69909-7_1303-2
Cyders, M. A., & Smith, G. T. (2008). Emotion-based dispositions to rash action: Positive and negative urgency. *Psychological Bulletin, 134*(6), 807–828. https://doi.org/10.1037/a0013341
Damasio, A. (2018). *The strange order of things: Life, feeling, and the making of culture [Kindle]*. Pantheon Books.
Damasio, A. (2021). *Feeling & knowing: Making minds conscious [Kindle]*. Pantheon.
Davidson, R. J. (2018). Reactivity, recovery, regulation the three R's of emotional responding. In A. S. Fox, R. C. Lapate, A. J. Shackman, & R. J. Davidson (Eds.), *The nature of emotion. Fundamental questions [Kindle]* (pp. 1–6). Oxford University Press.
Dawkins, R. (2016). *The selfish gene [Kindle]*. Oxford University Press.
Deci, E. L., & Ryan, R. M. M. (2008). Hedonia, eudaimonia, and well-being: An introduction. *Journal of Happiness Studies, 9*(1), 1–11. https://doi.org/10.1007/s10902-006-9018-1

Devlin, H. C., Zaki, J., Ong, D. C., & Gruber, J. (2014). Not as good as you think? Trait positive emotion is associated with increased self-reported empathy but decreased empathic performance. *PLoS ONE 9*(10), e110470. https://doi.org/10.1371/journal.pone.0110470
DeYoung, C. G. (2006). Higher-order factors of the big five in a multi-informant sample. *Journal of Personality and Social Psychology, 91*(6), 1138–1151.
DeYoung, C. G., & Weisberg, Y. J. (2018). Cybernetic approaches to personality and social behavior. *Oxford Handbook of Personality and Social Psychology*, 387–414.
Diener, E. (2006). Guidelines for national indicators of subjective well-being and ill-being. *Journal of Happiness Studies, 7*(4), 397–404. https://doi.org/10.1007/s10902-006-9000-y
Diener, E., Sandvik, E., & Pavot, W. (1991). Happiness is the frequency, not the intensity, of positive versus negative affect. In F. Strack, M. Argyle, & N. Schwarz (Eds.), *Subjective well-being*. Pergamon Press.
Diener, E., Scollon, C. N., & Lucas, R. E. (2009). The evolving concept of subjective well-being. The multifaceted nature of happiness. In E. Diener (Ed.), *Assessing well-being. The collected works of Ed Diener* (pp. 67–100). Springer.
Douglas, H. (2009). *Science, policy, and the value-free ideal [Kindle]*. University of Pittsburgh Press.
Elster, J. (2009). Excessive ambitions. *Capitalism and Society, 4*(2). https://doi.org/10.2202/1932-0213.1055
Ericsson, A., & Pool, R. (2016). *Peak: Secrets from the new science of expertise [Kindle]*. Houghton Mifflin Harcourt.
Field, J. (1981/1934). *A life of one's own*. J. P. Tarcher. (Original work published in 1934).
Flanagan, O., LeDoux, J., Bingle, B., Haybron, D., Moody-Adams, M., Mesquita, B., Ren, S., Sun, A. X., & Wilson, Y. (2023). *Against happiness [Kindle]*. Columbia University Press.
Frankl, V. (1945). *Man's search for meaning. An introduction to logotheraphy*. Washington Square Press.
Frankl, V. (1970). *The will to meaning*. Plume.
Fredrickson, B. L., & Kahneman, D. (1993). Duration neglect in retrospective evaluations of affective episodes. *Journal of Personality and Social Psychology, 65*(1), 45–55.
Frijda, N. H. (1986). *The emotions*. Cambridge University Press.
Gilbert, D. (2006). *Stumbling on happiness*. Harper Press.
Ginsburg, H., & Opper, S. (1969). *Piaget's theory of intellectual development. An introduction*. Prentice-Hall.
Glatz, C., & Eder, A. (2020). Patterns of trust and subjective well-being across Europe: New insights from repeated cross-sectional analyses based on the European social survey 2002–2016. *Social Indicators Research, 148*(2), 417–439. https://doi.org/10.1007/s11205-019-02212-x
Glatzer, W. (1984). Life-satisfaction and alternative measures of SWB. In W. Glatzer & W. Zapf (Eds.), *Quality of life in Germany* (pp. 177–191). Campus.
Goetz, J. L., Keltner, D., & Simon-Thomas, E. (2010). Compassion: An evolutionary analysis and empirical review. *Psychological Bulletin, 136*(3), 351–374. https://doi.org/10.1037/a0018807
Gopnik, A. (2009). *The philosophical baby: What children's minds tell us about truth, love and the meaning of life [Kindle]*. Farrar, Straus and Giroux.
Greene, J. D. (2013). *Moral tribes: Emotion, reason, and the gap between us and them [Kindle]*. Penguin.
Gross, J. J. (2015). Emotion regulation: Current status and future prospects. *Psychological Inquiry, 26*(1), 1–26. https://doi.org/10.1080/1047840X.2014.940781
Gruber, H. E. (1974). *Darwin on man. A psychological study of scientific creativity*. Wildwood House.
Heintzelman, S. J. (2018). Eudaimonia in the contemporary science of subjective well-being: Psychological well-being, self- determination, and meaning in life. In E. Diener, S. Oishi, & L. Tay (Eds.), *Handbook of subjective well-being*. DEF Publishers. https://doi.org/nobascholar.com
Held, V. (2006). *The ethics of care: Personal, political, and global*. Oxford University Press.
Helliwell, J. F., Layard, R., & Sachs, J. (Eds.). (2019). *World happiness report 2019*. http://worldhappiness.report/

Henrich, J., McElreath, R., Barr, A., Ensminger, J., Barrett, C., Bolyanatz, A., Cardenas, J. C., Gurven, M., Gwako, E., Henrich, N., Lesorogol, C., Marlowe, F., Tracer, D., & Ziker, J. (2006). Costly punishment across human societies. *Science, 312*(5781), 1767–1770. https://doi.org/10.1126/science.1127333

Hofer, B. K., & Pintrich, P. R. (2012). *Personal epistemology: The psychology of beliefs about knowledge and knowing*. Routledge. https://doi.org/10.4324/9780203424964

Holyoak, K. J., & Morrison, R. G. (2005). Thinking and reasoning: A reader's guide. In K. J. Holyoak & R. G. Morrison (Eds.), *The Cambridge handbook of thinking and reasoning* (pp. 1–9). Cambridge University Press.

Hsee, C. (1996). The evaluability hypothesis: An explanation for preference reversals between joint and separate evaluations of alternatives. *Organizational Behavior and Human Decision Processes, 67*(3), 247–257.

Hurka, T. (1993). *Perfectionism*. Oxford University Press.

Izard, C. E., & Ackerman, B. P. (2000). Motivational, organizational, and regulatory functions of discrete emotions. In M. Lewis & J. M. Haviland-Jones (Eds.), *Handbook of emotions* (pp. 253–264). The Guilford Press.

Jasanoff, S. (2019). *Can science make sense of life? [Kindle]*. Wiley.

Jensen, K., Call, J., & Tomasello, M. (2007). Chimpanzees are rational maximizers in an ultimatum game. *Science, 318*(5 October), 107–109.

Johnson, W. (2014). *Developing difference [Kindle]*. Palgrave Macmillan.

Kahneman, D. (2003). A psychological perspective on economics. *The American Economic Review, 93*(2), 162–168.

Kahneman, D., Wakker, P. P., & Sarin, R. (1997). Back to Bentham? Explorations of experienced utility. *Quarterly Journal of Economics, 112*(2), 375–405.

Keltner, D. (2009). *Born to be good: The science of meaningful life [Kindle]*. Norton.

Kiley, K., & Vaisey, S. (2020). Measuring stability and change in personal culture using panel data. *American Sociological Review, 85*(3), 477–506. https://doi.org/10.1177/0003122420921538

Kuhn, T. S. (1970). *The structure of scientific revolutions*. The University of Chicago Press.

Kushlev, K., Drummond, D. M., Heintzelman, S. J., & Diener, E. (2020). Do happy people care about society's problems? *The Journal of Positive Psychology, 15*(4), 467–477. https://doi.org/10.1080/17439760.2019.1639797

Kwak, J. (2017). *Economism: Bad economics and the rise of inequality [Kindle]*. Pantheon.

Lercher, M. (2018). Homeostasis. In J. Brockman (Ed.), *This idea is brilliant. Lost overlooked and underappreciated scientific concepts everyone should know [Kindle]* (pp. 120–121). Harper Collins.

Lewis, R. (2018). What actually is a belief? And why is it so hard to change? *Psychology Today*. https://www.psychologytoday.com/us/blog/finding-purpose/201810/what-actually-is-belief-and-why-is-it-so-hard-change

Longino, H. E. (1979). Evidence and hypothesis: An analysis of evidential relations. *Philosophy of Science, 46*(1), 35–56. http://www.jstor.org/stable/186801

Longino, H. E. (2008). Values, heuristics, and the politics of knowledge. In M. Carrier, D. Howard, & J. Kourany (Eds.), *The challenge of the social and the pressure of practice: Science and values revisited* (pp. 68–85). University of Pittsburgh Press. http://ebookcentral.proquest.com/lib/tromsoub-ebooks/detail.action?docID=2038168

MacIntyre, A. (2007). *After virtue [Kindle]* (3rd ed.). University of Notre Dame Press.

Marcel, A. J. (2003). Introspective report. In A. Jack & Roepstorff (Eds.), *Trusting the subject? The use if introspective evidence in cognitive science* (Vol. 1, pp. 167–186). Imprint Academic.

Mayr, E. (1982). *The growth of biological thought. Diversity, evolution, and inheritance*. Harvard University Press.

McGilchrist, I. (2012). *The divided brain and the search for meaning: Why we are so unhappy [Kindle]*. Yale University Press.

Mill, J. S. (1859). *On liberty [Kindle]*.

Møller, V. (2001). Happiness trends under democracy: Where will the new South African set-level come to rest? *Journal of Happiness Studies, 2*(1), 33–53.
Murphy, G. L. (2002). *The big book of concepts*. The MIT Press.
National Academy of Sciences, N. A. (2009). *On being a scientist: A guide to responsible conduct in research*. National Academies Press (US). https://www.ncbi.nlm.nih.gov/books/NBK214568/
Neiman, S. (2015). *Why grow up?: Philosophy in transit [Kindle]*. Penguin.
Nurse, P. (2020). *What is life?: Five great ideas in biology [Kindle]*. Norton.
Oatley, K. (1992). *Best laid schemes*. Cambridge University Press.
Oatley, K. (2004). Emotional intelligence and the intelligence of emotions. *Psychological Inquiry, 15*(3), 216–236.
Oatley, K. (2018). *Our minds, our selves: A brief history of psychology [Kindle]*. Princeton University Press.
OECD. (2013). *OECD Guidelines on measuring subjective well-being*. https://doi.org/10.1787/9789264191655-en
Offer, A., & Söderberg, G. (2016). *The Nobel factor: The prize in economics, social democracy, and the market turn [Kindle]*. Princeton University Press.
Oishi, S., & Westgate, E. C. (2022). A psychologically rich life: Beyond happiness and meaning. *Psychological Review, 129*(4), 790–811. https://doi.org/10.1037/rev0000317
Oishi, S., Choi, H., Buttrick, N., Heintzelman, S. J., Kushlev, K., Westgate, E. C., Tucker, J., Ebersole, C. R., Axt, J., Gilbert, E., Ng, B. W., & Besser, L. L. (2019). The psychologically rich life questionnaire. *Journal of Research in Personality, 81*, 257–270. https://doi.org/10.1016/j.jrp.2019.06.010
Oishi, S., Choi, H., Koo, M., Galinha, I., Ishii, K., Komiya, A., Luhmann, M., Scollon, C., Shin, J.-E., Lee, H., Suh, E. M., Vittersø, J., Heintzelman, S. J., Kushlev, K., Westgate, E. C., Buttrick, N., Tucker, J., Ebersole, C. R., Axt, J., Besser, L. L., et al. (2020). Happiness, meaning, and psychological richness. *Affective Science, 1*(2), 107–115. https://doi.org/10.1007/s42761-020-00011-z
Oreskes, N. (2019). *Why trust science? [Kindle]*. Princeton University Press.
Panksepp, J. (1998). *Affective neuroscience. The foundations of human and animal emotions*. Oxford University Press.
Parducci, A. (1968). The relativism of absolute judgments. *Scientific American, 219*, 84–90.
Pennebaker, J. W. (2012). *Opening up: The healing power of expressing emotions*. Guilford Press.
Perry, W. G. (1999). *Forms of ethical and intellectual development in the college years. A scheme*. Jossey-Bass.
Phillips, J., De Freitas, J., Mott, C., Gruber, J., & Knobe, J. (2017). True happiness: The role of morality in the folk concept of happiness. *Journal of Experimental Psychology: General, 146*(2), 165–181. https://doi.org/10.1037/xge0000252
Pross, A. (2016). *What is life?: How chemistry becomes biology*. Oxford University Press.
Rodolfo, K. (2000). What is homeostasis? *Scientific American*. https://www.scientificamerican.com/article/what-is-homeostasis/
Romero, A. (2012). When whales became mammals: The scientific journey of cetaceans from fish to mammals in the history of science. *New Approaches to the Study of Marine Mammals*, 3–30.
Ryan, R. M. M., & Deci, E. L. D. (2001). On happiness and human potentials: A review of research on hedonic and eudaimonic well-being. *Annual Review of Psychology, 52*, 141–166. http://psych.AnnualReviews.org/cgi/reprint/52/1/141.pdf
Sandel, M. (2011). *What money can't buy [Kindle]*. http://www.justiceharvard.org/watch/
Sapolsky, R. M. (2017). *Behave. The biology of humans at our best and worst [Kindle]*. Penguin Press.
Schimmack, U. (2008). The structure of subjective well-being. In M. Eid & R. J. Larsen (Eds.), *The science of subjective well-being* (pp. 97–123). Guilford Press.

Schimmack, U., & Oishi, S. (2005). The influence of chronically and temporarily accessible information on life satisfaction judgments. *Journal of Personality and Social Psychology, 89*(3), 395–406.

Schimmack, U., Oishi, S., Diener, E., & Suh, E. (2000). Facets of affective experiences: A framework for investigations of trait affect. *Personality and Social Psychology Bulletin, 26*, 655–668.

Schrödinger, E. (2010/1946). What is life? (selections). In C. E. Cleland & M. A. Bedau (Eds.), *The nature of life: Classical and contemporary perspectives from philosophy and science* (pp. 50–69). Cambridge University Press. (Original work published in 1946). https://doi.org/10.1017/CBO9780511730191.007

Schwartz, B., & Wrzesniewski, A. (2016). Internal motivation, instrumental motivation, and eudaimonia. In J. Vittersø (Ed.), *Handbook of Eudaimonic well-being* (pp. 123–134). Springer International Publishing. https://doi.org/10.1007/978-3-319-42445-3_8

Sen, A. (2009). *The idea of justice*. Harvard University Press.

Silvia, P. J. (2006). *Exploring the psychology of interest*. Oxford University Press.

Singer, T. (2015). *How to build a caring economy*. World Economic Forum. https://www.weforum.org/agenda/2015/01/how-to-build-a-caring-economy/

Sirgy, J. M. (2012). *The psychology of quality of life. Hedonic well-being, life satisfaction, and eudaimonia* (2nd ed.). Springer. https://doi.org/10.1007/978-94-007-4405-9

Small, D. M., Zatorre, R. J., Dagher, A., Evans, A. C., & Jones-Gotman, M. (2001). Changes in brain activity related to eating chocolate. From pleasure to aversion. *Brain, 124*, 1720–1733.

Smith, C. A., Tong, E. M. W., & Ellsworth, P. C. (2014). The differentiation of positive emotional experience as viewed through the lens of appraisal theory. In M. M. Tugade, M. N. Shiota, & K. N. Kirby (Eds.), *Handbook of positive emotions* (pp. 11–27). Guilford.

Southward, M. W., Wilson, A. C., & Cheavens, J. S. (2021). On what do therapists agree? Assessing therapist evaluations of emotion regulation strategy effectiveness. *Psychology and Psychotherapy: Theory, Research and Practice, 94*(2), 231–246. https://doi.org/10.1111/papt.12302

Steger, M. F., Frazier, P., Oishi, S., & Kaler, M. (2006). The meaning in life questionnaire: Assessing the presence of and search for meaning in life. *Journal of Counseling Psychology, 53*(1), 80–93. https://doi.org/10.1037/0022-0167.53.1.80

Sumner, L. W. (1996). *Welfare, happiness, and ethics*. Clarendon Press.

Taplin, J. (2017). *Move fast and break things: How Facebook, Google, and Amazon have cornered culture and what it means for all of us [Kindle]*. Pan Macmillan.

Tan, H. B., & Forgas, J. P. (2010). When happiness makes us selfish but sadness makes us fair: Affective influences on interpersonal strategies in the dictator game. *Journal of Experimental Social Psychology, 46*(3), 571–576. https://doi.org/10.1016/j.jesp.2010.01.007

Thagard, P. (1992). *Conceptual revolutions*. Princeton University Press.

Thagard, P. (2012). *The cognitive science of science*. The MIT Press.

Tomasello, M. (2016). *A natural history of human morality [Kindle]*. Harvard University Press.

Tomasello, M. (2018). The origins of morality. *Scientific American, 319*(3), 70–75. https://doi.org/10.1038/scientificamerican0918-70

Tomasello, M. (2019). *Becoming human: A theory of ontogeny [Kindle]*. Belknap Press.

Tov, W., & Lee, H. W. (2016). A closer look at the hedonics of everyday meaning and satisfaction. *Journal of Personality and Social Psychology, 111*(4), 585–609. https://doi.org/10.1037/pspp0000081

van der Horst, F. C. P., LeRoy, H. A., & van der Veer, R. (2008). "When strangers meet": John Bowlby and Harry Harlow on attachment behavior. *Integrative Psychological and Behavioral Science, 42*(4), 370–388. https://doi.org/10.1007/s12124-008-9079-2

Vittersø, J. (2016). The feeling of excellent functioning: Hedonic and eudaimonic emotions. In J. Vittersø (Ed.), *Handbook of eudaimonic well-being* (pp. 253–276). Springer International Publishing. https://doi.org/10.1007/978-3-319-42445-3_17

Von Devivere, B. (2018). *Meaningful work: Viktor Frankl's legacy for the 21st century*. Springer.

Wilson-Mendenhall, C. D., Barrett, L. F., & Barsalou, L. W. (2013). Neural evidence that human emotions share core affective properties. *Psychological Science, 24*(6), 947–956. https://doi.org/10.1177/0956797612464242

Wojcik, S. P., Hovasapian, A., Graham, J., Motyl, M., & Ditto, P. H. (2015). Conservatives report, but liberals display, greater happiness. *Science, 347*(6227), 1243–1246. https://doi.org/10.1126/science.1260817

A Very Brief Epilogue

Everything begins with creation. Even wellbeing. Our ability to value started with the origin of life and is rooted in biological structures. But human values are sophisticated by culture, and it is our social humanness that enables us to reflect upon what wellbeing is. Hence, the understanding and valuation of wellbeing change with culture and historical eras.

For some ancient Greeks, wellbeing was seen as the complete life and the highest good. Denying its ultimate value would be irrational because nothing can be better than complete goodness. Today, scientists no longer juxtapose wellbeing with completeness. The concept has been decomposed into separable dimensions of psychological states and processes, and the normative part of goodness has decayed. Most researchers seem to argue that science is objective and therefore value-free. Scientists deliver empirical facts and others must decide what to do with them.

The humanistic theory of wellbeing holds a different view. Rooted in feminist epistemology, it maintains that science is a social activity that achieves objectivity when a plurality of subjective perspectives is critically debated by a community of peers. Values can be objectified in the same manner, by surviving debates and open criticism provided by scientific institutions. The HTW therefore suggests that a moral value expressed as a background assumption can be supported by means of the same practices as other background assumptions are justified.

Like everyone else, scientists are committed to universal ethics and agree, I suppose, that living out such a morality will contribute to a better world. Humans need in other words morality to have good lives. The HTW takes this reasoning one step further and claims that people who like their lives for the right reasons lead lives that are closer to the notion of a good life than people who seriously violate moral commitments universally acknowledged. Humans are cultural beings and cannot perform their humanness well outside a social community or in the absence of morality.

In this book, I have adopted the view that knowledge grows by replacing inapt concepts with more fruitful ones. Steps toward a humanistic understanding of wellbeing have been offered in the hope of contributing to such developments. The promise of science is to provide knowledge that helps us to lead better lives. But

J. Vittersø, *Humanistic Wellbeing*, https://doi.org/10.1007/978-3-031-69292-5

knowledge alone will not change the world. The world itself must also accommodate new insights. If knowledge is an interactive and social activity, better ways of being human will generate improved understandings of what it means to be well. Hence, both the world and the way we see it must change together.

MIX
Papier aus verantwortungsvollen Quellen
Paper from responsible sources
FSC® C105338

If you have any concerns about our products,
you can contact us on
ProductSafety@springernature.com

In case Publisher is established outside the EU,
the EU authorized representative is:
Springer Nature Customer Service Center GmbH
Europaplatz 3, 69115 Heidelberg, Germany

Printed by Libri Plureos GmbH
in Hamburg, Germany